Shabbos Secrets
VOLUME II

The Significance and Spirituality of Traditional Jewish Foods

RABBI DOVID MEISELS

Shabbos Secrets
Volume II

Copyright © 2017 by
Rabbi Dovid Meisels
718-946-9831
ddmeisels@gmail.com

ISBN 978-1-60091-521-5

ALL RIGHTS RESERVED

No part of this publication may be translated, reproduced, stored in a retrieval system, or mechanical, photo-copying, recording, or otherwise, without prior permission in writing from both the copyright holder and publisher.

OTHER BOOKS BY THE AUTHOR
Seudah Secrets - III volumes
Shabbos Secrets
Seder Secrets
Shavuos Secrets
Rosh Hashana Secrets
Succos Secrets
Bris Milah Secrets
Bar Mitzva and Tefillin Secrets

DISTRIBUTED BY:
ISRAEL BOOKSHOP PUBLICATIONS
501 Prospect Street
Lakewood, NJ 08701
Tel: 732-901-3009
Fax: 732-901-4012
Email: info@israelbookshoppublications.com

Table of Contents

Introduction 9

Chapter 1
Shabbos Hayom laShem 11
Shabbos: The Chanukas Habayis of Hashem - 11 • The Shechinah Rests upon Us on Shabbos - 12 • The Shechinah's Presence at the Shabbos Seudah - 13 • Proper Comportment in the Presence of the Shechinah - 15 • Seudas Shabbos Arouses Simchah shel Mitzvah - 17 • Performing Mitzvos with Joy - 19 • Understanding the Shabbos Food - 19 • Discussing Shabbos Foods During the Seudah - 22

Chapter 2
V'karasa laShabbos Oneg— Delighting in the Shabbos 24
The Mitzvah of Oneg Shabbos - 24 • Oneg Shabbos—An "Investment" for the Future - 27 • The Purpose of Shabbos - 29 • Pleasure for Body and Soul - 30 • Pleasure for Hashem - 32 • The Power of Eating on Shabbos - 33 • "Eating" Shabbos - 39 • Delighting in Shabbos for the Sake of Hashem - 39 • Honoring Hashem - 41 • Eating with Joy - 41 • Being Mindful While Eating - 44 • Food Should Bring One to Teshuvah - 45 • Oneg Shabbos Leads to Yiras Shamayim - 45 • Eating L'shem Mitzvah - 47 • No Reason to Overindulge - 49

Chapter 3
Shabbos Food—A Different Dimension 52
Elevated Eating - 52 • A Seudah of Emunah - 55 • The Special Aroma and Taste of Shabbos Food - 56 • Shabbos Food Is Uplifted - 59 • Comparable to Korbanos - 66 • Shabbos Food Sanctifies a Person - 68 • Differentiating between Shabbos and Weekday Food - 70 • Eating Fish during the Week - 74 • Saying L'kavod Shabbos Kodesh - 75 • Curative Food - 76 • Shabbos Food Does Not Cause Harm - 79 • Shabbos Food Brings Parnassah - 80 • Praising Shabbos Food - 81 • Eating on Shabbos Is Different - 82

Chapter 4
Preparing for Shabbos 84
Purchasing Shabbos Food - 84 • Fish at Any Price - 84 • Shabbos Requires Preparation - 86 • Cooking in Honor of Shabbos - 87 • Preparing the Fish - 88 • Peppery Shabbos Food - 90 • Bread for Two Days - 91 • Hafrashas Challah - 92 • Baking Challah - 94 • Preparing the Shabbos Table - 95

Chapter 5
Erev Shabbos—A Prelude to Shabbos Kodesh..................98
The Amount One Should Eat on Erev Shabbos - 98 • Thursday Night L'chaim - 100 • Eating a Seudah on Erev Shabbos - 101 • Tearing Apart the Challah - 102 • Eating Dairy on Erev Shabbos - 106 • Eating Meat on Erev Shabbos - 108 • Drinking Mead - 111 • Drinking Wine on Erev Shabbos - 111 • Russil - 111 • Tasting the Shabbos Food - 113 • Tasting Each Dish or Specific Dishes - 114 • Tasting the Fish - 115

Chapter 6
Seudas Shabbos..................117
Eating Three Seudos - 117 • Three Meals Are Compared to... - 119 • Requirements for the Seudos - 121 • Extra Food on Shabbos - 124 • Eating Shabbos Food with One's Hands - 126

Chapter 7
Friday Night—Beginning the Meal and Kiddush..................129
Seeing the Shabbos Food - 129 • Not Eating before the Meal - 129 • Sending Away the Angels - 130 • Hastening to Recite Kiddush - 130 • Reciting Kiddush on Wine - 130 • Wine Brings Healing - 137 • A Full Glass - 139 • The Kiddush Cup - 139 • Rinsing the Cup - 140 • Borei Pri Hagafen - 140 • Sitting While Drinking - 141 • Drinking Kiddush Wine - 141 • Leaving Over Kiddush - 142

Chapter 8
Hamotzi on Friday Night..................143
Challah - 143 • Lechem Mishneh - 145 • Shape of the Challos - 147 • Twelve Challos - 152 • Loaves of Equal Size - 153 • Different Types of Bread - 153 • Topping the Challah - 154 • Appealing, Tasty Challos - 154 • Setting the Challos on the Table - 154 • Covering the Challos - 156 • Marking the Challah - 156 • Holding the Challah - 157 • With Ten Fingers - 158 • A Whole Loaf - 159 • Reciting the Brachah - 159 • Removing the Challah Cover - 162 • Holding the Challah While Cutting It - 162 • Cutting One or Both Challos - 163 • Slicing the Challah - 164 • Distributing the Challah - 166 • Dipping the Challah into Salt - 168 • Dipping the Challah Three Times - 173 • Sugar Instead of Salt - 174 • Not Dipping in Salt - 174 • Eating the Hamotzi - 175 • Crumbs of Hamotzi - 177 • The Power of Crumbs - 178 • Dipping the Hamotzi into the Kiddush Wine - 179 • Delicious Taste of Challah - 180 • Challah as a Segulah - 181 • Eating Challah with Each Dish - 181

Chapter 9
The Friday Night Seudah..................182
Eating the Seudah in its Proper Order - 182 • Friday Night Foods - 184 • Hot Food - 185

Chapter 10
Not Just an Appetizer— The Significance of Fish **188**
Reasons for Eating Fish on Shabbos - 188 • The Significance of Fish - 191 • Fish as the First Course - 194 • Segulos from Eating Fish - 196 • Varieties of Fish - 200 • Large Fish - 205 • Placing Fish on the Reverse Side of the Plate - 206 • The Order of Eating the Fish - 207 • The Head of the Fish - 207 • The Eyes of the Fish - 208 • Not to Insult the Slices of Fish - 209 • Warm Fish - 209 • Challah with Fish - 210 • Weekday Bread with Fish - 210 • Dipping Challah into Fish Sauce - 212 • Pepper in the Fish - 214 • Eating Other Foods with Fish - 215 • Separating between Fish and Meat - 216 • Drinking Whiskey after Fish - 217 • Drinking Wine after the Fish - 219

Chapter 11
Splendid Soup **221**
Soup from Mashiach's Bowl - 221 • Soup with Lokshen - 221 • Square Noodles - 223 • Beans in the Soup - 224 • Spices and Salt in the Soup - 226 • Challah in the Soup - 227 • How to Eat Soup - 228

Chapter 12
The Main Course **231**
Meat on Shabbos - 231 • Not Eating a Lot of Meat - 234 • Meat with Challah - 235 • All Parts of the Chicken - 235 • Chrein with the Meat - 236 • Meat with Compote - 237 • Kugel on Friday Night - 237 • Drinking after Eating - 238 • Drinking Wine during the Seudah - 238 • Tzimmes - 240 • Farfel - 242 • Stuffed Cabbage - 245 • Gedishachtz - 246 • Gelingelech - 246 • Liver - 246 • Liver with Challah - 248 • Karsh - 249 • Garlic - 250 • Compote - 250 • Apples - 252 • Eating Challah at the End of the Meal - 255 • Leaving over Shabbos Food - 256 • Eating in Order to Recite Birkas Hamazon - 256 • Reciting Birkas Hamazon over a Cup of Wine - 256

Chapter 13
After the Meal—Friday Night Oneg **258**
Shehakol Cake after Birkas Hamazon - 258 • Eating Fruit for 100 Brachos on Shabbos - 258 • Beans - 259 • Whiskey on Friday Night - 260 • Friday Night Cholent - 260

Chapter 14
Shabbos Morning and Kiddush **261**
Drinking Coffee Early in the Morning - 261 • Preparing the Challos before Mussaf - 261 • Pas Shacharis on Shabbos - 261 • Kiddusha Rabba - 262 • Kiddush over Whiskey - 262 • Amount of Whiskey and Time Allotted for Drinking It - 264 • Kiddush over Wine - 265 • Participants Drinking from Kiddush - 266 • Not Wishing L'chaim - 267 • Covering the Cake - 267 • Pastries after Kiddush - 267 • Whole Cookie - 269 • Lechem Mishneh on

Pastries - 270 • Cake - 270 • Seudas Rabbi Chidka - 271 • Compote before the Meal - 272 • Yerushalmi Kugel - 272 • Shalom Bayis Kugel - 273 • Eating Fish Prior to the Seudah - 274 • Meat Prior to the Seudah - 275 • Brachah Acharonah after Kiddush - 275

Chapter 15
The Shabbos Day Seudah 276
Being Ma'avir Sedrah Before the Seudah - 276 • Eating Right after Davening - 276 • The Honor of the Day Seudah - 277 • Reciting Kiddush a Second Time - 278 • Drinking before Washing - 279 • Covering the Challos - 279 • Challah for Shabbos Day Seudah - 280 • Menu and Order of Shabbos Day Seudah - 280 • Fish during the Day Seudah - 283 • Not Eating Fish at the Day Seudah - 283 • "Falshe" Fish - 284 • Garlic - 284 • Onions - 284 • Raw Onions - 287 • Cutting Onions - 288 • Eggs and Onions - 289 • Preparing the Eggs - 292 • Adding Fat to Eggs - 294 • Pepper and Salt - 295 • Liver - 295 • Eating Eggs with the Cholent - 295 • Galaretta and P'tcha - 296 • P'tcha as a Segulah - 300

Chapter 16
The Main Course—Cholent 302
Chamin—Hot Food on Shabbos - 302 • Cholent - 304 • The Word "Cholent" - 305 • The Angels Guard the Cholent - 306 • Cholent as a Segulah - 306 • Cholent Is Not Harmful - 307 • Liquid from the Cholent - 309 • Cholent with Beans - 310 • Cholent with Kasha - 312 • Kasha as a Segulah - 314

Chapter 17
Kugel—More Than a Side Dish 315
Preparation for Eating Kugel - 315 • Importance of Eating Kugel - 315 • Round Kugel - 317 • Lokshen Kugel - 318 • Mehl Kugel - 320 • Challah Kugel - 320 • Potato Kugel - 321 • Helzel Kugel - 321 • Number and Types of Kugels - 321 • Gezunter Kugel - 322 • Kugel as a Segulah - 322 • Flipping over the Kugel - 325 • Eating Kugel with One's Hands - 325 • Kugel as Hachnasas Orchim - 327 • Meat after Kugel - 328

Chapter 18
Dessert and Shabbos Afternoon Treats 329
Drinking Tea - 329 • Compote - 329 • Oneg Shabbos for Children - 330 • Eating Fruits before Minchah - 330

Chapter 19
Shalosh Seudos—Equal to All Three Meals 331
Shalosh Seudos—the Importance of the Third Meal - 331 • Shalosh Seudos as a Segulah - 334 • Eating Shalosh Seudos with Others - 334 • The Proper Time for Eating Shalosh Seudos - 335 • Minimizing the Amount Eaten at

Shalosh Seudos - 336 • Reciting Shehakol Prior to Shalosh Seudos - 338 • Covering the Challos - 339 • Braided Challos - 340 • Salt at Shalosh Seudos - 340 • Crumbs of Hamotzi - 340 • Wine at Shalosh Seudos - 340 • Fish at Shalosh Seudos - 342 • Eggs and Onions - 344 • Herring - 344 • Meat at Shalosh Seudos - 344 • Dairy at Shalosh Seudos - 346 • Pomegranates and Plums - 347 • An Additional Kezayis at Shalosh Seudos - 347 • Shalosh Seudos—a Segulah for Livelihood - 347 • Drinking Wine after Birkas Hamazon - 348

Chapter 20
Havdalah—Marking the Separation 350
No Eating before Havdalah - 350 • A Separation - 350 • Not Reciting Havdalah Individually - 351 • The Havdalah Cup - 351 • Raising the Cup - 352 • Havdalah over Wine - 352 • Besamim - 353 • The Brachos of Havdalah - 355 • Looking at One's Reflection in the Wine - 355 • Drinking the Whole Cup of Havdalah - 357 • Giving Havdalah Wine to Others - 357 • Women Drinking Havdalah Wine - 358 • Water in the Havdalah Cup - 360 • Water from the Well of Miriam - 360 • Havdalah Wine on Back of Neck - 361

Chapter 21
Escorting the Queen—Melaveh Malkah 362
Importance of Melaveh Malkah - 362 • Reasons for Melaveh Malkah - 365 • The Seudah of the Naschoy Bone - 367 • The First Melaveh Malkah - 370 • The Seudah of Dovid, Melech Hamashiach - 372 • Segulos of Melaveh Malkah - 374 • Timing of the Seudah - 379 • Fresh Food - 381 • Shabbos Leftovers - 383 • Hot Food - 385 • Lechem Mishneh - 386 • Fish - 387 • Drinking Liquor - 388 • Drinking Wine - 389 • Soup - 389 • Borscht - 390 • Meat - 391 • Kugel - 391 • Garlic - 392 • Radishes - 393 • Dairy Foods - 393 • No Eggs - 395 • Coffee or Tea - 395 • Kos shel Brachah - 396 • Not Eating Melaveh Malkah - 396

Chapter 22
Yom Tov, Shabbos Yom Tov, and Other Special Shabbasos—an Added Dimension 397
The Difference between Shabbos and Yom Tov Meals - 397 • Yom Tov that Falls out on Shabbos - 400 • Shabbos Yom Tov—Three Seudos - 401 • Minhagim for Special Shabbasos - 401

Chapter 23
In Honor of a New Month— Shabbos Mevarchim or Rosh Chodesh 403
Shabbos Mevarchim - 403 • Eating Shalosh Seudos on Shabbos Erev Rosh Chodesh - 403 • Shabbos Rosh Chodesh - 404

Chapter 24
Shabbasos in Elul/Tishrei.. *406*
Shabbos before Rosh Hashanah - 406 • Shabbos Rosh Hashanah - 407 • Shalosh Seudos - 408 • Shabbos Shuvah - 409 • The Shabbos between Yom Kippur and Sukkos - 410 • Shabbos Chol Hamoed - 411 • Shabbos Bereishis - 412

Chapter 25
Shabbos Chanukah.. *415*
Additions and Changes to the Seudos - 415 • Eating Olive Oil on Shabbos Chanukah - 417 • Extra Kugels - 421

Chapter 26
Shabbos Shirah and Tu B'Shevat.. *422*
Shabbos Shirah - 422 • Eating Wheat - 423 • Throwing Food to the Birds - 424 • Shabbos Tu B'Shevat - 427 • Shabbos Aseres Hadibros - 428

Chapter 27
Shabbasos in Adar.. *429*
Shabbos Zachor - 429 • Shabbos Erev Purim - 429 • Seudas Purim on Erev Shabbos - 429 • Shabbos of Purim Hameshulash - 431 • Parshas Parah - 433 • Shabbos Hachodesh - 433

Chapter 28
Shabbos Hagadol, Pesach, and the Shabbos after Pesach....... *434*
Shabbos Hagadol - 434 • Challos for Shabbos Hagadol - 434 • Three Types of Kugels - 435 • Purim Leftovers - 436 • Afikoman in the Cholent - 436 • Erev Pesach that Falls out on Shabbos - 436 • Eggs - 436 • Shalosh Seudos - 437 • Shabbos Chol Hamoed Pesach - 439 • Galaretta - 439 • Kugel for Shabbos Chol Hamoed - 440 • Shabbos "Gella" (Yellow) Matzos - 440 • Shlissel Challah - 447

Chapter 29
Shabbos Shavuos.. *453*
Erev Shavuos That Falls out on Shabbos - 453 • Second Day of Shavuos on Shabbos - 453 • Second Day Yom Tov—a Different Type of Kedushah - 453

Chapter 30
Shabbasos during the Three Weeks.. *455*
Shabbos Rosh Chodesh Av - 455 • Shabbos Chazon - 455 • Shalosh Seudos of Shabbos Chazon - 456 • Motza'ei Shabbos Chazon - 462 • Shabbos Nachamu - 463

Introduction

Blessed is Hashem who has granted us the tremendous gift of Shabbos!

It is with great gratitude to Hashem that I present the second volume of Shabbos Secrets. The first volume discusses the different aspects of the holiness of Shabbos—baruch Hashem, that book was very enthusiastically received. In the second volume of Shabbos Secrets, the many customs and ideas related to the foods eaten on Shabbos are presented and explained.

There are deep reasons for each dish eaten on Shabbos; all of them are significant and elevated, and they all stem from a holy source. Our *tzaddikim* have revealed to us some of the lofty secrets that are concealed within the essence of our Shabbos food. These ideas are treasures, small glimpses of *Olam Haba*; a special gift to allow us to tap into the greatness and depth of *seudos Shabbos*. Understanding these ideas allows us to experience a taste of Divine pleasure, as delighting properly in Shabbos—the beautiful, precious gift bequeathed to us by Hashem Himself—is truly one of the highest forms of becoming close to Hashem.

This work is an accumulation of many years of toil and effort. The concepts and stories presented here are taken from the words of *Chazal* and midrash, and from our *tzaddikim* throughout the generations. Although this *sefer* is a comprehensive work, it is not all-inclusive, since there are countless ideas that lie behind each custom, and it would be impossible to enumerate them all.

The Meiri writes that if a person is sitting and learning Torah, and a mitzvah comes his way, he should perform the mitzvah only after he finishes learning. This is because the more a person learns, the more enhanced his mitzvah performance will be, since it will now be done with greater understanding. Similarly, if we understand the reasons for the Shabbos foods we eat, our eating will be on an entirely different level.

The *Mesilas Yesharim* states that his work is not complete, since there is no limit to that which one can learn. However, he says, learning a bit about each topic can be the beginning of greater knowledge. So, too, it is my hope that this *sefer* will spur greater growth and knowledge beyond that which is written in these pages.

It is my fervent wish and prayer that this *sefer* help us all comprehend the greatness and the splendor of *seudos Shabbos*. May my work be an inspiration to others, and thereby increase the honor of Shabbos.

We should merit to receive the holy Shabbos properly, and indeed to be redeemed in its merit, speedily and in our days.

***

I would like to take this opportunity to thank Hashem for all of the kindness He has done for me and for my family, especially in regard to seeing this *sefer* through to completion. I humbly request of Hashem that He help me further in my efforts to inspire Jews and bring more meaning into their lives.

Rabbi Dovid Meisels
Adar 5777

Chapter 1
Shabbos Hayom laShem

Shabbos: The Chanukas Habayis of Hashem

When a person builds a house, he celebrates its completion with a *chanukas habayis*. Similarly, when Hashem finished the creation of the world, He made a day of celebration and rejoicing.

This day was called Shabbos.

Hashem instructed us to rest on Shabbos, just as He rested on Shabbos (*Sheiltos D'Rav Achai Gaon, Bereishis*). Moreover, because Shabbos is like a *chanukas habayis,* and a *chanukas habayis* is a day of rejoicing, all authorities agree that Shabbos is *chetzyo lachem*; one must take pleasure in it (*Pesachim* 68b). When a person comes to his friend's *chanukas habayis*, he tours the house, inspecting and examining each detail to express his admiration of how much wisdom and thought were put into it. Similarly, at Hashem's *chanukas habayis,* we must appreciate the greatness of the world that He created for us and take pleasure in it.

Additionally, the purpose of the mitzvah of *oneg Shabbos* is to constantly remind us that Hashem created the world, and to strengthen our *emunah* in Hashem. We must be continually grateful that there is a Creator in the world Who commanded us to keep Shabbos in order to create a bond between Him and us. This is one of the fundamental foundations of belief in Hashem (*Ramban, Shemos* 20:8), and it is this *emunah* that leads to true *oneg Shabbos*.

The Midrash Rabbah (*Bereishis* 9:4) states that this is compared to a king who built a palace that pleased him. He said, "Palace, palace, if only you should find favor in my eyes all the time, as you do now." After creating the world, Hashem said, "My world, My world, if only you always find favor in My eyes as you do now." Rabbi Yonasan further compared this to a king who married off his daughter. He gave her a house that he plastered, ornamented, and decorated with beautiful pictures. He told her, "My child, if only this home will always find favor in my eyes as it does at this time."

This midrash demonstrates that Hashem, so to speak, derived pleasure from the creation of the world. This is clearly stated in the *pasuk*, as it says: *And Hashem saw all that He made and, behold, **it was very good**. And it was evening, and it was morning, the sixth day. And [Hashem] rested...and He blessed... and He sanctified...* After Hashem realized that the world He created was "very good," He rested and designated Shabbos as a day of happiness. Our mitzvah of *oneg Shabbos* reflects this, and requires us to rejoice in Hashem's world and His control over it.

The Shechinah Rests upon Us on Shabbos

The essence of Shabbos is that the *Shechinah* rests upon us. We find that Shabbos is referred to as *kallah* (bride) and *malkesa* (queen). The Gemara (*Shabbos* 119a) states that when Rabbi Chanina would go out to greet the Shabbos, he would say, "Come, let us go out and greet the Shabbos queen." Rabbi Yannai would say, "Come bride, come bride." The words *kallah* and *malkesa* also refer to the *Shechinah*.

Rabbi Yosef Gikatilla writes in the *Sefer Sha'arei Orah*: *Know that a person who keeps Shabbos properly becomes, so to speak, like a throne for Hashem.* This means that such a person becomes a place for the *Shechinah* to rest, which is why Shabbos is called "*menuchah*" (rest). Similarly, the Pri Tzaddik writes that by keeping Shabbos, a person becomes a suitable vessel for the *Shechinah*. By refraining from desecrating the Shabbos, his heart is sanctified to be able to receive the *Shechinah*. Indeed, the *Zohar* states that the main time in which the *Shechinah* rests upon a person is on Shabbos.

The holiness of Shabbos is comparable to the holiness of the Beis Hamikdash, which was the main place where the *Shechinah* rested, as it says: *And they shall make Me a sanctuary and I will dwell in their midst* (Shemos 25:8). *Chazal* state that there was a mitzvah to kindle lights in the Menorah in the Beis Hamikdash (*Shabbos* 22b), since the Menorah testified that the *Shechinah* rested upon Bnei Yisrael.

The *Shechinah* was revealed specifically through the Menorah because the main place where the *Shechinah* rests is in our souls. The soul of a person can be referred to as *ner* (candle), as it says: *Ner Elokim nishmas adam*—"[A] candle of G-d [is the] soul of man" (Mishlei 20:27). This is also why, nowadays, we light candles at the Shabbos table. Just as in the Beis Hamikdash, the Menorah testified that the *Shechinah* rested upon Bnei Yisrael, lighting Shabbos candles is a sign that the *Shechinah* rests upon us at our tables on Shabbos.

The Shechinah's Presence at the Shabbos Seudah

Seudas Shabbos is also termed *seudasa d'Malka kaddisha* (the *seudah* of the holy King) and is considered to be the *seudah* of Hashem. Shabbos is a time when the King of kings comes to live in our homes, and we merit sitting at His table with Him. The midrash states that Shabbos is compared to a king sitting with his queen across from him. At this time, any person who would come between them would be deserving of death. Such intense closeness is the essence of *seudas Shabbos*.

If *seudas Shabbos* is the *seudah* of Hashem, then eating Shabbos food is like partaking from Hashem's table, which is like eating from the *korbanos* (see *Asarah Ma'amaros, Ma'amar Chikur Din*, vol. 1, ch. 21). Moreover, when we sit at Hashem's table, the food we eat is food that Hashem, so to speak, paid for. This explains the dictum expressed in the Gemara: *All the livelihood of a person is decreed for him on Rosh Hashanah, except the expenses of Shabbos and Yom Tov* (Beitzah 16a).

Furthermore, we find in the *Zohar* (Pekudei, p. 252b) an explanation of the greatness of setting the Shabbos table. On Shabbos, everyone's table, together, ascends to a special place in the Upper Worlds. Tens of thousands of angels are appointed over these tables. One angel blesses each table, and all the angels answer "amen." These angels protect us from harm.

The Gemara also states: *Rabbi Yosi Bar Yehudah said that two angels accompany a person on Friday night from the* beis haknesses *to his house, a good angel and a bad angel. When the angels arrive at his house and they find lit candles, a set table, and a prepared bed, the good angel says, "May it be so the coming Shabbos," and the bad angel is forced to respond, "Amen"* (Shabbos 119b).

The *Zohar* explains the words from *Shemos* (31:16) *La'asos es HaShabbos l'dorosam*—"[And Bnei Yisrael should observe the Shabbos] to make the Shabbos an eternal covenant for their generations" (Bamidbar, p. 332, Midrash Hane'elam). *L'dorosam* has the same root word as *dirah* (dwelling) to teach us that when Shabbos comes, the *Shechinah* comes to dwell among us. If we are honoring the Shabbos properly, it remains among us. If not, it will depart.

As long as the *Shechinah* rests among Klal Yisrael, no nation can have any power over us. This is clear from the *Midrash Rabbah* (Eichah, intro. 27) that before the *Churban*, Hashem said, "I will take away my *Shechinah* and there will be a *Churban*." We also find that immediately after Bnei Yisrael went out to gather the *mann* on Shabbos, Amalek came and waged war with them. This was because by desecrating Shabbos, Bnei Yisrael caused the *Shechinah* to depart and they lost their

Divine protection. The Yismach Moshe writes (*Va'eschanan*) that the cause of all tragedies is the departure of the *Shechinah*, as the *pasuk* in *Devarim* (31:17) states: *Is it not because our G-d is no longer among us that these evils have befallen us?* Conversely, the presence of the *Shechinah* is the source of all blessing.

Proper Comportment in the Presence of the Shechinah

Bearing these concepts in mind, one must sit at the table in a respectful manner during the *seudah* in honor of the *Shechinah* that rests there. If he does so, he will merit great blessings.

Similarly, a person should be careful with his speech while sitting at the table of the King. The Yismach Moshe (*She'eilos Uteshuvos Heishiv Moshe*, sec. 1) compares this to a person who has a great and awesome king come to lodge by him. This person needs to constantly remember how great the king is and that in the presence of such greatness, even a small flaw would be considered a large offense. He needs to be exceedingly careful to act properly at all times and accord the king his due honor. If he does so, the king will honor him as well.

Similarly, one must give proper honor to the King of the world, Hashem. One should not speak of mundane matters that are not appropriate in the presence of the holy *Shechinah*, as *Chazal* have said (*Shabbos* 113b) that one's speech on Shabbos should not be like his speech during the week. Additionally, one should be careful with the purity of his thoughts. The Reishis Chachmah writes that a person's heart needs to be ready for the *Shechinah* to rest there; it should be like the Holy of Holies. If a person allows a flaw into his heart, it is like bringing an idol into the Beis Hamikdash. If that is the case during the week, how much more so on Shabbos, when the presence of the *Shechinah* is much stronger; one must be careful not to banish the Divine Presence from his midst through improper thoughts.

The Torah instructed us: *And you should guard the Shabbos* (*Shemos* 31:14). This means that we must guard the *Shechinah* and be careful of our actions, speech, and thought, because by acting, speaking, or thinking of mundane matters on Shabbos we can cause the Divine Presence to depart.

The *Zohar* states that by eating *seudos Shabbos* we are recognizable as children of Hashem. One who omits one of the *seudos* demonstrates that he is not one of the children of the King and his punishment is great. If a person is careful to eat three *seudos* throughout Shabbos, he will surely be a fitting receptacle for the *Shechinah* and blessing will rest upon him.

It is therefore self-understood that the purpose of *seudas Shabbos* is not merely to satiate ourselves; each is a *seudah* of the Holy King at Whose table we are dining. As such, it is appropriate that the entire household sits together around a beautifully set Shabbos table, sings *zemiros* and hears *divrei Torah*, *mussar*, or stories of *tzaddikim*. There is no better way to strengthen *Yiddishkeit* than when there is a pleasant atmosphere at the Shabbos table, where one can sense the presence of the *Shechinah* and feel the joy of Shabbos.

Parents should educate their children from when they are young about the greatness and preciousness of our holy Shabbos, so that they have the ability to take pleasure in it. They should also teach them to respect the *Shechinah* that rests on the Shabbos table during the *seudah* by sitting throughout the entire meal in a manner befitting the honor of the *Shechinah*. In this way, they too will merit having the *Shechinah* rest upon them.

The Chafetz Chaim once told someone, "It is not enough that you are careful to keep Shabbos, since in the Torah it says, … *you should perform no labor, neither you, your son, your daughter…* (*Shemos* 20:10). We do not find such instructions with any other mitzvah. The Torah does not state, *Do not eat meat and milk, neither you, your son, your daughter…* It is only in regard to Shabbos that this phrase is used, since a father is responsible for his children and family, and he can only receive the blessings of Shabbos if he ensures that they observe Shabbos properly. This seems to be the reason that fathers in earlier generations insisted that the children not leave the table during the *seudah* and they remain seated in honor of the *Shechinah*.

It is written in the name of Reb Levi Yitzchak of Berditchev (in his *sefer Zavas Abba*, p. 29, sec. 8) that on Shabbos and Yom Tov, when the *Shechinah* sees the tables of Bnei Yisrael prepared with delicacies and families sitting together in holiness, rejoicing and eating in honor of Shabbos, the *Shechinah* ascends to Hakadosh Baruch Hu with great joy and proclaims, "*Meine kinderlach essen shoin* (My children are eating already)*!*"

Seudas Shabbos Arouses Simchah shel Mitzvah

Physical joy brings spiritual joy, so if someone is lacking physical necessities it will be difficult for him to become elevated spiritually. The goal of taking pleasure in the Shabbos with food and drink is to lift the spirits to a state of *simchah*, so that one can have peace of mind and be able to elevate his soul to delight in Hashem.

Indeed, Rabbeinu Bacheye writes in his commentary on the Torah (*Bereishis* 1:21): *It is known that by eating and drinking, which arouse the forces of one's body, the spiritual powers of a person are also aroused and strengthened. Food and drink bring a person to happiness and distance him from sadness and worry. It is known that when there is* simchah, *one's spiritual powers are strengthened, and he has a greater ability to reach higher levels of understanding.*

The obligation of *simchah* on Shabbos is found in the *tefillah* of *Yismichu B'malchuscha shomrei Shabbos*—"They rejoice in your sovereignty, those who keep the Shabbos." The *Zohar* states (as written in *Zemiros Shabbos*) that a voice announces each Shabbos that the Jews, "should bring joy to Hashem and arouse themselves to joy and prepare themselves with the three *seudos*, of the three *Avos*, for *emunah*."

The reason why there is an obligation to have joy is that, as we have seen, during the *seudos* the *Shechinah* rests on us. The Gemara states (*Pesachim* 117a) that the *Shechinah* only rests on a person who is in a state of *simchah shel mitzvah*, as we find that Elisha requested that music be played for him in order that he be a fitting receptacle to receive prophecy (*Melachim II* 3:15). When a person performs a mitzvah with joy, he becomes close to Hashem and is purified and becomes filled with *yiras* and *ahavas Hashem*. This causes him to become a fitting vessel for the *Shechinah*. Indeed, we find that *Chazal* say that a person receives greater reward for *simchah shel mitzvah* than for performing the mitzvah. Therefore, it is imperative that we keep Shabbos with great joy and festive singing. This is also a reason for lighting Shabbos candles. *Neiros Shabbos* increase *shalom bayis,* so that the home is happy and the *Shechinah* can rest there.

The Gemara states (*Moed Katan* 9a) that Reb Yochanan says that in the year that Bnei Yisrael celebrated the *chanukas Beis Hamikdash* they did not fast on Yom Kippur. They then worried that they would be destroyed. A Heavenly voice called out, "All of you are destined for *Olam Haba*." The Gemara asks why Bnei Yisrael needed to eat and drink on that Yom Kippur; couldn't they have sufficed with sacrificing *korbanos* and not eating from them? The Gemara answers that there is no joy without food and drink.

The mishnah explains that the words, *and the day that His heart rejoiced* (*Shir Hashirim* 3:11) refer to the building of the Beis Hamikdash (*Megillah* 10a). The Gemara states that the day of *chanukas haMikdash* was a day of *simchah* to Hashem like the day that He created the heaven and earth. Shlomo Hamelech saw with *ruach hakodesh,* and understood with his great wisdom that this long-awaited day when Hashem would rest His *Shechinah* among the Jews was a time of such great joy for Hashem that it was appropriate that Klal Yisrael rejoice together with Him. This required sacrificing *korbanos* and eating them, and was a greater mitzvah than fasting on Yom Kippur.

Similarly, on Shabbos, Hashem rests his *Shechinah* on Bnei Yisrael, and it is a time of great joy for Hashem. Therefore, it is a mitzvah for us to rejoice with Him by eating the *seudos*.

Performing Mitzvos with Joy

Although *seudas Shabbos* has several parts to it, including *zemiros* that bring a person to *simchah* and love for Hashem, and *divrei Torah* that sanctify the *seudah* and elevate it to be a table of Hashem (see *Pirkei Avos* 3:4), one should know that the goal of eating itself is also to achieve *simchah shel mitzvah*. A person who fulfills the obligation of eating *seudas Shabbos* without thinking about this is therefore missing its main purpose, which is a great loss.

Indeed, the Rambam states that *simchah shel mitzvah* is a great service, and one who performs a mitzvah without *simchah* is liable to be punished, as it says, *because you did not serve Hashem with happiness and with gladness of heart when [you had an] abundance of everything* (*Devarim* 28:47). The Maggid Mishneh explains this Rambam as follows: A person should not perform a mitzvah in a manner which demonstrates that he is forced to do it. Rather, he should understand that he was created for the purpose of serving Hashem with joy, and he should perform every mitzvah with *simchah*.

Understanding the Shabbos Food

The Shabbos foods eaten by Jews throughout the world have trustworthy sources from previous *tzaddikim* and were handed down from generation to generation. Each of these foods contains deep and hidden reasons, some of which are stated clearly in *sefarim* and some of which are concealed, but every custom was instituted by *gedolei Yisrael* with *ruach hakodesh*.

We see that although they were not generally involved in food and drink, our *tzaddikim* were very careful to eat the accepted Shabbos foods and discuss the reasons for eating them. They explained that the source of these foods is rooted in spiritual ideas, since Shabbos food is really a spiritual entity. They gave reasons that were straightforward, as well as reasons based on *mussar*, Kabbalah, or allusions, and they understood that Shabbos food leads a person to have a greater ability to understand the Torah and mitzvos, and reach loftier heights.

The *Sefer Mishmeres Shalom* (Koidonov 28:7) explains at length that our Shabbos food reaches very elevated upper worlds and alludes to the ten *sefiros* (Kabbalistic attributes of Hashem). It is praiseworthy if one knows the proper hidden intentions while eating Shabbos food, but even if he does not understand the hidden meanings, if he can grasp even part of a reason for a certain food, he should have that reason in mind while eating it. And even if one does not understand any reason at all, if he has in mind to fulfill the mitzvah of *oneg Shabbos*, that also has great value and will bring him holiness and purity.

The previous generations clearly recognized the power hidden within the traditional Shabbos foods, and they were aware that these foods have the ability to effect blessing. Today we do not possess this understanding, but we must follow what our ancestors did with the clear belief that it was all for good reason. The Gemara in *Pesachim* states that one is not permitted to change the *minhag* of his parents, as it says: *Listen, my son, to the discipline of your father, and do not forsake the instruction of your mother* (Mishlei 1:8). A person should not veer from that which his parents did, nor let go of any *minhag*.

Today, however, many traditional Shabbos foods are disregarded, and people do not value the importance of these *minhagim*. This is caused by a lack of knowledge that has led people to believe that there is no difference between eating one dish and another, and that they may eat whatever they like.

This attitude is sadly misguided. The Ya'avetz (*Avos* 3:4) writes that the holiness of Klal Yisrael depends on the food they eat. Food has a tremendous power to lead either to holiness or the opposite. Pure food leads to a pure body, and this will positively affect the spirituality of the person.

The Chavas Da'as writes in his *sefer, Nachalas Yaakov* (*Bereishis, Beha'aloscha*), that the more elevated a species is in creation, the more refined is its food. Animals, which are physical, earthly beings, eat straw. A snake, which is a coarser animal, eats earth. A person, who is more refined, eats more delicate foods. The people who lived in the times of Moshe Rabbeinu, who were on such a lofty level that they were more spiritual than physical, ate the *mann*, a spiritual food referred to as, "bread of the angels."

On Shabbos, the soul is sanctified and elevated, as stated in the *Zohar* (vol. 2, p. 205a), and by eating Shabbos food, the body is sanctified and purified from its physicality as well. Thus, Shabbos foods need to be more spiritual than physical, and the Shabbos foods that the previous generations instituted are the proper spiritual foods to nourish the soul.

Rashi cites the following midrash on a *pasuk* in *Devarim* (33:19): *Gentile merchants came to Eretz Yisrael. While they were standing at the border they decided that since they expended so much effort in reaching Eretz Yisrael they may as well travel to Yerushalayim and observe the Jewish nation. They went and saw that the Jews all serve one G-d and eat one food, unlike the gentiles who have many different gods and their foods are all different. This inspired the merchants to convert to Judaism.*

Tzaddikim explain that "one food" refers to Shabbos foods. On Shabbos, all Jews eat similar foods according to the traditions that were handed down to us, because these specific foods bring us to a lofty, more spiritual level.

Discussing Shabbos Foods During the Seudah

The Gemara *(Sanhedrin* 101a) states that Hakadosh Baruch Hu said to the Torah, "My daughter, at the time that Bnei Yisrael eat and drink, with what should they occupy themselves?"

The Torah answered, "Ribono Shel Olam, if they are people who are knowledgeable in Tanach, they should occupy themselves with learning Tanach. If they have knowledge of Mishnayos, they should occupy themselves with learning Mishnayos, *halachos*, and *aggados*. If they know Talmud, they should occupy themselves on each Yom Tov by learning its *halachos*; on Pesach, they should learn *hilchos Pesach*; on Shavuos, *hilchos Shavuos*; and on Sukkos, *hilchos Sukkos*."

Reb Shimon ben Elazar said in the name of Reb Shimon ben Chananyah that one who reads a *pasuk* in its [proper] time brings good to the world, as it says: *He has made everything beautiful in its time (Koheles* 3:11). Rashi explains that if a person says words of Torah in their time during a meal (i.e. on Yom Tov, he speaks of matters pertaining to that Yom Tov), he brings good to the world. Rabbeinu Yonah explains that discussing something in its time is good, because it is applicable immediately and has an immediate effect *(Talmidei Rabbeinu Yonah, Brachos* 31).

From this we see that in addition to the general obligation to speak words of Torah at each meal, as explained in *Pirkei Avos*, there is an obligation to speak words of Torah relevant to that time. Such words elevate a person's heart to sense the greatness of the time and ultimately bring good to the world. We can conclude from here that it is appropriate and fitting to discuss Shabbos foods on Shabbos.

The Gemara states (*Sotah* 40a) that Reb Avahu and Reb Chiyah bar Abba once came to a certain place. Reb Avahu gave a discourse on *aggados* (stories and allusions from *Chazal*), while Reb Chiyah bar Abba discussed *halachos*. The participants all left Reb Chiyah bar Abba's discourse and went to hear Reb Avahu. Reb Chiyah bar Abba was distressed, but Reb Avahu consoled him with a parable: *There were once two peddlers who sold wares. One sold expensive gems, and the other sold small items and trinkets. Which peddler had more customers? The one who sold cheaper items, since people could afford them.* Reb Avahu explained to Reb Chiyah bar Abba that people came to hear his discourse on *aggadah* since they gravitate more toward lighter ideas than to halachah, but that didn't mean that his discourse had less value than Reb Avahu's; on the contrary, perhaps it was more valuable.

Furthermore, the *pasuk* states: *Ko somar l'veis Yaakov v'sagid l'vnei Yisrael*—"So shall you say to the house of Yaakov and tell the sons of Yisrael" (*Shemos* 19:3). Rashi explains that "Beis Yaakov" refers to the women, who should be spoken to in a softer manner. Bnei Yisrael refers to the men, who should be spoken to in a harsher manner. This demonstrates that one needs to speak to each person in a suitable way.

Since the Shabbos table generally includes men, women and children, one should speak in a pleasant manner, discussing lighter ideas that are suitable for everyone, and that will hold their interest. One should definitely discuss the greatness of the Shabbos *seudos* and its foods, so that his family gains the proper understanding and attitudes, but he should do so in a way that is palatable to all those present.

If a person can give over these ideas successfully, his family will come to understand the significance of the Shabbos food and will eventually delight in true closeness to Hashem at the Shabbos table, which is a semblance of the World to Come.

Chapter 2
V'karasa laShabbos Oneg—Delighting in the Shabbos

The Mitzvah of Oneg Shabbos

The *pasuk* in *Yeshayah* (58:13) states: *V'karasa laShabbos oneg*—"and you should call the Shabbos a delight." We learn from here that it is a mitzvah to delight in the Shabbos with sweet and fine foods.

When one makes Shabbos different from the other days of the week and eats finer foods, a person will come to contemplate the fact that Hashem created the world and rested on Shabbos. He will then praise Hashem with his entire being, and his *neshamah* will take pleasure in Shabbos.

(*Radak, Yeshayahu* 58:13)

Every person is required to take pleasure in the Shabbos through eating and drinking. Women are also included in this commandment, as any mitzvah given for *simchah* and *oneg*, women are considered equal to men (*Pri Megadim* 280, *MZ* 1; *Klei Chemdah, Vayakhel*), and *Chazal* state: *Rabbah said that all agree that on Shabbos, part of the day should be for you* (*Pesachim* 68b).

One should eat delectable and fine foods on Shabbos, as the Gemara states that one should delight in Shabbos with spinach, large fish and heads of garlic, which Rashi explains to mean choice foods. (*Shabbos* 118b)

How should a person take pleasure on Shabbos? Each

person should prepare a dish of choice meat and fine drinks, according to his means. One who spends a large amount on Shabbos food and prepares many fine dishes is praised.

(Rambam, Hilchos Shabbos 30:7)

The mitzvah of *oneg* applies throughout Shabbos. It does not refer only to the *seudos*, or to the challah that one is required to eat. We see in the Rambam that one should cook a fine dish and prepare a sweet drink. Every food eaten in honor of Shabbos contributes to *oneg Shabbos*.

The *Shulchan Aruch* states that there were those who permitted telling a gentile to carry food needed for Shabbos through an area where carrying is prohibited *d'Rabbanan*, since telling a gentile to do a *melachah* is permitted in order for one to be able to fulfill a mitzvah.

The *Mishnah Berurah* states that, practically, this is only permitted if it is needed to fulfill a mitzvah, such as if one needs wine for Kiddush or *chamin*, a warm dish to eat. However, if one sees a person ask a gentile to carry other Shabbos food for him, he should not object.

This proves that *oneg Shabbos* refers to any food eaten throughout Shabbos, not just the three *seudos*. Even after a person has finished all three *seudos*, he still fulfills the mitzvah of *oneg Shabbos* by eating other foods.

Additionally, the Gemara states that whatever one spends for Shabbos is not determined in his yearly income. The Gemara does not say "whatever one spends on the Shabbos **seudos**." It seems from these words that *oneg Shabbos* refers to any food eaten during Shabbos. *(Lev Banim 17:2)*

How should a person take pleasure in Shabbos? Each person should act according to the custom in the place where he lives and according to his own preference. One should prepare many fine dishes with a good fragrance for the *seudah*.

One who spends a large amount of money on Shabbos food and gifts for the poor on Erev Shabbos is praised.
(Shulchan Hatahor 242:2-3)

The mitzvah of *oneg Shabbos* is clarified in the *Navi*, as it says: *And you should call Shabbos a delight.* There are *poskim* who hold that the basic mitzvah is written in the Torah: *Shabbos Shabbason mikra kodesh* (*Vayikra* 23:3). *Chazal* explain this to mean that one should sanctify and honor the Shabbos with clean clothing, food and drink. *Chazal* have praised this mitzvah and extolled the greatness of its reward. One who delights in the Shabbos is given an unlimited portion, is spared from being subjugated by the nations, and will merit wealth and additional blessings. *(Mishnah Berurah 242:1)*

Conversely, the *Sefer Hachinuch* and the Beis Yosef hold that *mikra kodesh* refers to sanctifying the Shabbos by refraining from doing *melachah,* and is not a reference to eating and drinking at all. *(Sefer Hachinuch*, mitzvah 297; *Beis Yosef* 287)

The Gemara states that one who takes pleasure in the Shabbos is granted all his heart's desires *(Shabbos* 118b), as the *pasuk* in *Tehillim* (37:4) states: *And you will take pleasure in Hashem and He will grant all your heart's desires.*

The *Bnei Yissaschar* cites the Alshich who asks why the above Gemara says *kol hame'aneg es HaShabbos*—"one who gives pleasure *for* the Shabbos." Why doesn't the Gemara say *kol hamisaneg*—"one who has pleasure *on* Shabbos"?

The Alshich explains that the intended meaning of *oneg Shabbos* is not to derive pleasure from lightheartedness, walks, speaking nonsense, etc., because Shabbos does not have any pleasure from these activities. Therefore, *Chazal* use the phrase of one who gives pleasure *for* the Shabbos; *oneg* on Shabbos must be something from which the Shabbos itself will have pleasure. *(Dvar Tzvi, Shabbos* 118)

The *Zohar* states that during the week, the *Shechinah* gets pleasure from one's *Birkas Hamazon*, but on Shabbos it gets pleasure from the actual *seudah* that he eats to fulfill *oneg Shabbos*, because any form of pleasure on Shabbos is a mitzvah. (*Zohar, Parshas Vayakhel*, p. 218)

By eating meat and drinking wine on Shabbos one fulfills the mitzvah of *oneg Shabbos*. (*Rambam, Hilchos Shabbos* 30:10)

The *kohanim* were permitted to eat the *korbanos* in different forms—roasted or cooked, either with spices that were holy (*terumah*) or unsanctified spices. This teaches us that the *kohanim* did not have to eat the *korbanos* purely for the sake of Heaven; they were permitted to derive pleasure from them as well, by making the meat taste good.

Similarly, if one enjoys the food, the pleasure he derives from it does not take away from the mitzvah. (*Zevachim* 90b)

Shabbos is a foretaste of the World to Come, where there is pleasure hidden for the *tzaddikim*. Therefore, it is fitting for a person to compare Shabbos in This World to the eternal Shabbos, and to delight in all kinds of pleasures. Just as Hashem will prepare a *seudah* for the *tzaddikim* in the World to Come with meat, fish, and wine that were created at the time of the creation of the world for this purpose, a person should do the same at his Shabbos *seudah* and eat these three foods. (*Mateh Moshe* 404; *Toras Chaim, Eiruvin*, ch. 2)

Oneg Shabbos—An "Investment" for the Future

One should do whatever he can to increase his *oneg Shabbos*; for example, he should spice his food with various kinds of spices. This is because in the future, for every flavor he ate on Shabbos, he will merit a different kind of spiritual light.

(*Mateh Moshe*, sec. 404)

One who delights in the Shabbos with eating and drinking eats the fruit, but the seeds are reserved for *Olam Haba*.

(*Nefesh Yeseirah, Ma'areches* 300, sec, 10)

The *pasuk* states, *va'achaltem achol*—"and you should eat, eating" (Yoel 2:26). The *seudah* of the *Livyasan*, after Mashiach comes, will consist of what the Jews ate at their Shabbos and Yom Tov *seudos*, when hosting guests, and at other *seudos mitzvos*. Thus, the *pasuk* means that in the future you will eat that which you already ate. *(Kedushas Levi, Likutim)*

Chazal say that one who takes pleasure in Shabbos merits a long life. *Chazal* also say that one who recites Kiddush on wine on Friday night, which honors the Shabbos, will live a long life in This World and the Next World. The Seforno states (Shemos 20:12) that the assurance of a long life, which is stated in the fifth commandment (honoring parents), pertains not only to the commandment of honoring parents, but also to the rest of the first five commandments as well; thus, Shabbos is included in this blessing of long life.

It is written in the *Midrash Rabbah* (Bereishis 11:4) that Rabbi Yishmael ben Rabbi Yosi asked Rabbi Yehudah Hanasi how people in *chutz la'Aretz* merit long life. Rabbi Yehudah answered that it is in the merit of honoring the Shabbos and Yom Tov. This can be seen in the word Shabbos, which is an acronym of the words **Shanim B'zechuso Tarbeh**—in the *zechus* of Shabbos you will live many years, and also **Shanim Ba'avuro Tosif**—because of the Shabbos, your years will be increased. *(Nefesh Yeseirah, Ma'areches 300, sec. 13)*

When the Radvaz was still a young man, he became gravely ill. One Friday morning, he was drifting in and out of consciousness and he seemed to be nearing his end. Suddenly, his soul was called up to the Heavenly court and he was given the opportunity to plead his case.

At first, he tried to acquire more time in This World by mentioning that he had more Torah to learn, *sefarim* to write, *chessed* to do, and children to raise. To each claim, the answer was that someone else could do these tasks for him. Finally, he stated that every Thursday night, his wife would stay up all night preparing for Shabbos. Then, the two of them would sit down together and discuss how they could better enhance Shabbos, have more *oneg*, and thus bring more joy to Hashem.

This created a huge tumult in Heaven and it was finally able to overturn the decree against the Radvaz. He soon miraculously recovered and lived to be 110 years old—all in the merit of the exceptional honor that he accorded Shabbos, and his dedicated preparation for its arrival each week.

(*Sefer Be'er Haparshah*)

The Purpose of Shabbos

Rabbi Brachyah states in the name of Rabbi Chiya bar Abba that the Shabbos was given only to provide pleasure.

(*Pesikta D'Rav Kahana*, ch. 23)

The Yerushalmi cites two views regarding the purpose of Shabbos:

Rabbi Chagai says in the name of Rabbi Shmuel Bar Nachman: The Shabbasos and Yamim Tovim were given only for eating and drinking, i.e. Shabbos and Yom Tov were given exclusively for pleasure and rest. However, *Chazal* were afraid that if a person would indulge in food and drink all day without learning Torah, he would come to frivolity or to use his mouth for forbidden speech. Therefore, *Chazal* permitted one to learn Torah.

Rabbi Brachyah states in the name of Rabbi Chiya Bar Abba, The Shabbasos and Yamim Tovim were only given to learn Torah, i.e. on Shabbos one should *only* learn Torah.

The Yerushalmi brings proof for both views and then concludes that one should use part of the day for learning and part for eating and drinking. (*Yerushalmi, Shabbos* 15:3)

A person should not think that by preparing fish, meat, and wine for Shabbos, he has fulfilled the mitzvah of Shabbos in its entirety. On Shabbos, a person needs to have more *yiras Hashem* and *ahavas Hashem* than during the week. To the extent that he increases these traits, he fulfills the mitzvah of Shabbos. One who does not do so has not fully fulfilled it.

We can learn this from the following *pasuk*: *Ri'u ki Hashem nasan lachem haShabbos, al kein hu nosen lachem bayom hashishi lechem yomayim, shevu ish tachtav al yeitzei ish mimkomo bayom hashvi'i*—"See that Hashem has given you the Shabbos. Therefore, on the sixth day, He gave you bread for two days. Let each man remain in his place; let no man leave his place on the seventh day" (*Shemos* 16:29).

Ri'u ki Hashem-A person should see how much *yiras* and *ahavas Hashem* he gained on Shabbos, and, according to that, *nasan lachem haShabbos*—you have fulfilled the mitzvah of Shabbos. *Shevu ish tachtav*—a person should sit under Hashem, and *al yeitzei ish mimkomo*—a person should not go out of his awareness of Hashem, who is the *Mekomo shel olam* (*Bereishis Rabbah* 68:9).

A person should therefore not forget *yiras* and *ahavas Hashem* for even a moment on Shabbos.

(*Ma'ayan Hachachmah, Beshalach*, s.v. *Ri'u*)

Pleasure for Body and Soul

The body and soul are opposites. The pleasure of one generally causes suffering to the other, except for pleasure that is derived from a mitzvah. With this we can explain the phrase from the Gemara (*Shabbos* 118a): *Kol hame'aneg es haShabbos, nosnin lo nachalah bli metzarim*—"One who delights in the Shabbos food [which is a mitzvah] will be given a portion without any *metzarim*." *Metzarim* can mean suffering, because *oneg* on Shabbos is pleasure for the body and the soul together, with no suffering. (*Toldos Yaakov Yosef, Parshas Va'eira*)

Kol hame'aneg es haShabbos, nosnin lo nachalah bli metzarim means that one who delights in the Shabbos is given a portion without any suffering. Eating is painful for the soul and fasting is painful for the body, except for on Shabbos and Yom Tov when they don't have that effect.

(*Tefillah L'Moshe, Tehillim*, 29:6)

The entire creation senses that it is Shabbos. Therefore, during *davening* on Shabbos we say *Nishmas kol chai*, every living being should bless Hashem, and...*yefa'aru v'yevarchu laKeil kol yetzurav*, they should bless Hashem, all His creations.

Reb Pinchas of Koritz says that even a pig enjoys his mud more on Shabbos than during the week. (*Ohr Ganuz*, p. 1)

The act of eating on Shabbos cannot be compared to eating during the week, because eating on Shabbos is a delight, *oneg*, which is an acronym for *eden, nahar,* and *gan,* referring to Gan Eden. (*Bnei Yisaschar, Ma'amarei HaShabbasos* 7)

Reb Yechiel, the son of Reb Elazar of Kozhnitz, once spent Shabbos in Neustadt at the home of Reb Yossele of Neustadt. When Reb Yechiel was served the Shabbos food, he ate a very small amount.

Reb Yossele commented, "Why will the *tzaddikim* eat the *shor habor* and the *livyasan* in *Olam Haba*? We would think that in *Olam Haba* there is no need for food. It seems to me that one who was holy and separated himself from the pleasures of This World will have pleasure from the *Shechinah* in *Olam Haba,* which is a tremendous pleasure that cannot be described. But since the *tzaddik* never tasted the pleasures of *Olam Hazeh* he does not know what is truly good. He may think that perhaps the pleasures of *Olam Hazeh* are just as good as, or even better than, the pleasure of *Olam Haba*. Therefore, he is first given the *seudah* of the *shor habor* and the *livyasan,* which includes all pleasures of This World, and then when he takes pleasure in the *Shechinah,* he knows the difference between the physical and spiritual pleasures.

"This concept also applies to Shabbos. Shabbos is *mei'ein Olam Haba.* Thus, our Sages have commanded us to take pleasure in the Shabbos with physical enjoyment, so that a person will be able to clearly differentiate between the pleasure of Shabbos food and the pleasure derived from recitation of *Nishmas Kol Chai, Hakol Yoducha,* etc.

"If the Rebbe does not taste the food at all, he will not know how to differentiate between spiritual pleasures and physical pleasures. The Rebbe might suspect that perhaps physical pleasures are better. Thus, it is proper for the Rebbe to partake of all the dishes." *(Gedulas Hatzaddikim,* p. 24)

Pleasure for Hashem

Shabbos provides Hashem with greater pleasure than any other mitzvah. This is comparable to a king who is celebrating an event and wishes to have all his subjects, acquaintances, relatives and, of course, his children, present to participate and rejoice with him, and enjoy the fine foods and wines that he prepared.

How much more so is the immeasurable joy of Hashem when we take pleasure in His day of happiness by partaking of fine foods three times. Hashem gives us a tremendous reward for doing so. One who eats three *seudos* will be spared from the birth pangs of Mashiach, Gehinnom, and the war of Gog and Magog. He will be given an unlimited reward and be freed from his *yetzer hara*. He will also be granted his heart's desires and given wealth, among other blessings *(Shabbos* 118a).

(Sidduro Shel Shabbos, vol. 1, *Shoresh* 5, section 3)

Just as a person is sustained by food and drink, Hashem gets "sustenance" from the mitzvos of Jews *(Zohar,* vol. 3, p. 7b). As we say during *zemiros, Askinu seudasa,* by preparing

seudos Shabbos, we bring *chedvasa l'Malka kaddisha*, joy to Hashem.
(Shloshah Sefarim Niftachim, s.v. *Askinu)*

The Yismach Yisrael cites the following explanation on the words of *Askinu Seudasa*: *Askinu seudasa dimheimenusa*, through the *emunah* that one attains from *seudos Shabbos*, *chedvasa l'Malka kaddisha*, one brings joy to Hashem.
(Yismach Yisrael, Chanukah, section 32)

Askinu seudasa dimheimenusa, through believing in the power of *seudas Shabbos*, i.e. that it contains lofty secrets above our understanding, *chedvasa l'Malka kaddisha*, one brings tremendous pleasure to Hashem.
(Yismach Yisrael, Parshas Tazria, section 6)

The Power of Eating on Shabbos

The light of Shabbos is stronger than that of any other day, including Yom Tov, because Shabbos is an *isarusa dileila*—the awakening of spirituality is from Above; we do not need to invest effort in order for it to happen.

The source of every person's *neshamah* is Above and is connected to his *neshamah* down in This World. The light of Shabbos travels from up in the Heavens to one's *neshamah* down in This World and he is awakened and filled with joy according to how connected he is to the source of his *neshamah*. Even the weakest Jew is aroused on Shabbos because the tremendous light of Shabbos affects every *neshamah*, without the person needing to invest effort for it to happen. One who does not take pleasure in Shabbos and does not feel this light shows that he has [severely impaired] his connection to Above and has [weakened the] link to his source.

Therefore, eating on Shabbos is different from other mitzvos involving food. Most mitzvos involving food, such as eating matzah, eating on Erev Yom Kippur, or *korbanos,* are to awaken something Above. On Shabbos, though, the holiness is already there—we just need to bring it down. We do not need to do anything for *oneg Shabbos,* yet Hashem, in His great kindness, gives us an infinite amount of reward as if we deserve credit for it.

One who delights in the Shabbos will merit much good and happiness, and will rejoice in Hashem when Mashiach comes, as we say in the Shabbos *Shemoneh Esrei, Yismichu v'malchuscha shomrei Shabbos v'korei oneg*—"They will rejoice in Your kingdom, those who keep the Shabbos and call it a delight."

The mitzvah of *oneg Shabbos* is not written in the Torah because the spiritual pleasure of Shabbos is something one feels in his heart. He does not need to be commanded to do so. If he does not feel it, then Hashem does not want to command him to eat food that will just be consumed to fulfill his desires without a higher purpose.

The *Navi* does mention *oneg Shabbos*, but states, *If you will call the Shabbos oneg... then you will delight in Hashem (Yeshayahu* 58:13-14). The *Navi* is not commanding us to have *oneg Shabbos*, but rather is stating that if one feels the pleasure of Shabbos, and thus does actions that bring him more *oneg*, then he will merit to delight in Hashem.

Two people can eat a *Korban Pesach* and one will stumble from it and one will gain merit, depending on their intentions, as it says: *The ways of Hashem are straight; the righteous will walk in them and the wicked will stumble upon them (Nazir* 23a). If one eats the *korban* because he is hungry, even if he does not eat gluttonously, he is eating to satisfy his desires and thus stumbles in this mitzvah *(Rashi).* But one whose intentions are for the sake of Hashem gains merit. Likewise, Hashem knows a person's intentions when eating on Shabbos. He knows if it is to honor Shabbos or to satisfy his own desires.

(*Sidduro Shel Shabbos*, vol. 1, *Shoresh* 5, section 3)

Eating Shabbos food is the primary means through which we honor Shabbos. Eating on Shabbos is an act that is tremendously valued by Hashem because it is completely holy and the Satan has no part in it. Therefore, it is a great mitzvah to enhance our Shabbos food. Shabbos food nullifies all bad forces and it has the power to rectify *chillul Shabbos* (desecration of the Shabbos). (*Likutei Eitzos, Eirech Shabbos*, sec. 6, 15)

In *zemiros* we sing, *Yom kadosh hu, mibo'o v'ad tzeiso*—"[Shabbos is] a holy day, from when it arrives until it leaves. The children of Yaakov should honor it, like the words of the King and His commands that are written in the Torah, to rest on this day and to rejoice, and to have pleasure by eating and drinking."

This can be understood to mean that honoring the Shabbos is equivalent to fulfilling the entire Torah, as it says, *like the words of the King and His commands*. How does a person honor the Shabbos? The *zemer* continues by stating, *...to rest on this day and to rejoice, and to have pleasure by eating and drinking*. This demonstrates that by eating and drinking on Shabbos, it is as if a person fulfilled the entire Torah.

Eating the Shabbos *seudos* also helps a person keep the entire Torah. The pleasure of eating on Shabbos is the link between mundane eating and fulfilling mitzvos, because it is eating that can bring a person to fulfill Torah and mitzvos. If this is what eating Shabbos food can accomplish, how much more so will keeping the Shabbos help a person fulfill all of Torah and mitzvos! (*Ateres Yisrael, Parshas Kedoshim*)

During the week, the foods one eats become part of him. It is separated into its parts and enters his bloodstream, which is his life force. The liver receives the blood containing the nutrients and then sends it to the heart and brain. Thus, food is used to create the cells which make up the heart and the brain of a person.

A person's heart and brain are thus strengthened in *avodas Hashem* through eating during the week because the heart is awakened to serve Hashem and the brain becomes strengthened to contemplate Hashem's greatness.

On Shabbos, however, *borer* (separating) is forbidden, so eating must be for a different, higher and holier purpose; it is to have *oneg* with Hashem. *(Torah Ohr, Chayei Sarah)*

If a wise person does not take pleasure in Shabbos, his wisdom will depart from him. *(Tikkunei Zohar, Tikkun 19, p. 31a)*

Shabbos demonstrates that the Jewish nation is not under the influence of *mazel*. We see in the *Sefer Tikkunim* *(Tikkun 48, p. 85a)* that Shabbos is under the *mazel* of *shabsai* which represents sadness, mourning, and all evil in the world. However, we rejoice on Shabbos and are not afraid of the nations. This is what *Chazal* say *(Shabbos 118a)*: *One who delights in the Shabbos will be given an unlimited portion, as the pasuk states: Then, you shall delight with Hashem, and I will cause you to ride on the high places of the land, and I will give you to eat the heritage of Yaakov, your father...* *(Yeshayahu 58:14)*. This means that one who delights in the Shabbos and rejoices with food, drink, and clean clothing, will be elevated above the *mazel* of Shabbos that symbolizes suffering. When we take pleasure in Shabbos we do not need to fear the nations, and no nation will have power over us.

If we act according to what the *mazel* symbolizes and don't honor the Shabbos—we don weekday clothes and eat weekday food—then the nations will be able to rule over us and subjugate us under the influence of the *mazel* of Shabbos. Therefore, on Shabbos one should wear different clothes, light candles, and eat better food than one eats during the week. This shows the nations of the world that, unlike them, we are not under the power of the *mazel* of Shabbos, and they will be incapable of harming us. *(Nefesh Yeseirah, Ma'areches Shin, sec. 100)*

Rabbi Shimon ben Pazi said in the name of Rabbi Yehoshua ben Levi, in the name of Bar Kapara, that one who eats three *seudos* on Shabbos is spared from three evil happenings: the birth pangs of Mashiach, Gehinnom, and the war of Gog and Magog.

Rabbi Yochanan said in the name of Rabbi Yosi that one who delights in the Shabbos is given an unlimited portion, as the *pasuk* in *Yeshayah* states: *...and you call the Shabbos a delight...and I will cause you to ride on the high places of the land, and I will give you to eat **the portion of Yaakov**, your father...* (*Yeshayah* 58:13-14).

Unlike Avraham, to whom Hashem said, *Rise, walk in the land, to its length and to its breadth* (*Bereishis* 13:17), or Yitzchak, to whom He said, *To you and your children I will give all these lands,* Hashem said to Yaakov, *and you shall gain strength westward and eastward and northward and southward* (*Bereishis* 28:14). Avraham's and Yitzchak's portions were defined and limited, but the *pasuk* indicates that Yaakov's portion had no boundaries. Therefore, when the *pasuk* in *Yeshayah* refers to the portion of Yaakov, it is referring to an unlimited portion.

Rabi Nachman bar Yitzchak states that one who delights in the Shabbos will be spared from being subjugated by the nations.

Rav Yehudah states in the name of Rav: *One who delights in the Shabbos will be granted his heart's desires, as the pasuk in Tehillim states*: "*So shall you delight in Hashem, and He will give you what your heart desires* (*Tehillim* 37:4)."

(*Shabbos* 118a)

Through *oneg Shabbos* one merits *Olam Haba*, because one who eats for the sake of Hashem is serving Hashem through eating, just as he is when he learns Torah or *davens*.

(*Yisa Brachah, Parshas Balak*, s.v. *Ne'um*)

A chassid once complained to Reb Simchah Bunim of Peshischa that he was beset by many problems. He and his wife were both ill, he had no *nachas* from his children and they did not respect him, and he was earning a meager income.

Reb Simchah Bunim opened up the *sefer* that he had been learning, immersed himself in it for a moment, and then told the chassid, "Our sages teach that one who sees that his *tefillos* are not being answered should take a resolution upon himself. The *sefer* that I was just learning explains that if a person begins to honor the Shabbos more, he will merit life, children and sustenance, and his *tefillos* will be answered."

The chassid assured the Rebbe that from that day and on he would honor the Shabbos more than in the past. After he kept his word, he and his wife were healed, his children improved their ways and started honoring him, and their livelihood improved. Just as his situation changed, so did his relationship with Shabbasos and Yamim Tovim. He invited guests to his Shabbos table and honored them greatly.

(*Kitzur Shulchan Aruch Im Sippurim Chasidi'im*, p. 195)

The Friday night *tefillos* and *seudah* influence Sunday and Monday of the following week, Shacharis and the day *seudah* influence Tuesday and Wednesday, and Minchah and *shalosh seudos* influence Thursday and Friday.

(*Yalkut Reuveini, Parshas Beshalach*, s.v. *V'hayah*)

Alternatively, the Sfas Emes says that the Friday night *seudah* influences Sunday and Friday of the following week, the day *seudah* influences Monday and Thursday, and *shalosh seudos* has an effect on Tuesday and Wednesday.

(*Sfas Emes, Parshas Vayakhel* 5651)

The Apter Rav said that through eating Shabbos food one can accomplish what he can achieve with his *tefillos* during the Yamim Noraim. (*Magen Avos*, p. 218)

"Eating" Shabbos

The Torah states: *Ichluhu hayom ki Shabbos hayom laHashem, hayom lo simtza'uhu basadeh*—"And Moshe said, 'Eat [the *mann*] today, for today is Shabbos for Hashem; today you will not find it [*mann*] in the field'" (*Shemos* 16:25). Just like the food a person eats enters him and becomes part of him, we should "eat" the day, i.e. Shabbos; we should ensure that the Shabbos enters our very essence and becomes a part of us.

(Be'eiros Mayim)

Chazal say that word *hayom* appears three times in this *pasuk* (*Ichluhu hayom...*) to correspond to the three *seudos* Shabbos.

The letters that form the word *hayom*—*heh, yud, vav* and *mem*—appear most often in the Torah. The letter *vav* appears in the Torah 76,922 times, the letter *yud* appears 76,500 times, the letter *mem* appears 52,805 times and the letter *heh* appears 47,754 times. All other letters of the *aleph-beis* appear fewer times; *peh* is the least common letter, appearing only 1,975 times. The Torah alludes to *seudos Shabbos* with the word *hayom* to show us that just as the letters of the word *hayom* appear most often in the Torah, it is fitting for a person to enhance his Shabbos table to the greatest extent that he is able. *(Benayahu Ben Yehoyadah, Shabbos* 117b)

Delighting in Shabbos for the Sake of Hashem

The Gemara states on the *pasuk, Remember the Shabbos day* (*Shemos* 20:8), that because the Torah tells us to remember Shabbos, it means that a person is liable to forget it. The Dubno Maggid explains that since body and soul both have a part in the mitzvos of Shabbos, one can forget why he is eating bread and delicacies on Shabbos and just eat for physical pleasure. Therefore, the Torah tells us to remember the Shabbos—remember that you are eating in honor of Shabbos. Engrave it in your memory because it is possible to forget that the main mitzvah of *oneg Shabbos* is not for one's personal pleasure but rather to fulfill the will of Hashem. If we do so, then Hashem will redeem us for our sake. *(Yitev Lev, Parshas Bo,* p. 23)

One who eats for his own pleasure only has pleasure from the food while eating. But one who eats for the sake of a mitzvah, his happiness lasts even after he has finished eating, as it says in *Tehillim* (19:9): *The mitzvos of Hashem are upright, causing the heart to rejoice.* *(Yitev Panim, Shabbos Hagadol,* sec. 9)

The Gemara states: *One who delights in the Shabbos will be granted his heart's desires, as it says, And you will delight in Hashem and He will grant you your heart's desires* (Tehillim 37:4). *Chazal* explain that the delight, [*oneg*] in this *pasuk* refers to Shabbos, as the *pasuk* in *Yeshayah* (58:13) states: *I will call Shabbos a delight.*

The Geon Yaakov explains that the reward of being granted one's heart's desires is given to those who call the Shabbos delight, i.e. they delight in and honor the Shabbos. However, those who celebrate the Shabbos for their own physical pleasure do not merit this reward. *(Ein Yaakov, Shabbos* 118)

When eating and drinking on Shabbos, one should have in mind that he is doing so because Hashem commanded him to take pleasure in the Shabbos, to come close to Him even through physical deeds. *(Yishrei Lev, Remazei Kedushas Shabbos)*

Reb Aharon Eisenberg of Zhitomir once made a resolution to break his desire for food. On Shabbos morning, when the kugel was distributed, he cut it into small pieces and ate it very slowly. Inside, he discovered a rusty nail. He saw that in the merit of eating Shabbos food slowly, solely for the sake of Heaven, he merited being saved from swallowing the nail.

(Siddur Tzelusa D'Aharon, Pinsk Karlin)

It is a mitzvah on Shabbos Kodesh to increase one's menu, yet this pleasure should only be for the sake of Hashem, as we say *Shabbos Hayom LaHashem*: *You should keep the Shabbos because Hashem commanded so.*   (*Imros Tehoros*)

The Gemara in *Shabbos* (118b) states that *One who delights in the Shabbos will be granted his heart's desires*. The reason for this is because he takes pleasure in the Shabbos to fulfill Hashem's will and not to fulfill his own desires. Thus, he will merit that Hashem will grant him his heart's desires.

(*Levush* 242)

Honoring Hashem

Remember the Shabbos day to sanctify it (*Shemos* 20:8). With what should one sanctify the Shabbos? By learning Torah, eating and drinking, wearing clean clothing, and resting. One who takes pleasure in the Shabbos, it is as if he honors Hashem. As it says, *You should call the Shabbos a delight, for the Holy Hashem that is honored* (*Yeshayahu* 58:13). It can be understood from this *pasuk* that one who delights in the Shabbos honors Hashem.

Although Rabbi Akiva said that it is preferable to eat weekday food on Shabbos than to take charity, one should still accept a small amount of meat and wine for Shabbos if he does not have any, but he should not take more than necessary.

(*Tanna D'vei Eliyahu Rabbah*, ch. 26)

Tosafos writes that one honors Hashem more through keeping Shabbos than other mitzvos, because through keeping Shabbos he is testifying that Hashem created the world (*Yevamos* 5b, s.v. *Kulchem*).

Another reason is because Shabbos is equated with keeping all the mitzvos of the Torah.

(*Nefesh Yeseirah, Ma'areches Shin*, sec. 79)

Eating with Joy

One should be extremely careful to be happy and in good spirits on Shabbos, because we fulfill the mitzvah of honoring the Shabbos mainly through joy. One should not exhibit any sadness or worry, and he should increase his *oneg Shabbos* in whatever manner possible, whether with food, drink, or clothing. (*Nefesh Yeseirah, Ma'areches Shin*, section 180)

The Sifri states that the *pasuk* in *Bamidbar* 1:10, *On the days of your rejoicing,* refers to Shabbos. About the days of the week, the *pasuk* states: *With toil, you will eat* (*Bereishis* 3:17), but about Shabbos it says the opposite: *Go, eat your bread joyfully...* (*Koheles* 9:7).

The *pasuk* in *Koheles* 4:6 states: *Better is a handful of ease than two handfuls of toil and frustration*, meaning it is better to have a small amount of tranquility than a large amount achieved through toil. *Handful of ease* refers to Shabbos, and *two handfuls of toil and frustration* refers to the six days of the week (*Midrash Rabbah, Vayikra* 3:1). The Imrei Emes explains that during the week we need to toil for our food, but Shabbos is the source of all blessing, and therefore no work is necessary.

We can see this concept with the *mann*. The Jews in the *midbar* needed to gather the *mann* every day of the week, but on Shabbos they already had it prepared from Friday.

(*Imrei Emes*)

One may wonder how a person can enjoy a lavish feast on Shabbos if he knows that he has committed sins. The Gemara explains that one who keeps Shabbos properly, even if he worships *avodah zarah* like the generation of Enosh, will be forgiven (*Shabbos* 118b). Therefore, every person can eat the Shabbos *seudah* joyously. (*Rabbi Dovid Meisels*)

The main time that one's food is elevated is on Shabbos and Yom Tov. These are days of rejoicing, because there is tremendous joy in the upper worlds.

(*Likutei Halachos, Hilchos Basar V'chalav*, halachah 4, sec. 9-10)

The Gemara states (*Beitzah* 16a) that all mitzvos were given publicly except Shabbos. Shabbos was given privately, between Hashem and Bnei Yisrael. The Gemara then asks why gentiles are punished for not keeping Shabbos if the mitzvah wasn't given publicly. The answer is that the gentiles were informed about Shabbos, but they were not informed about the *neshamah yeseirah*. Rashi explains *neshamah yeseirah* to mean an expansive heart for tranquility and joy; a person's heart is open wide to be able to eat and drink.

Hashem did not inform the gentiles about the *neshamah yeseirah* because to the gentiles, eating is purely physical. It is not possible for them to eat in a holy manner and experience the joy that comes from that holiness.

(*Gilyonei Hashas, Beitzah* 16a, s.v. *Neshamah yeseirah*)

Chazal say that *zachor* and *shamor* were uttered simultaneously. *Shamor* refers to keeping Shabbos by refraining from *melachah*. *Zachor* symbolizes happiness, because it refers to Kiddush recited on wine, which brings a person to a happy state of mind.

A person can think that he is losing out by not working on Shabbos, and this can cause him to be unhappy. He may think that one who does not keep Shabbos should be joyful since he is earning more money. But the Torah tells us the opposite—a person who keeps Shabbos is one who can truly be happy because he has faith in Hashem, that He will provide him with whatever he needs.

Zachor and *shamor* were said simultaneously to show that only through *shamor* (keeping Shabbos) can there be *zachor* (can a person be truly happy). With this we can understand *Chazal's* words: *If the Jews will keep two Shabbasos, they will be redeemed immediately.* "Two Shabbasos" refers to the two mitzvos of Shabbos, *zachor* and *shamor*.

Therefore, the Gemara states that all opinions agree that on Shabbos one must eat a *seudah*. This is because by eating a Shabbos *seudah* one demonstrates that although he is refraining from work, he is still happy.

(She'eilos Uteshuvos Ksav Sofer, Orach Chaim 78)

Being Mindful While Eating

One should sit at the Shabbos table with awe and respect. He should be dressed in white and wear a hat in honor of the Shabbos table. One should remember the words of *Askinu Seudasa* that express the tremendous holiness of the Shabbos table. A righteous person should know before Whom he is sitting and should sit in a manner that befits sitting before a king. *(Chemdas Hayamim, p. 172)*

The Even Ezra writes on the topic of *nezirus* that most people are enslaved to earthly desires, except those who free themselves from them. They are kings with crowns on their heads.

We can apply this concept to the Shabbos *seudah*. If one eats the Shabbos *seudah* with the proper intent, without being drawn after the physical pleasures, he is sitting at the *seudah* with a crown on his head. Every person should ensure that his eating is to derive pleasure from Shabbos and not just from the food. *(Shem Mishmuel, Parshas Chukas 5680)*

The Erloier Rebbe and the Yad Sofer would eat with a *shinui* (in a different manner than usual) on Shabbos, so that if they, Heaven forbid, came to *chillul Shabbos* while eating (with *borer, tochen,* or any of the other *melachos* that are related to food) they had not transgressed a *d'Oraisa*. *(Beis Sofreihem, issue 12)*

It is incredible that one can atone for his sins and is considered as if he fulfilled all 613 mitzvos simply by eating, drinking, and having pleasure on Shabbos! But a person can also desecrate Shabbos with mundane speech or by carrying an object outside when it is forbidden. With one such small action a person can relinquish all the benefits of Shabbos, and it is considered as if he transgressed all the mitzvos in the Torah. *(Kisei Dovid of the Chida, Drush 26)*

Food Should Bring One to Teshuvah

One who sinned can do *teshuvah* on Shabbos through eating Shabbos food. This can be seen in the *zemer, Shabbos Hayom LaHashem,* from the words *mei'avor derech ugevulim*—"one who transgressed the ways and the boundaries of the Torah," *mei'asos hayom pe'alim*—"instead of fasting and doing acts of affliction to rectify his deeds," *le'echol v'lishtos behilulim*—"he should eat and drink and praise Hashem," *ki zeh hayom asah Hashem*—"because Shabbos is a day that Hashem gave us to rejoice."

(Pri Hakerem, issue 2, in the name of Reb Mendele of Riminov)

A person experiences a stronger awakening to *teshuvah* during *seudas Shabbos* than while *davening*.

(Beis Aharon, in the name of Reb Asher Stoliner)

Oneg Shabbos Leads to Yiras Shamayim

Eating meat, fish, and wine at all three *seudos* on Shabbos is a *segulah* for *yiras Shamayim*.

(Zemiros Shabbos Kadshecha, p. 71)

The Torah states that the purpose of *ma'aser sheini* (ma'aser that a person was required to separate that could only be eaten in Yerushalayim) was that, *you may learn to fear Hashem, your G-d, all your days (Devarim* 14:23). *Chazal* say that, *all your days* refers to Shabbasos and Yamim Tovim. However, this seems contrary to the *pasuk* which appears to be including all days of the year.

There are two categories of food: food that is eaten during the week for the purpose of serving Hashem and food that is eaten on Shabbos and Yom Tov. The second type of food is a purpose in and of itself, because it fulfills the mitzvah of *oneg Shabbos*.

Likewise, eating *ma'aser sheini* in Yerushalayim is itself a mitzvah and is similar in this respect to Shabbos food. The purpose of *ma'aser sheini* was that a person should see the *kohen's* holy manner of eating and then be able to emulate it once he returned home. Thus, the *pasuk* states that one should fear Hashem, *kol hayamim*, all the time, which means even at home.

One cannot compare eating weekday food, which is just a means to a goal, to eating *ma'aser sheini*, which is an end in and of itself. Thus, *Chazal* say that *"all your days"* refers to Shabbos and Yom Tov because eating on Shabbos and Yom Tov is also a goal in and of itself, and is therefore comparable to *ma'aser sheini*. *(Chamishah Ma'amaros, Parshas Re'eh)*

Reb Tzvi Hersh of Riminov asks: How is Shabbos compared to *Olam Haba*? In *Olam Haba* there is no eating and drinking, whereas the mitzvah of *oneg Shabbos* is fulfilled mainly through food and drink. He explains that the pleasure of *Olam Haba* is achieved by reaching a level of pure *yiras Shamayim*. Similarly, the Shabbos food can bring a person to true *yiras Shamayim* as well. *(Be'eiros Hamayim, Yikavu Hamayim)*

The Chiddushei Harim says that eating Shabbos food brings a person to *yiras Shamayim*, as the *pasuk* states in regard to *ma'aser*, *Ve'achalta lifney Hashem Elokecha bamakom asher yivchar*, "And you will eat before Hashem, your G-d, in the place that He will choose..." *(Devarim 14:23)*. *Tzaddikim* instituted that Jews should gather together to eat *seudos Shabbos* (as is customary in certain circles where the Rebbe eats the Shabbos *seudah* at a *tish*), which is comparable to gathering on a fast day. It is actually greater if one is spiritually aroused from *oneg Shabbos* than if he is aroused through fasting.

(Siach Sarfei Kodesh, vol. 1, p. 168, sec. 55)

There is a well-known concept that the world consists of three components: *olam*, *shanah*, and *nefesh*—place, time, and person.

In the Beis Hamikdash, which is in the realm of place, the *korbanos* connected the lower and upper worlds. Through the influence of the Beis Hamikdash, the entire world was connected to its source.

Shabbos, which represents the realm of time, elevates all the points in time of the entire year. The Shabbos *seudah* connects the physical food of This World to the upper worlds and elevates the food of the entire week.

The *pasuk* states that one who eats *ma'aser sheini* will learn to have *yiras Shamayim* (Devarim 14:23). The Chiddushei Harim points out that we learn from this that all *seudos mitzvah* bring a person to *yiras Shamayim*.

In truth, it can be understood from the words of *Chazal* that the *pasuk* really refers to Shabbasos and Yom Tovim (see above). *Chazal* want to demonstrate that just like eating *ma'aser sheini* in Yerushalayim helps a person eat with *yiras Shamayim* in any place in the world, eating Shabbos and Yom Tov food helps a person eat with *yiras Shamayim* on all the days of the year. (*Sfas Emes, Parshas Tzav*, 5651)

Chazal say that *ma'aser sheini* teaches a person to have *yiras Shamayim*. Through eating *ma'aser sheini* in the Beis Hamikdash, a person's body was purified to the point that he was able to break his desire for food and elevate food even when he was at home. Just like *ma'aser sheini* was eaten in the holiest place in the world, Shabbos and Yom Tov are the pinnacles of holiness in the realm of time.

(*Yismach Yisrael Likutim*, s.v. *Vayochal k'negdo*)

Eating L'shem Mitzvah

With every mitzvah which involves physical pleasure, such as *oneg Shabbos*, one should be extra careful to have in mind that he is eating for the sake of the mitzvah, because Hashem commanded him to do so. Since a person eats every day of the week without these thoughts, if he does so on Shabbos as well, it remains just a physical act, and he will not fulfill the mitzvah of *oneg Shabbos*.

(She'eilos Uteshuvos Ksav Sofer, Orach Chaim 39, 107:16)

It is said in the name of the Ba'al Shem Tov that there are three mitzvos that even if one does them without having in mind the deeper meanings, they are still considered mitzvos: immersing in the *mikvah*, eating on Shabbos, and giving *tzedakah*.

(Chamishah Ma'amaros)

The Imrei Elimelech said that his father once rebuked a certain person who devoured his food, stating that he was eating it in honor of Shabbos. He told him that since he obviously had not yet rectified his character traits, in which case physical pleasures would be repulsive to him, he was clearly not eating in honor of Shabbos.

(Imrei Elimelech, Parshas Mishpatim, s.v. Ki sikneh)

If someone ate on Shabbos but did not have in mind to fulfill the mitzvah of *oneg Shabbos*, some opinions hold that he has nevertheless fulfilled the mitzvah. This is in accordance with the principle that it is not imperative to have in mind the mitzvah when fulfilling a mitzvah which requires pleasure, because the person did experience the requisite pleasure. If one has in mind both to honor the Shabbos *and* his own pleasure, his mitzvah is certainly on a higher level, but it is still not the ultimate level of fulfilling the mitzvah.

(Ben Ish Chai, Shnei Eliyahu, p. 20b)

Even if one eats more than usual on Shabbos, unless he is overeating, it is considered a mitzvah.

(Mosach HaShabbos HaYa'avetz, Mattan Shabbos 1:40)

There are several mitzvos in the Torah which sanctify the physical, such as the mitzvah of *oneg Shabbos*. By eating special foods and wearing nice clothing a person should realize that Shabbos is great and elevated. This is the main goal of this mitzvah.

However, the *yetzer hara* misleads a person to desire only the physical pleasures and to delude himself into thinking that he is fulfilling a mitzvah. In fact, however, this person is turning holiness into impurity. Thus, Reb Yisrael Salanter said, "People consume the Shabbos with *tzimmes*," meaning they becomes so immersed in their food that they forget about Shabbos itself. *(Michtav M'Eliyahu, vol. 1, p. 226)*

No Reason to Overindulge

Although it is viewed as meritorious to increase one's menu on Shabbos, one should take care not to overindulge, especially with a large variety of foods.

(Siddur HaYa'avetz Seudas Halailah, sec. 5)

We eat three meals on Shabbos because generally, one who overeats needs to wait a long time until he can consume another meal. Since it is a mitzvah to eat three *seudos* on Shabbos, one will make sure not to overeat so that he can still partake of the next *seudah*. Thus, all his *seudos* will be for the sake of Hashem and his heart will remain available to learn Torah. He will also conquer his evil inclination by refraining from eating all the food that he desires. If he does this on the day of rest, he will definitely do so during the week so that overeating does not cause him to decrease his productivity.

(Avudraham)

Although eating and drinking on Shabbos is a mitzvah, one should still be careful to minimize the amount that he eats, and it should all be for the sake of Heaven.

(Kaf Hachaim 242:105)

The *pasuk* states regarding *ma'aser*: *You should eat it...so that you will learn to fear Hashem (Devarim 14:23)*. The Gemara explains that this refers to having *yiras Shamayim* when eating on Shabbos and Yom Tov.

We can explain this Gemara according to how the Likutim Yekarim explains another Gemara in *Kesubos* (110b) which states that all the days of a poor person are bad. The Gemara asks, how can we say that *all* the days of a poor person are bad, when surely on Shabbos and Yom Tov even a poor person has food to eat? The Gemara answers that the change in the poor person's diet when he increases his food on Shabbos can lead to digestive problems.

The Likutim Yekarim explains that this Gemara can be understood to refer to someone who is poor in knowledge and spirituality. Throughout the week his spiritual level is minimal, but on Shabbos and Yom Tov, every person receives holiness and his spiritual level is increased. However, by eating more than usual a person can become haughty and lose his spirituality.

One needs to know that although *oneg Shabbos* is a mitzvah, if a person overindulges he can become coarsened and pulled to negative desires. In that case, even the light of Shabbos and Yom Tov will not penetrate his soul. The Chernobyler Rebbe writes that one who is a glutton and drunkard on Shabbos has no connection to the spirituality of Shabbos.

Thus, when *Chazal* say that the *pasuk* refers to eating on Shabbos and Yom Tov, it means that a person *should learn* how to have *yiras Shamayim* even when fulfilling the mitzvah of *oneg Shabbos*. Otherwise, he may lose the special gift of spirituality granted on Shabbos. (*Yatzav Avraham*)

The Ruzhiner Rebbe ate a very minimal amount at the Shabbos *seudah,* whereas the Apter Rav would make long *seudos* and eat a large amount of food. The Ruzhiner Rebbe was once a guest at the Apter Rav's *seudah* and he observed that the Apter Rav ate only a small amount. The Ruzhiner

Rebbe asked the Apter Rav why he was deviating from his usual custom.

The Apter Rebbe replied that the six days of the week host the Shabbos as a guest. Thus, we prepare all week for the Shabbos guest. When Yom Tov falls on Shabbos, the Shabbos hosts the Yom Tov and we add another special dish in honor of the Yom Tov. But when the holy day of Yom Kippur occurs on Shabbos, the Shabbos refrains from eating altogether in honor of the holy guest, Yom Kippur.

"Likewise," he explained, "since I am now hosting a holy guest of your stature, I am giving deference to your custom. Therefore, I am minimizing the amount of food I eat."

(*Imrei Tzaddikim, Likutei Omrim,* sec. 9)

Chapter 3
Shabbos Food—A Different Dimension

Elevated Eating

The main time that one feels the *kedushah* of Shabbos is during the *seudos*. One who does not eat a Shabbos *seudah* turns Shabbos into a weekday. *(Poked Ikarim Likutim)*

Reb Yitzchak of Vorka explains that Jews are on a higher spiritual level than the angels, since the angels do not have the ability to elevate food. We see this from the midrash *(Shemos Rabbah* 28:1), that when Moshe Rabbeinu came up to receive the Torah, the *malachim* (angels) argued that they should be the ones to receive it. Hashem then showed them an image of Moshe Rabbeinu looking like Avraham Avinu, to remind them that they ate dairy and meat together in Avraham's home. Avraham, however, did not eat meat and dairy together. This proved that humans can reach a higher level of *kedushah* than *malachim* through eating. (Even though the *malachim* didn't really eat, it was still considered a *chillul Hashem*—desecration of Hashem's name—since it looked like they ate forbidden foods.)

When we sit down to our Shabbos meal, we are displaying this high level of *kedushah*. Therefore, we say *"Tzeischem l'shalom"* and tell the *malachim* to leave before the *seudah,* so they shouldn't feel bad when they see the tremendous holiness that the Jews achieve by eating *seudas Shabbos*.

(Ohel Yitzchak, sec. 165)

During the time that they eat and drink, which normally can bring one to frivolity and lightheadedness, Jews become elevated. They praise and bless Hashem and learn Torah, instead.

Food and drink expand the heart and can cause one to understand concepts that he would not grasp at any other time. The storehouses of spiritual treasures and Heavenly lights open up before a person, and anyone who wants can acquire eternal assets. The gentiles misuse this time of eating and drinking, and involve themselves in nonsense, but the Jews elevate this time and use it to delve into *avodas Hashem* and praise of Hashem.

Chazal compare this to the following parable: *A king once made a feast to which he invited guests. Some of the guests ate and drank and then blessed the king, and some of them partook of the food and then cursed the king.*

The king saw this and wanted to interrupt the festivities to punish the offenders. One minister came to their defense and said, "Do not look at those who eat and drink and curse you, look at those who eat and drink and bless you."

When the Jews eat and drink and then bless Hashem, Hashem listens to their requests. When the non-Jews eat and drink and anger Hashem, Hashem considers destroying the entire world. The Torah then enters as a defense and says, "Hashem, don't look at those who anger You, look at the Jews who bless and praise Your great name and learn Torah after eating." A Heavenly voice then announces that Hashem should escape from the gentiles and cleave to the Jews.

(*Midrash Rabbah, Shir Hashirim* 8:19)

It is written in the *Zohar* (vol. 2, p. 205a) that Shabbos is a day that is entirely for the *neshamah* and not for the body. One would think, therefore, that we should not eat on Shabbos. However, on Shabbos, eating is also an act of holiness and serving Hashem. This is what the *pasuk* states: *Therefore, keep the Shabbos, for it is a sacred thing for you* (*Shemos* 31:14). "For you" shows us that even our physical needs on Shabbos are elevated and holy. (*Toras Avos*)

The Ba'al Shem Tov explained to the Maggid of Mezritch that if people would know to what extent Shabbos purifies the *neshamah* and sanctifies the body, they would be involved in eating and drinking the entire day, without stopping for even a moment. (*Kitzur Shulchan Aruch im Sippurim Chassidi'im,* p. 186)

Today, the holiness of the Beis Hamikdash is concealed within the Shabbasos and Yamim Tovim. If one honors the Shabbasos and Yamim Tovim, it is like he built the Beis Hamikdash and its holy vessels. Shabbos is parallel to the *Kodesh Kadashim* because it is the holiest of all times. The *Aron* in the *Kodesh Kadashim* was comprised of three boxes, one inside the other, that correspond to the three *seudos* of Shabbos and the three *Avos*. On top of the *Aron* was the *zeir zahav*, a gold rim, which corresponds to Dovid Hamelech and *seudas melaveh malkah*. The two *Badim*, poles, which carried the *Aron* correspond to the two Shabbos candles.

Chazal state that for each generation during which the Beis Hamikdash is not built, it is considered as if it was destroyed in their days. "Days" refers to the holy days of the year. Therefore, if one does not honor these days properly, it is as if he destroyed the Beis Hamikdash. (*Agra D'bei Hilula,* p. 31)

The Arizal sates that one can reach greater heights through eating Shabbos and Yom Tov food than he can through *tefillah*. (*Toras Avos L'Shabbos*)

Eating and drinking on Shabbos elevates a person because there is a holy angel that is appointed over Shabbos food. When a person takes pleasure in the Shabbos by eating and drinking, he becomes elevated through that angel.

(*Davar Shebakedushah,* p. 4)

A Seudah of Emunah

The *Zohar* states that *seudas Shabbos* is *seudasa dimheimenusa*, a *seudah* of *emunah*. The Chiddushei Harim explains that the word *seudah* comes from the base word *so'ed*, which means to support, since the Shabbos *seudah* supports our *emunah*.

Every one of our Shabbos foods is from the table of Hashem, similar to the *korbanos* and *terumos*. Just as *korbanos* bring a person to greater levels of *yiras Shamayim* (see *Devarim* 14:23), Shabbos foods bring a person to stronger *emunah*. Also, just as *korbanos* atone for a person's sins, Shabbos food can atone for sins.

According to this, it is clear that all the *minhagim* associated with Shabbos food have a holy source. (*Birchas Avraham*, ch. 18)

Every *seudah* can increase *emunah* and *yiras Shamayim* when one recognizes Who gave him the food. This is why Avraham Avinu told his guests to bless Hashem after they ate. Our Shabbos *seudah* is called *seudasa dimheimenusa*, a *seudah* of *emunah*, since it has the ability to influence every person, great or simple, to have *emunah*.

(*Chiddushei Harim, Likutim Shabbos*, s.v. *Kol seudah*)

The entire week derives its blessing from Shabbos. However, we do not see this openly, just like the *mann* in the *midbar* did not fall on Shabbos.

The Shabbos *seudah* has the ability to impart *brachah* into our week, relative to how much *emunah* we have in the power of Shabbos. The Shabbos *seudah* is therefore called *seudasa dimheimenusa*, because *seudah* can also mean to influence.

(*Sfas Emes, Vayeira*, 5652, s.v. *B'midrash ve'achar*)

Seudas Shabbos is called *seudasa dimheimenusa* since it supports and strengthens the *emunah* that is hidden within each person, unlike a weekday meal which pulls a person toward the physical world.

(Chiddushei Harim, Likutim Shabbos, s.v. Omrim)

The Special Aroma and Taste of Shabbos Food

The Gemara states that the Emperor asked Reb Yehoshua ben Chananyah, "Why does the Shabbos food have a good fragrance?"

Reb Yehoshua replied, "We have one spice that we put into the food which gives it a good fragrance and Shabbos is its name."

The emperor told him, "Give me some of this spice."

Reb Yehoshua replied, "For one who keeps the Shabbos, this spice is effective; for one who does not keep the Shabbos, it is ineffective."

Why is the holiness of Shabbos experienced specifically as a fragrance? Shabbos is like the World to Come. There is no eating or drinking in Gan Eden, but the *neshamos* bask in the pleasure of a good fragrance. Therefore, the holiness of Shabbos that comes into the food is experienced as a fragrance.

Since only our Shabbos foods have that special aroma, it proves that Shabbos is specifically for the Jews and not for the gentiles. The word *tavshil* (dish) reads backwards as *li Shabbos* (Shabbos is for me, meaning for the Jews).

(Ben Yehoyadah, Shabbos 119, s.v. Tavlin echad)

And Hashem blessed the seventh day and He sanctified it (*Bereishis* 2:3). Rashi states that Hashem blessed the Shabbos and sanctified it with the *mann*.

The Gemara states that an ignoramus is forbidden to eat meat. Meat can arouse in a person evil desires, and an ignoramus does not have Torah learning with which to fight those desires, as it says: *I created the* yetzer hara *and I created the Torah as an antidote.*

The *mann* did not arouse evil desires since it was entirely spiritual. So too, the holiness of Shabbos generates holiness in our Shabbos food, and therefore it does not arouse evil desires.

This explains why a person's sustenance is decreed for him from the beginning of the year, except for the expenses of Shabbos and Yom Tov. Shabbos and Yom Tov food are not governed by the laws of nature because they do not contain any physical components. Hence, our Shabbos food is similar to the *mann.*

With this we can understand the Gemara which states that the Emperor asked Rabbi Yehoshua ben Chananyah why his Shabbos food had such a good fragrance. Rabbi Yehoshua replied that we have one spice that we put into our food to give it a good fragrance and its name is Shabbos. The Emperor requested that Rabbi Yehoshua give him the spice. Rabbi Yehoshua replied that this spice only works for one who keeps Shabbos.

Fragrance is something from which the *neshamah* gets pleasure. The Emperor understood that this was a spiritual fragrance, and he was asking Rabbi Yehoshua why Shabbos food is so elevated. Rabbi Yehoshua replied that Shabbos only works for one who keeps Shabbos, because then he possesses the merit which will protect him from any evil desires which could be aroused from the Shabbos food.

The *neshamah yeseirah* delights in the Shabbos food, unlike during the week when the *neshamah* does not enjoy food. Therefore, Hashem gave us a mitzvah of *oneg* on Shabbos and Yom Tov. However, if one does not keep Shabbos, his food will obviously not have the holiness and special fragrance of Shabbos. (*Ma'aglei Tzedek, Parshas Pinchas*, s.v. *Midrash*)

The Kli Yakar states on the *pasuk* in *Shemos* (16:15), *And a man told his brother "This is mann,"* that the reason they called it *mann* is because the sounds of the letters of the word *mann*, *mem* and *nun*, are formed using one's nose. When a person's nose is closed, he cannot enunciate these letters clearly. They called it *mann* to demonstrate that the significance of the *mann* was only when one could smell it.

However, *Chazal* say that the *mann* also had the taste of all foods (*Yoma* 75a). *Mann* can mean a "prepared portion," so perhaps they called it that because they were able to use it to prepare all types of food. However, they hadn't yet officially called it *mann*, but only told each other that it was *mann*, meaning a food that encompasses all foods. It was only after Shabbos that they named it *mann*, because on Erev Shabbos they received a double portion of *mann*, and the letters that form the word *mann* allude to this: When spelling the words *mem* and *nun*, the letters are doubled (the word *mem* is spelled *mem* and *mem*; the word *nun* is spelled *nun* and *nun*).

According to the abovementioned *Kli Yakar*, we can say that they named the *mann* after Shabbos because on Shabbos they realized that the fragrance of the *mann* was doubled.

(*Kli Yakar, Shemos* 16:15)

Rashi explains *neshamah yeseirah* to mean that a person has a hearty appetite and will not be repulsed by eating more food than usual. What is the connection between eating and drinking and the *neshamah*?

Every food contains a spiritual component which provides the *neshamah* with sustenance. Since on Shabbos we have a *neshamah yeseirah*, an extra *neshamah*, one needs to eat and drink more than during the week.

An aroma is something from which the *neshamah* has pleasure. Since the purpose of eating on Shabbos is not for the body, but rather for the *neshamah*, Shabbos foods have a pleasant smell. (*Yisrael Kedoshim*, chap. 5)

The closer something is to holiness, the better it tastes. Therefore, our Shabbos food has a good fragrance and its taste greatly surpasses weekday food. *Chazal* have said that on Shabbos we possess the spice called Shabbos; Shabbos enhances the taste of our food.

(*Likutei Halachos, Hilchos Nosen Ta'am L'fgam*, Halachah 2)

Reb Tzvi Hersh of Ziditchov would say, "One who merits experiencing the taste of Shabbos in his *tefillos* will merit tasting Gan Eden in his food, too."

(*Be'er Yaakov Chaim, Maseches Shabbos*)

One who keeps Shabbos senses a special taste in the Shabbos food and also experiences one-sixtieth of *Olam Haba*.

(See *Brachos* 57b; *Taharas Yisrael, Hakdamah*, sec. 30)

Shabbos Food Is Uplifted

When one sets aside food for Shabbos during the week, that food is imbibed with the holiness of Shabbos. If one then finds something superior and puts the finer food aside for Shabbos and eats the first dish during the week, then even his eating during the week is elevated and is a mitzvah. We see this from the Gemara that tells us when Shammai Hazakein would come across a choice meat, he would set it aside for Shabbos. If he later found meat that was superior, he would put that aside for Shabbos and eat the first piece of meat during the week.

One who only derives pleasure from food eaten during a *seudas mitzvah* or on Shabbos and Yom Tov acquires merit that will prevent his body from being consumed by worms after his death. One who always has Shabbos in mind, as described above, is always eating *seudos mitzvah* and the worms will have no effect on him.

(*Reishis Chachmah, Sha'ar Hakedushah*, ch. 15)

Hashem created the world to exist for only six days. Shabbos gives it the ability to exist for another six days. Hence, Shabbos has a special significance because on Shabbos the world receives a renewed strength to exist for another week.

Since on Shabbos a new spiritual strength descends to the world, the Shabbos food is also blessed and provides the *neshamah* with new pleasure. *(Oheiv Yisrael L'Shabbos)*

The Shabbos food we eat becomes completely elevated and holy, without any physical components. One can merit defeating his enemies through *oneg Shabbos*, just as he would merit it through fasting. Thus, the day is called Shabbos, because it has the power to be *mashbis*, subjugate, our enemies and take revenge on them. *(Likutei Moharan 57:5)*

When the abundance of blessings and holiness descends from the Heavens on Friday night, it enters the Shabbos food. When one eats the food, he receives light and holiness from Above. *(Olas Tamid)*

A Jew who is on a lofty level can merit to experience the taste of the *mann* in his Shabbos food.

(Shulchan Menachem, Parshas Beshalach)

After reciting *Hamotzi* on *lechem mishneh* during the Shabbos day *seudah*, the Berditchever Rebbe once cried out, "*Oneg Shabbos!*" over and over again with tremendous fervor. A coarse peasant heard this and saw the tremendous amount of pleasure that the Rebbe was experiencing. He said to the Rebbe, "I can't understand this. I spend so much effort and money in order to experience pleasure and enjoyment, and I never reached this level of pleasure. How can that be?"

The Rav replied that true pleasure is only spiritual pleasure. When a person has pleasure from the physical aspects of this world, his body has pleasure from it, but the spiritual part of him does not. From spiritual acts, the spiritual part of a person also has pleasure, and this is true pleasure.

(Ohr HaShabbos, vol. 1, p. 175)

Before Adam Harishon sinned, the world and everything in it was entirely good. It was only after the sin that good and bad were combined. On Shabbos, the food we eat is completely holy and good, like the world during the first days of creation; thus, Shabbos commemorates the six days of creation.

The *pasuk* states: *And Hashem blessed the seventh day* (*Bereishis* 2:3). *Chazal* explain that this refers to the *mann*. This is difficult to understand since the Jews had the *mann* for only 40 years. How has Shabbos been blessed with the *mann* since then?

The *mann* symbolizes something that is entirely good and completely spiritual, as it was completely absorbed into the body and did not produce any waste. Similarly, our Shabbos food is completely holy and spiritual, just like *mann* and the food in the world before Adam Harishon sinned.

(*Chessed L'Avraham*)

Shabbos symbolizes the state of Adam Harishon before the sin, and also the End of Days. Therefore, the *Korban Mussaf* brought on Shabbos is the only *Mussaf* that did not have a *Korban Chatas* sacrificed with it to atone for the sins of the Jews—with the clarity of Shabbos there is no sin.

The Ramban writes (*Bereishis* 2:17) that we can understand from the words of *Chazal* (*Shabbos* 55b) that if Adam Harishon would not have sinned, he would have lived forever. His *neshamah*, which comes from Above and is eternal, would have been attached to him and would have sustained him for eternity.

Before Adam sinned, eating was only for pleasure and not for sustenance. The fruits of Gan Eden were absorbed into Adam's body like the *mann*. When it was decreed upon Adam that he should eat the grass of the field and the bread of the earth, his food then began to contain physical components, whereas before it was entirely spiritual. Since Adam was created from earth and he was eating earth, he would eventually return to earth and die, as the *pasuk* states: *But from the Eitz Hada'as of good and evil you shall not eat, for on the day that you eat thereof, you shall surely die* (Bereishis 2:17).

We see from the words of the Ramban that the purpose of food before the sin was not to keep body and soul together, because at that point Adam's body and soul were one. Eating was simply for pleasure. Since Shabbos is a symbol of Adam Harishon before the sin, and at that time Adam did not need food for sustenance, one might think that on Shabbos we don't need food to sustain us either and we should refrain from eating.

Indeed, on Shabbos, the food we eat is different; we do not eat to sustain our bodies, but the delicacies we eat are purely for the pleasure and enjoyment of the soul, like Adam's eating before he sinned. One who thinks that the Shabbos food sustains him physically is missing a basic understanding of a foundation of his knowledge regarding the holiness of Shabbos.

With this we can understand that on Shabbos we are given *a neshamah yeseirah,* which Rashi explains as serenity to eat and drink *(Beitzah* 16a). Eating on Shabbos is possible only with peace of mind; otherwise a person would need to fast on Shabbos. Thus, *oneg* is necessary for the *neshamah yeseirah,* and not to sustain us physically.

(*Ma'amarei Pachad Yitzchak,* p. 222)

In general, when a person eats, nothing remains from the food he has eaten. However, when a person eats for the sake of Hashem, he elevates the spark of holiness in the food that gives the food existence. This holiness lasts forever, just like the Name of Hashem is forever.

(*Oheiv Yisrael, Likutim Drush Shabbos*)

An *ishah sotah* who was accused of sinning was forced to drink holy water in which the Name of Hashem was erased. If she remained alive, thus proving that she was innocent, the Torah blessed her that she would have children easily (*Bamidbar* 5:28).

Rebbe Yechezkel of Kuzmir explains that because the Name of Hashem entered the woman's innards and purified her body, she was blessed and helped from Above with everything she needed, despite the fact that her intentions had been impure and she had secluded herself with a strange man.

Similarly, when Shabbos food enters a person, it can accomplish a tremendous amount. Shabbos is one of the names of Hashem (*Zohar*, vol. 2, ch. 1), and if one prepares for Shabbos with the intent of honoring it, and doing so for the sake of Hashem, then Hashem's name is inscribed on his food, so to speak. When this food enters him, he will be blessed with everything good.

This is the reason that there is a custom to travel to *tzaddikim* for Shabbos. *Tzaddikim* bring down the Name of Hashem into their Shabbos food with their holy *kavanos* during their Shabbos preparations. Those who eat for the sake of Hashem are helped and blessed with everything good through the food they eat. All this only applies to one who eats with the intention of "ingesting" the holiness of Shabbos; if one eats gluttonously, to satisfy his desires, then even if he is at the table of a *tzaddik*, the *tzaddik's* merit will not influence him. (*Divrei Yisrael, Parshas Mikeitz*, p.83)

Shabbos is called *kodesh,* which means separate; it is a day that is separate from the rest of the week. Similarly, the Jews are called *kodesh* because we are separate from the gentiles. This is why in Havdalah on Motza'ei Shabbos we state that Hashem separates between holy and mundane, light and dark, the Jews and the nations.

There have been pious people who were therefore careful not to give Shabbos food to non-Jews, and it is correct to do this, if possible. Shabbos food will not be beneficial for a gentile. It is an elixir for life for Jews but has the opposite effect on gentiles. *(Bnei Yissaschar, Ma'amarei HaShabbasos* 1:12)

Shabbos food is completely spiritual and holy. During the week, the *Shechinah* only derives pleasure from our *brachos* of *Hamotzi* and *Birkas Hamazon*. On Shabbos, however, the *Shechinah* takes pleasure in our actual eating, as explained in the *Zohar* (*Parshas Vayakhel*, p. 218a).

On Shabbos, the food itself ascends to a holy place in the upper worlds to be blessed, and all the worlds take pleasure in it. This is what the *pasuk* alludes to with the words: *And the seventh day should be holy for you* (*Shemos* 35:2). On Shabbos, even the *"for you,"* i.e. the physical eating and drinking, is holy. The reward of one who eats *seudos Shabbos* is far greater than that of one who eats during the week, and his reward will be in accordance with how much pleasure it provides Hashem. Therefore, a person should be filled with great joy on Shabbos, without any worry or sadness. He should take pleasure in Hashem and fulfill as much *oneg Shabbos* as possible, with all types of pleasures for the sake of Hashem—eating, drinking, wearing nice clothing—according to his ability.

(*Sidduro Shel Shabbos*, vol. 1, ch. 5, section 3)

On Shabbos, we eat food that is physical but has spiritual powers. *Chazal* say that one can only recite Kiddush in the area where he is eating his *seudah*. Because the *seudah* is holy (*kodesh*), we recite Kiddush there to demonstrate its holiness. This is why it is called "Kiddush" and not "Zechirah" (remembrance), although the *pasuk* states, *Zachor es yom haShabbos l'kadsho* (*Shemos* 20:8), which *Chazal* explain to mean that we should remember the Shabbos with wine when Shabbos begins. (*Zera Shimshon, Parshas Eikev*, p. 130a)

Shabbos Secrets • *Shabbos Food—A Different Dimension*

Eating Shabbos food is a mitzvah that connects the spiritual and physical components of a person. We learn this from the concept found in the words of the Rema (*Orach Chaim* 6:1). He cites the words *umafli la'asos*—"and performs wonders," in the *brachah* of *Asher Yatzar* and explains that the wonder is the fact that Hashem keeps a spiritual *neshamah* together with a physical body. Since on Shabbos there is an extra level of *neshamah*, a person is required to eat more in order to connect with that spiritual part of him. (*Rabbi Dovid Meisels*)

The Ba'al Shem Tov states that a person who merited to participate in his *seudah* would be spared from falling prey to his evil desires, and the food that he ate would influence him to act properly even once he returned home.
(*Tiferes Shlomo, Parshas Yisro*, s.v. *Vayikach*)

Every Shabbos food and *minhag* of Jews on Shabbos contains extremely lofty, mystical secrets.
(*Nesiv Mitzvosecha*, p.87)

On Shabbos, we are commanded to take pleasure in physical food, to demonstrate that even in our physical world down here, we need to feel the holiness of Shabbos.
(*Vayidaber Moshe L'Shabbos*)

Since one eats on Shabbos to fulfill the mitzvah of *oneg Shabbos*, one may think that he can eat any food to fulfill this mitzvah. However, if one delves into the reasons behind the Shabbos foods traditionally eaten by Jews, he'll see that everything has a reason and deep concepts concealed within it.

The Arizal alludes to this in *Askinu Seudasa*: *We will crown the table with precious secrets*. One can understand from this that even the way in which one sets the table has deep meaning. (*Siach Zekeinim*, vol. 4, p. 96)

Whatever one eats during the week, aside from the food that is essential to keeping him alive, increases the strength of the *yetzer hara*. Conversely, everything eaten on Shabbos is entirely spiritual, even if one eats more than necessary.

(*Nagid Umitzvah Devarim Hashayachim L'seudah, Minchas Shabbos* 72:31)

When a person eats during the week, and subsequently learns and *davens* with the strength he receives from the food, the food he ate is sanctified. But on Shabbos, all food is elevated, even that which is eaten solely for pleasure and is not needed to give strength. Therefore, on Shabbos, it is a mitzvah to eat delicacies and increase one's consumption of meat and wine, even though during the week one who does so is considered a glutton and a drunkard.

(*Likutei Amarim Tanya, Iggeres Hakodesh* 26)

Comparable to Korbanos

Seudas Shabbos is the *seudah* of our King, Hashem. It says in the *Zohar*, *askinu seudasa d'Malka*; *Malka*, the king, refers to Hashem. We, Bnei Yisrael, are the queen and we dine together with Hashem, so to speak, at the Shabbos *seudah*. Therefore, our Shabbos food is food from Hashem's table and comparable to eating *korbanos*, and it follows that one's house can be compared to the Beis Hamikdash.

(See *Asarah Ma'amaros, Ma'amar Chikur Din*, vol. 1, ch. 21)

Hashem commanded us to have pleasure on Shabbos by eating and drinking; these acts are as holy as sacrificing *korbanos*. (*Aderes Eliyahu, Bereishis* 2:9)

It is often asked why on Shabbos we do not read the Torah portion concerning the *korbanos* that were brought on Shabbos. The Gemara states that nowadays a person's food takes the place of *korbanos*. We refrain from reading the portion of *korbanos* to show that since our *seudos Shabbos* are like actual *korbanos*, we do not need to read about them.

(*Devarim Yekarim V'sippurim Niflaim*, p. 6)

Shabbos food is as significant as the *matanos kehunah*, the 24 gifts that the *kohanim* received. Rebbe Mendel of Riminov said that the Shabbos food is likened to the *Korban Minchah*.

(*Divrei Binah, Parshas Vayeitzei*, s.v. *V'chol Asher Titen Li*)

The holiness of Shabbos food is comparable to the holiness of *korbanos*. There were *gedolim* who said that the holiness of Shabbos food is even greater than that of *korbanos*, because something that is physical and elevated is holier than something that is essentially spiritual and holy.

When a person brought a *korban* to the Beis Hamikdash, the holiness of the Beis Hamikdash caused him to strip away from himself every vestige of physicality. Thus, the *korban* he sacrificed was purely spiritual. Shabbos food is essentially physical, but the holiness of Shabbos rests upon it. Thus, Shabbos food is more elevated than *korbanos* since it is something physical that is elevated.

(*Avodas Yissachar, Likutim*, section 9, p. 23b)

The Arizal states that Shabbos and Yom Tov food, and any food eaten for a mitzvah, are not physical at all; they are entirely holy and similar to *korbanos*. Even if one ate a large amount of meat from a *korban*, it was considered holy and not gluttonous. Likewise, if one eats with the proper intent on Shabbos, then even the mundane food that he eats becomes a mitzvah and his food is likened to a *korban*.

(*Machshavos Charutz*, section 9)

When eating cholent, there are those who move the spoon downwards, upwards, and then to each side, as an allusion to the *avodah* of the *kohen gadol* on Yom Kippur when he sprinkled blood on the *Mizbe'ach* downward and upward, and moved the coals to the side. (*Minhag Tzaddikim*)

Chazal say that if one gives food to a *talmid chacham*, it is as if he sacrificed *korbanos*. On Shabbos, all Jews are like *talmidei chachamim* and our eating is comparable to eating *korbanos*. *(Pri Tzaddik, Parshas Toldos,* sec. 3)

Shabbos Food Sanctifies a Person

In addition to Shabbos being a day during which the *neshamah* is sanctified and elevated to tremendous heights (*Zohar*, vol. 2, p. 205a), one should elevate his body as well. Through eating Shabbos food, a person's body is sanctified and elevated; on Shabbos one merits to rectify his body and soul.   (*Leket Imrei Kodesh,* in the name of Rebbe Yissachar Dov of Belz)

One of the Gerrer Rebbes would cry every Erev Shabbos and beseech Hashem that he should merit to enter the Shabbos and that the Shabbos should enter him.

(Shulchan Menachem, Addenda)

One of the *tzaddikim* said that everyone can recognize the pleasure of Shabbos, but not everyone merits to recognize its holy essence. *(Shulchan Menachem, Addenda)*

The *pasuk* in *Shemos* (16:23) states: *Shabbason Shabbos kodesh.* The three words correspond to the three levels of holiness that exist throughout Shabbos. At the night *seudah* the first level of holiness descends, during the day *seudah* it increases to the second level, and *shalosh seudos* is the highest point of Shabbos. *(Alshich, Shemos* 16:11)

One should prepare himself to welcome the King on Shabbos. Each food that he eats on Shabbos for the sake of Hashem, attains holiness that enters his body, and he receives a spiritual light from Above. Indeed, Shabbos is *mei'ein Olam Haba*; on Shabbos, we receive a semblance of the spiritual goodness that exists in *Olam Haba*.

(Olas Tamid, Shiniva, Hanhagos Erev Shabbos, p. 1)

The midrash states that the *pasuk: And Hashem blessed the seventh day* (*Bereishis* 2:3) refers to a new countenance which a person receives on Shabbos. One cannot compare a person's countenance during the week to his countenance on Shabbos. It has been said that the *Lechem Hapanim* were called by that name because they transformed the faces of the *kohanim*. Since it rested on the *Shulchan* from the previous Shabbos, it contained the holiness of Shabbos and every *kohen* who partook of it was filled with holiness and his face was transformed.

The challah we eat on Shabbos is compared to the *Lechem Hapanim*, so one who eats *seudos Shabbos* is filled with holiness and receives a new countenance. (*Sha'arei Aryeh*)

We cover the challah and eat kugel which has dough beneath and over it in order to symbolize the *mann* which fell, with dew beneath and above it. Just like the *mann* was an elevated food which purified a person, Shabbos food sanctifies and purifies a person.

The commentaries ask why we remember the *mann* on Shabbos, if no *mann* fell on Shabbos. They answer that just like the *mann* purified Klal Yisrael, Shabbos food purifies us.
(*Rav Tov, Parshas Behar*, s.v. *Oh Yomar*)

It is well known that the holiness of Shabbos brings physical and spiritual blessings to the world.
(*Imrei Noam, Parshas Toldos*, s.v. *Oh yomar mah zeh miharta*)

The Bas Ayin writes: *One can reach great heights of holiness by eating the fruits from Eretz Yisrael. Outside of Eretz Yisrael, Shabbos is in the realm of Eretz Yisrael because by eating Shabbos food, one can attach himself to an exalted holiness just like he can by eating fruits from Eretz Yisrael.*

In a different place the Bas Ayin writes: *I instruct you that eating the fruits of Eretz Yisrael should be like eating Shabbos food, meaning you can attach yourself to holiness and awaken the six spiritual* middos *through the seven species with which Eretz Yisrael is blessed.* (*Bas Ayin, Parshas Behar*)

The holiness of Shabbos is manifested on Friday night through the food, and on Shabbos day it is manifested through resting and refraining from *melachah*. The holiness of resting from work is more apparent during Shabbos day than on Friday night, because nighttime is always a time for rest. However, the *kedushah* of Shabbos is very apparent on Friday night through the food.   (See *Pri Tzaddik* 4:12)

Differentiating between Shabbos and Weekday Food

V'karasa laShabbos oneg (*Yeshayah* 58:13) means that one's Shabbos food should not be similar to the food he eats during the week; it should bring him extra pleasure. Those who eat such foods will merit basking in the pleasure of closeness with Hashem.   (*Tanchuma Bereishis* 2)

A wealthy person who eats on a high standard during the week should make sure that his Shabbos food is different from his weekday food. If it is not possible for him to do so, then he should eat his Shabbos meals earlier or later in the day than he does during the week so that there is a noticeable difference.   (*Rambam, Hilchos Shabbos* 30:8)

One should not prepare the foods that are specifically eaten on Shabbos for a weekday meal.
(*Ohr Hayashar, Amud Ha'avodah*, p. 17; *Minhagei Chasam Sofer*)

The Mechaber writes (*Shulchan Aruch, Orach Chaim* 249:2) that one may not eat a *seudah* on Erev Shabbos that is more lavish than his usual weekday meal, even if it is a wedding meal. This prohibition applies to the entire Friday, and the reason is that one should enter Shabbos with an appetite for the *seudah*.

The Biur Halachah (ibid., s.v. *Mipnei*) quotes the Pri Megadim who cites a different reason: One is lessening the respect for Shabbos by eating the same foods on Erev Shabbos as he does on Shabbos.

This is an explicit reproach against the contemporary custom of serving Shabbos food at every significant occasion. Many *gedolim* decry the fact that we make weekday meals comparable to Shabbos *seudos*. Similarly, the Magen Avraham writes *(Siman* 262*)* that one should not wear his Shabbos clothing during the week, since a weekday should not be similar to Shabbos in any aspect.

(Darchei Halachah, Hilchos Shabbos, addendum 249, p. 64*)*

The Chasam Sofer once visited the author of the *Sefer Tiv Gittin*. The Tiv Gittin's wife had prepared delicacies, including *tzimmes* (sweet, cooked carrots some eat on Friday night) in honor of the Chasam Sofer. When the *tzimmes* was placed before the Chasam Sofer, he stated that it is a Shabbos food and one should not eat Shabbos foods on a weekday.

The Rebbetzin replied that since they merited hosting such a worthy guest it was like Shabbos for them. The Chasam Sofer was very pleased with her answer. He stated that this was the first time that a woman triumphed over him and he partook of the food. (Interestingly, the Chasam Sofer later married this woman after the Tiv Gittin was *niftar*. The Chasam Sofer and the Tiv Gittin both passed away on 25 Tishrei, 11 years apart.) *(Minhagei HaChasam Sofer)*

It is appropriate for a person who has fear of Heaven, even if he is tremendously wealthy, to refrain from eating one specific fine food on a weekday and only eat that food on Shabbos or Yom Tov, in order to honor Shabbos and Yom Tov.

(Tikkunei Shabbos 159*)*

It seems that one who uses the same tablecloth on Shabbos as during the week, or who eats Shabbos foods on a weekday or weekday foods on Shabbos, is transgressing the positive commandment of *mikra kodesh (Vayikra* 23:2*)*. The Ramban quotes the Sifri *(Parshas Pinchas* 147*)* who explains *mikra kodesh* to mean that one's food, drink, and clothing should be different on Shabbos than during the week.

(Ramban, Vayikra 23:2; see *She'eilos Uteshuvos Maharshag* 2:82*)*

Reb Itzikel of Pshevorsk once participated in a Rosh Chodesh *seudah* during which eggs with onions were served. Reb Itzikel related that the Tzieshenover Rebbe was once served this food on a weekday and he refrained from eating it, relating the following story:

Reb Moshe of Ostrow once set the table, lit candles, and donned Shabbos clothing on a weekday. One of his young granddaughters asked him why he was doing this. Reb Moshe replied that they were expecting a great visitor, the Ba'al Shem Tov, in whose honor he was making preparations. When the Ba'al Shem Tov came, the young girl was eating eggs with onions. The Ba'al Shem Tov went over to her and told her, "My dear child, this food is eaten by Jews only on Shabbos."

(*Zemiros L'ateir Pesora*)

The Divrei Shalom stated in the name of his father, the Ba'al Divrei Yechezkel of Shiniva, that one is required to have one food that is special for Shabbos that he will not eat during the week. Reb Yechezkel fulfilled this with eggs with onions.

(*Zemiros Shabbos Shalom Umevorach*, p.73)

Tzaddikim were careful not to eat foods that are specifically eaten on Shabbos, such as fish or eggs with onions, on a weekday unless it was during a *seudas mitzvah* or Chol Hamoed. (*Zemiros Tiferes Tzvi*, p. 258)

Rashi cites the following midrash on a *pasuk* in *Devarim* (33:19): *Amim har yikra'u sham yizbichu zivchei tzedek*—"Nations shall assemble at the mountain; there they will slaughter righteous offerings."

Gentile merchants came to Eretz Yisrael. While they were standing at the border they decided that since they expended so much effort to reach Eretz Yisrael they may as well travel to Yerushalayim and observe the Jewish nation. They went and saw that the Jews all serve one G-d and eat one food, unlike the gentiles who have many different gods and their foods are all different. This inspired the merchants to convert.

It is difficult to understand the meaning of the phrase that the Jews all ate one food. This could be understood as referring to the fact that on Shabbos all Jews eat similar, traditional foods: fish, cholent, soup, etc. Therefore, it is improper that recently people have started adding many other foods and dips to their Shabbos *seudos*. There is no source for these foods to be eaten on Shabbos, and they are considered weekday foods.

(*Zichron Yehudah* 25)

The more spiritual a person is, the more refined his eating is. The generation of the *Midbar* ate *mann*, which was very fine. On Shabbos, when they were on a greater spiritual level, their food was even more refined (on Shabbos they ate *lechem mishneh*, which is explained as *meshunah b'ta'am*, having a better taste). During the week, we eat dairy, and on Shabbos, when we are more elevated and refined, we eat meat and fish.

(*Imrei Pinchas Hachadash*)

Conversely, a food that a person is unaccustomed to eating can upset his stomach. The Gemara in *Kesubos* (110b) states that all the days of a poor man are bad because if he eats more food on Shabbos than he does during the week he may feel sick. Therefore, if one can afford to, he should eat some Shabbos foods, such as meat and wine, during the week. If he does so, it's considered *oneg Shabbos* even during the week, because it will cause him to have more pleasure on Shabbos.

(*Imrei Yosef, Parshas Re'eh*, s.v. *Ki yarchiv*)

If someone received food for Shabbos as a gift, he should make sure to eat it on Shabbos and not save it for during the week. This concept is found in the *Yerushalmi* (*Nazir* 5:1) that if someone promised to bring a *Korban Minchah* on Yom Tov, he is required to bring it specifically on Yom Tov. Because of the importance of Yom Tov, he may not choose to bring it a different day. (*Be'er Heitev*, in the name of the *Sefer Chassidim* 242:1)

Eating Fish during the Week

One should not eat fish during the week, because on a weekday one does not have the ability to elevate the *nitzotzos* that are contained in the fish. One is only able to do this when he has the merit of Shabbos.

(Ohr Tzaddikim, Amud Ha'tefillah 28:66; Yafeh L'lev 134:4)

The Avnei Nezer once said that since *tzaddikim* are *megulgal* in fish, one should only eat fish on Shabbos and not during the week. *(Avir Haroim 375; Sefer Teshuvos Avnei Nezer, Notes)*

Another reason one should eat fish only on Shabbos is that fish are associated with Shabbos, as the word *dag* (fish) has a numerical value of seven, which corresponds to Shabbos, the seventh day of the week. *(Tehillos Chaim, p. 305)*

The Tchechenover Rebbe did not eat fish during the week except when partaking in a *seudas mitzvah*, so that fish would be special for Shabbos.

The Maharshal writes that he did not eat fish on Friday night *(Yam Shel Shlomo, Gittin, Perek Hasholeiach)* in order that his day *seudah* should be more special than the night *seudah*, as instructed by *Chazal*. Fish is a significant food, so even if one serves many fine foods at night, the day *seudah* will still be more honored if it contains fish and the Friday night meal does not.

Since the Maharshal did not eat fish on Friday night, we can assume that he definitely did not eat fish during the week, even during a *seudas mitzvah*. *(Vaya'as Avraham)*

Reb Meir of Premishlan only ate fish from Sunday through Wednesday, but not on Thursday or Friday.
(Ta'amei Haminhagim, Shabbos, Kuntris Acharon 41; Divrei Meir, p. 175)

The Chasam Sofer did not eat fish during the week, only on Shabbos and Yom Tov. *(Tomer Devorah 1:9)*

Reb Elazar Mendel of Lelov did not eat fish or herring during the week.   (*Tefillah L'Dovid*, p. 213)

Saying L'kavod Shabbos Kodesh

The *Zohar* states that when the Jews praise Hashem with song in their *batei midrash* and then arrive home and set the table, and say that it is all *l'kavod* Shabbos and Yom Tov, the angels say, "Praised is the people who do so" (*Zohar, Parshas Emor*).   (*Kav Hayashar*, ch. 86)

Before eating on Shabbos, it is fitting that one should say, "I am eating *l'kavod Shabbos*, for the sake of Hashem."
   (*Yesod V'shoresh Ha'avodah*, chap. 8)

Many blessings descend on the world together with the holiness of Shabbos. One who wishes to receive this Heavenly bounty should say "*l'kavod Shabbos Kodesh*" before eating.
   (*Mishnah Berurah* 250:102; *Siddur Ya'avetz, Seudas Halailah*, sec. 5)

The pleasure derived from the Shabbos food brings material blessings, while singing *zemiros* brings spiritual blessings. A person should say, "This is *l'kavod Shabbos*," before every pleasure he enjoys on Shabbos.   (*Bais Yaakov*, s.v. *Hiluchach*)

The *minhag* is to say *l'kavod Shabbos Kodesh* quietly several times before partaking of the Shabbos food.

The Tiferes Shlomo states the following idea on the *pasuk* in *Vayikra* (1:2): *When a man from [among] you brings a sacrifice to Hashem*. When a person pronounces an animal to be designated for a *korban*, he elevates the animal to the highest level. Although the animal itself appears to be no different from what it was before, the words and breath that emanated from the person rest upon it, and the animal becomes sanctified. A person should realize from this how great is the holiness contained within him, and how great are his words of Torah and *tefillah*. Through speech alone, a person can imbue all of his actions with holiness. This is the reason we say *l'kavod*

Shabbos Kodesh before eating Shabbos food; we sanctify the food with these words. *(Orchos Dovid, Erech Achilah)*

There is a principle that thoughts are overridden by speech. Thus, even if one's intentions are to derive physical pleasure from the food, when he says *l'kavod Shabbos Kodesh,* these words override his thoughts. His food becomes elevated and infused with the holiness of Shabbos.
(Kitzur Shulchan Aruch Im Sippurim Chasidi'im, p. 185)

Many *tzaddikim* sing *zemiros* when the food is placed on the table. *Chazal* state that matzah is called *lechem oni* since the word *onin* can mean, "to recite." Matzah is bread that "*onin alav,*" because the Haggadah is recited upon it, and through this its holiness is increased. Similarly, we sing *zemiros* when the Shabbos food is served to increase the holiness of the food. *(Mishkinos Haroim; Sefer Ta'amei Haminhagim, p. 173)*

Curative Food

The Gemara states that on Shabbos, a person is allowed to eat any food for healing purposes *(Shabbos 109b).* This can be interpreted to mean that any food that one eats on Shabbos is therapeutic.

Similarly, *Chazal* say that one who visits a sick person on Shabbos says, "*Shabbos hi milizok urefuah krovah lavo*—'Today is Shabbos during which we don't cry out for a *refuah*, but we bless you that the cure will come soon.'" We can understand this on a deeper level: Since today is Shabbos, the cure will come soon because Shabbos food is the source of all healing. *(Tiferes Shlomo, Parshas Mishpatim, s.v. Rak shivto)*

The *sefarim* explain why Shabbos has a special power to heal, based on the following midrash. Every two days of the week are paired together, but Shabbos was left without a partner. So, Shabbos came before Hashem and said, "Every being in creation has a partner, but I have no partner."

Hashem replied, "*Knesses Yisrael* will be your partner."

Just as when a woman falls ill, her husband is obligated to do whatever he can so that she should be healed (*Shabbos* 109b), Shabbos is obligated to heal Bnei Yisrael, its "spouse."

(*Yalkut Me'orei Ohr*, p. 283)

Shabbos food has therapeutic value. This is alluded to by the fact that the Ten Commandments parallel the ten utterances with which Hashem created the world (*Avos* 5:1). Accordingly, the commandment to keep Shabbos corresponds to the utterance, "*Let the earth sprout vegetation*" (*Bereishis* 1:11).

The earth sprouted various types of vegetation, as it says: *The earth sprouted vegetation...to its kind* (ibid. 1:12). There was no specific commandment to sprout various types of vegetation but the vegetation itself inferred a *kal v'chomer*: Since the large trees were instructed to be distinct by growing as different types, all the more so the small grasses.

Kal v'chomer is the first of the 13 rules by which the Torah is interpreted. These 13 rules correspond to the 13 attributes of Hashem's mercy. The first of the 13 attributes is *Keil*, (*aleph-lamed*), so *kal v'chomer* corresponds to *Keil*. *Keil* is also the Name of Hashem used to beseech Him for good health, as Moshe Rabbeinu prayed for Miriam's recovery with the words, "*Keil na refa na lah*."

Therefore, Shabbos food brings good health. This is proven from the fact that the commandment to keep Shabbos corresponds to the creation of the vegetation. At their creation, the vegetation used a *kal v'chomer* which corresponds to the Name of Hashem, *Keil,* that is used to pray for health.

(*Ohr L'Meir, Parshas Emor*)

The Rebbe of Rodishitz would distribute the leftover bread on which he had recited *Hamotzi* to those who came to him with various illnesses. To some people, he gave a glass of water which was taken from the well near his house and they were cured immediately. People saw this as a tremendous miracle, but the Saba Kaddisha explained that this is alluded to in the Torah, as it says in *Parshas Shemos* (23:25): *And you shall worship Hashem, your G-d, and He will bless your bread and your drink, and I will remove illness from your midst.* If one serves Hashem as the Torah directs him, then Hashem will bless his bread and water and they will have the capacity to heal.

This seems to be the reason why Shabbos brings healing: Hashem blessed the Shabbos, and therefore the blessing rests on the foods that are prepared in honor of Shabbos. Just as in the abovementioned interpretation, if there is blessing in the food, it removes illness. (*Dvar Tzvi, Kedushah Shabbos*, section 84)

The Ba'al Birchas Chaim was informed by doctors that he could not eat salt, as it was detrimental to his health. On Shabbos night, when the food was placed before him, he mentioned the words of the Rashba, that if we have a tradition that was handed down throughout the generations, it takes precedence over our own reasoning because it dates back to Moshe Rabbeinu or the *nevi'im*.

The Ba'al Birchas Chaim continued that women say, "Why is it called *heiliger* Shabbos (holy Shabbos)? Because Shabbos *heilt* (Shabbos heals)." He then filled his hand with salt and sprinkled it generously on his food. (*Kovetz Eitz Chaim*, year 4, p. 317)

A guest once went to the Rebbe, Reb Avraham Yosef of Zhilin, for Shabbos Shirah. An ill, weak person also came to the Rebbe that Shabbos.

Friday night, after *davening*, the Rebbe commanded the ill guest to make Kiddush. In a weak, faint voice, the man replied that he did not have the strength to do so and he was not allowed to drink wine. The Rebbe once again instructed him to make Kiddush. The guest mustered all his strength, quietly made Kiddush and slowly sipped the wine.

The Rebbe then instructed that they should bring the sick guest a small amount of chicken soup and said, "A bit of soup will be his cure." The Rebbe stood near the guest until he ate several spoonfuls, and then instructed that he should be given some chicken. The guest pleaded with the Rebbe not to command him to eat it, since he was afraid it would harm him. The Rebbe replied, "Shabbos food is the best medicine." The Rebbe stood near the guest until he ate a bit of chicken, and then the Rebbe instructed him to go to sleep in his room.

During the day *seudah* the Rebbe once again commanded him to eat. When the same guest came to the Rebbe again for Rosh Hashanah, the ill man was there too, but he was completely healthy. *(Toldos Avraham Yosef, Zhilin, Parshas Toldos)*

When the wife of the Darchei Teshuvah, the Munkatcher Rav, fell ill with a fatal illness, her husband commanded her to take upon herself that when she recovers, she will cook an additional dish each Shabbos. She recovered and added liver with chopped onions and stuffed neck to the day *seudah*. Their son, the Minchas Elazar, also did so.

(Darchei Chaim V'shalom, section 456)

Shabbos Food Does Not Cause Harm

The *pasuk* in *Bereishis* (2:3) states: *And Hashem blessed the seventh day.* The midrash states that Hashem blessed the seventh day with blessing in the food, because of people who are particular *(Bereishis Rabbah 11:4)*.

The Bnei Yissaschar explains that one who is particular and cannot tolerate food that is not fresh during the week, can eat meals that were prepared on Friday for Shabbos. Hashem blessed the Shabbos that the food served should be fine dishes with good fragrance, fit for a king.

(Bnei Yissaschar, Ma'amarei HaShabbos, 3:10)

The following incident was heard from Reb Yeshayah of Kerestir, in the name of Reb Hershele Lisker. A man once came to Reb Hershele Lisker and complained to him that the cholent on Shabbos was causing him digestive difficulties. Reb Hershele replied that it is not the Shabbos food that is causing him problems; rather, it was the weekday food. Shabbos food contains a blessing which enables it to satiate a person for a day or two after Shabbos. The damage to his stomach came from the excess food that he was eating on Sunday and Monday that his body did not need.

(Divrei Rabbeinu Tzvi Hersh, Liska, p. 160)

Rav Yehoshua Leib Diskin was once prescribed a strict diet for health reasons. According to the doctor's instructions, he was not served the cholent on Shabbos. Rav Yehoshua Leib requested that they should bring him the cholent and explained that Shabbos foods do not cause harm. Indeed, the Rav ate the cholent and was not harmed.

The following Shabbos, the attendants served the Rav the cholent right away. This time, however, Reb Yehoshua Leib refused it. He explained, "Last Shabbos I had faith in Hashem that the Shabbos food would not harm me. However, it is possible that this week I will rely on the fact that last week the cholent did not harm me and I will not place my *bitachon* entirely in Hashem. As soon as my *bitachon* is not complete, I am required to follow the instructions of the doctor."

(Sichos Harav Shimshon Pincus, Inyanei Chanukah, p. 97)

Shabbos Food Brings Parnassah

When a person rejoices with the spiritual pleasures of Shabbos, he draws down an abundance of spirituality for the entire week. When one rejoices with the physical pleasures of

Shabbos as well, and adds special food in honor of Shabbos, he is blessed with livelihood for the entire week.

(Toras Avos, Sha'arei Avodas Hashem, Mador Shabbos 2:94)

It is a mitzvah to eat on Shabbos; one who does so, brings down sustenance and blessings to the world.

(Tiferes Shlomo, Parshas Eikev)

Praising Shabbos Food

It was the *minhag* of chassidim to praise the Shabbos food and say that it is fit for the table of kings. The reason is written in the name of the Ba'al Chakal Yitzchak. In the *yotzros* on Shabbos Hagadol we say, *In the midbar they traveled 40 years and ate royal food*. The *Siddur Ya'avetz* explains this to mean that the *mann* tasted like royal food. Since Shabbos food has the taste of the *mann*, we praise the Shabbos food as royal foods.   *(Zemiros Tiferes Tzvi, p. 110)*

The Kedushas Levi explains that the *pasuk, Va'achaltem achol*—"and you should eat, eating" *(Yoel 2:26)*, is referring to when Mashiach will come. The midrash explains that in the future, after Mashiach comes, the Jews will eat *mann* like they did in the desert.

Every food has its distinct taste, but the *mann* did not; it tasted like whatever a person desired. Thus, the *mann* received its taste when it was eaten. This is how we can explain the above *pasuk*: *Va'achaltem*—during eating, *achol*—it will become a food.

The midrash states that Hashem blessed Shabbos that even a person who is very particular about his diet and most foods do not agree with him, can enjoy his food on Shabbos. Therefore, like the Kedushas Levi explains about the *mann*, by praising the Shabbos food and declaring that it is fit for a king, we create a new entity—tasty food which agrees with everyone, even the most particular person. *(Rabbi Dovid Meisels)*

Eating on Shabbos Is Different

Eating on Shabbos and Yom Tov is different from eating during the week, since eating during the week coarsens a person and removes his *yiras Shamayim,* as it leads to haughtiness. As the Gemara in *Brachos* (10b) states: One who eats and drinks and then *davens*, Hashem disapproves and says, "After this haughtiness he takes upon himself the yoke of Heaven?"

Tosafos writes in the name of the midrash that before a person *davens* that the Torah should enter within him, he should *daven* that delicacies should not enter his body (because indulgence in delicacies is a barrier to acquiring Torah). We find in the *Zohar* that through eating and drinking, the *yetzer hara* has the power to influence a person. But a *seudas mitzvah*, such as a meal eaten on Shabbos or Yom Tov, is a holy meal and can only bring a person to eat with *yiras Shamayim* and acccpt the yoke of Heaven. Rather than coarsening a person, eating on Shabbos leads him to holiness and purity.

The midrash states that if Jews fear Hashem, the nations of the world will fear the Jews, the animals will fear them, and even the water and fire will fear them. So too, during the *seudos* on Shabbos and Yom Tov, which bring *yiras Shamayim* into a person's heart, the impure powers are afraid to approach a person. *(Michael B'Achas, Michtav 40)*

Reb Yechezkel Halberstam, the Dikla Rav, once ate at the *seudah* of his brother, the Kalashitzer Rebbe. The question crossed his mind whether one is allowed to enjoy the taste of the food he eats on Shabbos, or if even on Shabbos he should not have pleasure from food and drink. Unexpectedly, the Kalashitzer Rav then mentioned the midrash that a person might think that Shabbos was detrimental for the Jews. The midrash concludes that is was given for our benefit. This is difficult to understand.

The Apter Rav would say that all the food he ate tasted bitter to him [during the week]. According to this, one may think that we were commanded to eat more on Shabbos so that we taste more bitterness. For this reason, the midrash says that Shabbos was given for our good, and even *tzaddikim* who don't have pleasure from food during the week taste the sweetness in the food and have pleasure from it on Shabbos.

(Divrei Chanah, Kuntris Divrei Torah)

Chapter 4
Preparing for Shabbos

Purchasing Shabbos Food

When one purchases food for Shabbos, he should do so when he is hungry so that he will buy a generous amount of food. During the week, one should do the opposite and buy food when he is satiated. It is a praiseworthy to fast on Erev Shabbos until one buys the necessary provisions for Shabbos.

Each time one spends money for the sake of a mitzvah (e.g. to buy food for Shabbos), he should do so with great joy and he will then merit wealth and wisdom. *(Shevet Mussar*, ch. 17)

Fish at Any Price

Merchants would often raise the price of fish before Shabbos since they knew that people needed it for Shabbos and would purchase it at any cost. If the price of fish became very expensive, then *beis din* could ration the fish, but they did not have the power to abolish the *minhag* of eating fish completely. This is because fish is a central component of *oneg Shabbos*, and *beis din* cannot nullify the mitzvah of *oneg Shabbos,* which is a positive commandment of the Torah.

(Shulchan Hatahor 242:7)

The first Tzemach Tzedek disagreed with the above ruling. He wrote that according to halachah, if the price of fish was raised by gentile merchants, it is appropriate to ban the purchase of fish in order to lower the price so that every person could afford fish in honor of Shabbos. This is similar to when Rabbi Shimon ben Gamliel, in order to benefit the poor women, worked towards lowering the price of the *korbanos* that a woman was required to bring after giving birth (*Mishnah Krisos*).

The Tzemach Tzedek's *talmidim* argued that Hashem repays a person for whatever he spends for the honor of Shabbos. The Tzemach Tzedek replied that since fish was so expensive, a poor person may not be able to borrow so much money, or may not have an item to use as collateral to buy on credit, and will be forced to welcome Shabbos with an empty table.

The Magen Avraham and the Pri Chadash agree with the Tzemach Tzedek's view. The Chida also agrees, since there are those who hold that one can fulfill the mitzvah of *oneg Shabbos* with other foods eaten in honor of Shabbos.

The Dzikover Rebbe once met the Sanzer Rav, his *mechutan*, and told him that he heard that the Sanzer Rav spent 70 golden dinars every week to buy fish in honor of Shabbos, and he wanted to know if this was true.

Indeed, at that time, there was no fish available in the vicinity of Sanz. The Sanzer Rav would send a special emissary by train to Cracow and he would purchase enough of whichever fish the Rebbe requested, even if it was expensive, for the entire city. Aside from the large expense of the fish itself, there were also travel expenses and the cost of transporting the fish back home.

The Dzikover Rebbe wondered if one had to expend such a tremendous amount of effort and expense to obtain fish for Shabbos.

The Sanzer Rav replied, "If there would be something that I like very much and something I dislike very much, to the extent that I cannot tolerate it, and a person came to me and told me, 'I will give you that which you like in exchange for that which you detest,' wouldn't I do so gladly? I very much like fish in honor of Shabbos, and I detest money. If someone will give me fish for Shabbos and is also willing to take a large amount of money from me, shouldn't I agree to such an exchange gladly?'" *(Olam Hachassidus)*

It is a great mitzvah to purchase fish in honor of Shabbos and to eat it at each of the *seudos*, especially *shalosh seudos*.
(Ohr Tzaddikim; Magen Avraham 242; Minchas Shabbos 72:28)

Shabbos Requires Preparation

We say in *Askinu Seudasa* that the *seudos* of Shabbos need preparation. They require one to contemplate before Whom he is eating and Who commanded him to eat. One should not rush to start the *seudah,* but should take the time to prepare himself for it.
(Chashavah L'tovah, Inyanei Shabbos, s.v. Seudas Shabbos)

The Shem Mishmuel explains the difference between Shabbos and Rosh Chodesh: Shabbos followed six days of creation and is the purpose of the whole creation, just like *Olam Haba* follows life in This World and is its purpose. *He who toils on Erev Shabbos will eat on Shabbos* (Avodah Zarah 3a) means that according to how much one exerts himself during the days of the week for Shabbos, he will reap the rewards on Shabbos. Similarly, since Shabbos is *mei'ein Olam Haba* (similar to the World to Come), according to how one exerts himself in This World, he will reap eternal reward in the Next World.

Therefore, *seudos Shabbos* need preparation and one may not prepare on Shabbos for the following week or for the Yom Tov which follows it, because Shabbos is an end itself.

Rosh Chodesh is the beginning of a new month. The month preceding it is not considered a preparation for the new month at all. Therefore, even if a person did not prepare himself beforehand, when Rosh Chodesh arrives, he has the ability to start anew.

Rosh Chodesh is the Yom Tov of Dovid Hamelech, because he taught that everyone can do *teshuvah*. Rosh Chodesh also shares the same root as the word *chiddush*, to renew, which refers to renewing our actions, as it says in the *midrash*, on the words *Bachodesh hazeh* (Parshas Emor), that we should renew our actions. *(Shem Mishmuel, Parshas Tazria, 5676)*

Chazal say if one keeps Shabbos properly in This World, then even if he is deserving of Gehinnom for his sins, he will not be punished on Shabbos in the Next World.

One of the *gedolei hador* explains that Shabbos will start for this person in the Next World from the time on Erev Shabbos when he began his Shabbos preparations while he was alive, because the merit of Shabbos will already protect him at that time. Therefore, one should make an effort to prepare for Shabbos early, to benefit him in This World and in the Next.
(Shem Olam, Sha'ar Shemiras HaShabbos, ch. 4)

Cooking in Honor of Shabbos

When the Toldos Yaakov Yosef and his wife once returned from a visit to the Ba'al Shem Tov, his wife was asked what she gained from the wife of the Ba'al Shem Tov. She replied, "I learned from her to think about the *Ketores* while preparing the kugel for Shabbos." *(Migdal Oz, p. 245)*

Reb Yaakov Yosef of Ostrow said, "I am unable to understand how Gehinnom can have an effect on the fingers of women who bake challos in honor of Shabbos." He felt that the merit of baking challos will definitely protect these women, and they will go to Gan Eden. *(Haparshah Bahalachah, Va'eschanan)*

The Gemara (Eiruvin 43b) states that Eliyahu Hanavi will not come on Erev Shabbos or on Yom Tov because it is then that the Jews are occupied with their preparations. It has been said in the name of a *gadol* that this refers to preparations of the kugel.

This demonstrates the greatness and holiness of the *minhag* of preparing kugel in honor of Shabbos. It is worth postponing the *Geulah* for two days so that we should be able to prepare the kugel in honor of Shabbos. (*Ohr HaShabbos*, p. 31b)

Women used to say, "A kugel must 'cry' because it contains so much oil." Perhaps the source for this is that which is written in the Rambam that on Shabbos one should prepare dishes with more fat than during the week. (*Rabbi Dovid Meisels*)

One should prepare Shabbos food generously and cook more than he needs (e.g. he should have large challos even if he only needs smaller ones). One should not limit the amount that he spends on Shabbos food, even if only a small amount of the food will be eaten. The angels come to see our Shabbos table and it is not respectful to prepare only a minimal amount of food. One who increases his *oneg Shabbos* is praised, and his reward is very great if his intent is to honor the Shabbos.
(*Magen Avraham* 249:102; *Otzar Halachos* 242: 106)

Preparing the Fish

Every week, Reb Aharon of Belz was particular that the fish for Shabbos should be brought to his house alive. At times, he instructed that each fish should be picked up separately, and he would discuss at length lofty concepts related to fish.

His chassidim stated that the reason for this *minhag* was simply to fulfill the Torah commandment of ensuring that the fish had the proper kosher *simanim* (see the Rambam's *Sefer Hamitzvos*, *Mitzvas Asei* 152; Rambam, *Hilchos Ma'achalos Assuros* 1:1; *Smag*, *Mitzvas Asei* 72). (*Halichos Hatzaddikim*, p. 284)

A chassid once traveled to Reb Aharon of Belz from a distant village and brought with him a live fish for Shabbos as a gift for the Rebbe. In order to keep the fish alive during the long journey, the chassid constantly fed it drops of whiskey. The chassid presented the fish to the Rebbe and related how he had kept the fish alive. The Rebbe responded in jest, "In general, we drink whiskey after eating the fish. Here there is no need for that, since the fish already drank the whiskey."

(Halichos Hatzaddikim, p. 286)

Reb Shimon of Yaroslav once ate the Shabbos *seudah* at the home of Reb Shalom of Belz. When Reb Shimon tasted the Shabbos food he was able to sense within it the righteousness of the Belzer Rebbetzin, who had cooked the food. Reb Shimon asked the Rebbetzin to tell him what was special about her food. She replied, "I put my whole heart into cooking my food." Reb Shimon then asked her in jest how the fish was so tasty, since she could not have put her heart into the fish (since one may not mix fish and meat). The Rebbetzin replied, "I put on a *fartech* (an apron)." The word *fartech* shares the same letters as the word *farcht*, which means to fear. The Rebbetzin was alluding to the *yiras Shamayim* with which she cooked her food.

We can see from this story that an elevated person can sense in his food the greatness of the person who cooked it. When Avraham Avinu served a meal to the angels who came to visit him, they sensed the holiness of Sarah Imeinu in their food and therefore they asked, "Where is Sarah, your wife?" They wanted to greet this holy woman. *(Mevaser Shalom, Avos 436)*

The Butchatcher Rebbe used to personally prepare the fish every week in honor of Shabbos. He would say that when one prepares the fish, it is an auspicious time to *daven* and merit great salvation. *(Eishel Avraham)*

There was a *minhag* in the large Jewish communities that the *shamash* would announce, a half an hour prior to Minchah, that everyone should cook the fish for Shabbos. *(Bach 256)*

Reb Aharon of Belz taught one of his attendants exactly how to cook the fish for Shabbos, including the precise amount of sugar and salt to use. Reb Aharon then told the attendant, "Don't think that I ever once watched this in the kitchen. I just envision that this is how it should be done."

On different occasions, he would instruct his attendant to cook the fish for different amounts of time. One time, he told him that the fish needed to be cooked for approximately two and a half hours; on a different occasion, he told him that less than three hours is not considered cooking. In another instance, he told him that the gefilte fish should cook for four hours and sliced fish for three hours; at a different time, he instructed him to cook all the fish for four hours.

He also instructed his attendant to put whole eggs into the fish as opposed to separating them, and that he should not put pepper into the fish. *(Halichos Hatzaddikim* 310, 311)

The Lelover Rebbe, Reb Dovid Tzvi Shlomo, was personally involved in both purchasing and cooking the fish for Shabbos. He cooked the fish for 18 hours, until the bones softened and tasted similar to the fish. *(Likutei Divrei Dovid)*

Peppery Shabbos Food

One should spice the Shabbos food, even if he is not accustomed to using spices during the week.

(Yosef Ometz, sec. 546)

Hashem commanded that the trees and the fruit they bear should taste alike. In actuality, most trees do not have a taste. The Gemara states that pepper is a tree that the taste of the tree and its fruits are the same *(Sukkah* 35a) The Tosafos Hashaleim states that because the pepper did not change the command of Hashem, it merited being used in Shabbos food. (The *esrog*, which also followed the precise command of Hashem, also merited being used for a mitzvah.)

(Tosafos Hashaleim, printed in *Chumash Otzer Harishonim, Bereishis)*

Bread for Two Days

The *pasuk* in *Shemos* (16:28-29) states: *Hashem said to Moshe, "How long will you refuse to observe My mitzvos and My Torah? See that Hashem has given you the Shabbos. Therefore, on the sixth day, He gives you bread for two days..."*

Whatever one prepares on Erev Shabbos, he will eat on Shabbos (i.e. he must prepare "bread for two days"), since on Shabbos he may not prepare anything new. These *pesukim* also serve as a reminder to exert effort in *Olam Hazeh,* which is compared to Erev Shabbos, so that the *neshamah* will have sustenance in *Olam Haba*, which is the eternal Shabbos.

In This World, people are very busy preparing on Erev Shabbos for Shabbos. How much more so does a person need to exert himself throughout life, which is the "Erev Shabbos" for the eternal Shabbos, *Olam Haba*. A person should constantly work towards *Olam Haba*; all his actions, even mundane ones, should be for the sake of Hashem.

This concept can be read into the *pesukim* above: Until when will you refuse to observe My Torah and mitzvos which will lead you to *Olam Haba*? I gave you the Shabbos to remind you of the eternal Shabbos, *Olam Haba*.

This also teaches us that one who invests effort on Erev Shabbos (i.e. *Olam Hazeh*, the world of accomplishment), will have "food" to eat on Shabbos (reward in *Olam Haba*). Additionally, it reminds us that just as we are occupied the entire Erev Shabbos with preparations, even when it is a long day, how much more time and effort must we invest in order to merit the eternal Shabbos, *Olam Haba*. The World to Come is spiritual pleasure filled with joy and holiness; one who prepares himself properly has no need to fear it.

This is also the meaning of the *pasuk*: *Remember the Shabbos day to sanctify it* (*Shemos* 20:8). The *pasuk* mentions Shabbos "day" to allude to the eternal Shabbos which is completely "day" and has no night. It reminds us to constantly keep *Olam Haba* in mind.

Chazal state: *If Bnei Yisrael will keep two Shabbasos then we will be redeemed immediately* (*Shabbos* 118b). The two Shabbasos refer to Shabbos in *Olam Hazeh* and *Olam Haba*; if Bnei Yisrael would observe Shabbos in This World and prepare for the World to Come as well, they would be redeemed immediately. (*Chiddushei Nishmas Tzvi, Beshalach*)

Hafrashas Challah

The mitzvah of challah is great and beloved, as the midrash states:

The world was created in the merit of three things: challah, ma'asros, *and* bikurim. *As the* pasuk *states: Bereishis bara Elokim.*

Rashi explains this to mean that because of the *"reishis"* the world was created. *Reishis* refers to challah, from the words *reishis arisoseichem*—"the first portion of your dough" (*Bamidbar* 15:20), to *ma'asros,* from the words *reishis degancha*— "the first of your grain" (*Devarim* 18:4), and to *bikurim* from the words *reishis bikurei admascha*—"the choicest first fruits of your land" (*Shemos* 23:19). (*Midrash Rabbah, Bereishis* 1:4)

One may wonder why *hafrashas challah* is so great that the entire world was created in its merit.

Hashem commanded us to separate the first portion of dough, which was created to sustain us, and to give it to the *kohen,* who symbolizes *chessed*. This is so that a person should not think that food sustains him, and the effort he invests in it is what brings him sustenance. One who thinks this way will come to forfeit his *Olam Haba,* because he will spend his time chasing after *Olam Hazeh* trying to earn a living. Giving away the first portion of the dough to the *kohen*, who symbolizes *chessed*, reminds a person that his income is in the hands of Hashem, who gives it to him as a *chessed*, not because he deserves it. A person who does more *hishtadlus* will not increase his wealth, and too much *hishtadlus* thwarts a person's *avodas Hashem*. If a person understands the mitzvah of challah properly, he will invest all his energies in Torah and *avodas Hashem*, for which the world was created.

(Agra D'kallah, Bereishis, Biurei Hamidrash Rabbah, p. 51)

Most people sustain themselves with bread. Hashem gave us this mitzvah that we constantly perform so that blessing should rest upon our bread, and our souls should receive merit. Thus, challah is sustenance for both body and soul.

(Sefer Hachinuch, mitzvah 385)

The reason for the mitzvah of *hafrashas challah* is to give the first of everything for Hashem, in order to strengthen our trait of giving and minimize our desire for food and money.

(Rambam, Moreh Nevuchim, vol. 3, ch. 39)

The words *"zu hi mitzvas challah"* have a numerical value of 613. If one is careful with the mitzvah of challah and fulfills it properly, it is as if he fulfilled all 613 mitzvos in the Torah.

(Hagahos Maimonios, end of Sefer Zeraim)

The main reason for the mitzvah of challah is to constantly bring one closer to Hashem. A person is surrounded by a physical body that prevents him from seeing the greatness of Hashem. Since the main physicality of this world expresses itself in the food that a person eats, which comes from the physical earth, Hashem commanded us to do a mitzvah with every food we eat in order to elevate it, so that it provides pleasure for the *neshamah*.

Since bread is the main sustenance of a person, Hashem gave us a special mitzvah of separating the first portion of dough in His honor, thus elevating the bread to a spiritual food. The bread is then considered like the remains of a *korban* that we merit to eat from the table of Hashem. This elevates a person's soul, increases his *yiras Shamayim*, and brings him closer to Hashem (see *Devarim* 14:23). (*Challas Lechem*, introduction)

The mitzvah of challah was given to women, and they were commanded to be careful with it, as the mishnah states: *It is because of these three sins that women die during childbirth: That they were not careful with* niddah, challah, *and* hadlakas neiros (*Shabbos* 31b).

These three mitzvos are all associated with women. We find that a woman is referred to as "bread," as it says about Potiphar: *So he left all that he had in Yosef's hand, and he knew nothing about what was with him except the bread that he ate* (*Bereishis* 39:6). Rashi states that "bread" refers to Potiphar's wife.

A woman is also referred to as a "house," as *Chazal* say that the *kohen gadol's korban* will atone for his house, which refers to his wife (*Yuma* 2a).

We also find in *Chazal: I never called my wife, "my wife" but rather, "my house"* (*Shabbos* 118b). Rashi explains that a woman is referred to as the house, because she is the mainstay of her house.

Therefore, a woman is commanded to fulfill these three mitzvos because that is how she elevates the three things that are associated with her. Through separating challah, she sanctifies the bread, through lighting candles she sanctifies her home, and through the laws of *niddah* she sanctifies her body.(*Nassan Piryo, Shulchan Aruch Hilchos Niddah, Pischa Zeirta*, p.4)

Baking Challah

The Rema writes that the *minhag* is to bake challos on Erev Shabbos, and one should not deviate from this *minhag*. The

Rebbe of Toldos Aharon was particularly meticulous with this, and he mentioned that he heard from one of his Rebbes that "one should not deviate from the *minhag*," means it should be performed even if it requires *mesiras nefesh*.

(*Zechor L'Avraham, Seder Hanhagos Erev Shabbos Kodesh,* section 8)

The Satmar Rebbe, Reb Yoel Teitelbaum, would say that if a woman would only know the greatness of the mitzvah of baking challos in honor of Shabbos, she would perform it with *mesiras nefesh*. (*Machmadei Shabbos*, p. 97)

Preparing the Shabbos Table

It is *oneg Shabbos* to adorn the Shabbos table with attractive tableware, as *Chazal* have said: *Rebbi asked Reb Yishmael ben Yosi, "How do the wealthy people in Eretz Yisrael merit wealth? ...And how do people in other lands merit wealth?"*

Reb Yishmael replied, "Because they honor the Shabbos."

Reb Chiya bar Aba once said that he was a guest at someone's house in Ludkia and they brought out a gold table that needed 16 people to carry it. It had 16 chains of silver attached to it. There were plates, glasses, bowls, and bottles on it. There were all kinds of food, delicacies, and fragrances. (*Shabbos* 119)

It is *oneg Shabbos* to adorn the Shabbos table with roses, as the midrash states: *Just as a rose is designated for Shabbos and Yom Tov, the Jews are designated for the* Geulah.

(*Midrash Rabbah, Shir Hashirim* 2:9)

One should make sure that he has food on his table both on Friday night and during the day, so that his table will be blessed with sustenance all week. This is because Shabbos is the source of *brachah*, and *brachah* does not take effect on an empty table. (*Shelah*, p. 139, in the name of the *Tola'as Yaakov*)

The Shabbos table should be positioned so that one end is facing north and the other end faces south. The candles should be placed on the southern end and the challah should be placed on the northern end.

This idea is found in the *zemer Azamer V'shvachin*, written by the Arizal: I *will place the menorah which contains deep mystical secrets on the south, and the table with the challos I will place on the northern side.* (*Zemiros Ateres Yehoshua*, p. 69)

The table that is used for the Shabbos *seudos* should have four legs, similar to the *Mizbe'ach* in the Beis Hamikdash.
(*Magen Avraham* 262)

One should be careful that the tablecloth on the Shabbos table should not be taken off all Shabbos. Reb Itzikel of Pshevorsk states in the name of the Chozeh of Lublin that one should be extremely careful not to take off the Shabbos tablecloth even partially, thus exposing the table. He compared an uncovered table on Shabbos or Yom Tov to the uncovered hair of a married woman.
(*Zemiros L'ateir Pesora; Zemiros Ateres Yehoshua*, p. 70)

The Biala Rebbe's table was set in a precise order and with specific intent. He set the cutlery in the following order: the knife (*sakin*), fork (*mazleig*), and then the spoon (the *kaf*). With this order, he alluded to the *pasuk* in *Tehillim* (145:14): *Somech Hashem l'chol hanoflim*—"Hashem supports all those who fall." The word *somech* is an acronym of the first letters of *sakin*, *mazleig* and *kaf*.

This demonstrates that even setting the table, when done with the proper intentions, can bring merit to a person.
(*Shiras HaShabbos*, p. 218)

When setting the Shabbos table one should ensure that there is a knife on the table with which to cut the challah. It says in *Mishlei* (23:1): *Ki seisheiv lilchom*—"when you sit to eat," and the next *pasuk* states *v'samta sakin*—"and you should place a knife." This can be explained homiletically to mean that when one sits down to eat bread he should place a knife on the table.

Another explanation is because, according to Kabbalah, there is a name for *seudas Shabbos* with the letters *ches, tav,* and *chaf*, which symbolizes *parnassah*. In the *pasuk: Posei'ach es yadecha umasbia l'chol chai*—"You open Your hand and satisfy every living thing" (*Tehillim* 145:16), the last letters of *posei'ach es yadecha* are also *ches, tav,* and *chaf*. These letters spell the word "*chasoch*," which means to cut. Therefore, we cut the challah with a knife and do not tear it.

(*Ramasayim Tzofim*)

In the Friday night *zemer* of *Azamer B'shvachin* we say: *Shechinta tisatar b'shisnahamai listar b'vavin tiskatar*. We ask Hashem that the *Shechinah* should rest on our table that has two *vavin*, six challos on each side, which correspond to the 12 loaves of *Lechem Hapanim* that were set upon the *Shulchan* in the Beis Hamikdash. Our Shabbos table should contain all the lofty concepts that were present in the Beis Hamikdash. (*Siddur HaYa'avetz*, s.v. *Shechinta*)

It is written in the *Zohar* (p. 252) that when Shabbos comes in, all the Shabbos tables from the entire world are brought to the Heavens. Thousands of angels are in charge of these tables and they check to see if they were properly prepared in honor of Shabbos. If so, the table and its owner are blessed and all the angels answer amen. If not, it is pushed aside and cursed, G-d forbid. Therefore, one who fears Hashem should put effort into preparing his Shabbos table.

(*Chareidim*, ch.14, *Mitzvos Asei Min HaTorah Hatluyos B'veishet*)

Chapter 5
Erev Shabbos—A Prelude to Shabbos Kodesh

The Amount One Should Eat on Erev Shabbos

People have more desire for food on Erev Shabbos than on Shabbos. This is because on Erev Shabbos we are still in the realm of This World, but on Shabbos, we are elevated to the higher worlds. *(Imrei Pinchas, Sha'ar HaShabbos 35)*

During the Erev Shabbos *seudah,* one should not eat to the point that he is completely satiated so that he has an appetite for the Shabbos *seudah*. There were *tzaddikim* who fasted every Erev Shabbos. Although we may not be on that level, we should at least eat less food than usual.
(Likutei Maharich, Hisnahagus Erev Shabbos; Mattan Shabbos 5:29)

Rabbi Yehudah says that a person should not eat on Erev Shabbos or Yom Tov from Minchah time so that he should enter Shabbos with an appetite *(Pesachim 99b)*. The Imrei Emes states on this Gemara: *One needs to be famished.*

The Pnei Menachem explains that the intent of the Imrei Emes was that one should have a strong desire for Shabbos.
(Pnei Menachem, Inyanei Shabbos)

One may not eat a *seudah* from the time of Minchah on Erev Shabbos until Shabbos, in order to come to the Shabbos *seudah* with an appetite and derive pleasure from the food.

There is a difference between eating on Erev Shabbos and eating on Erev Yom Tov. On Shabbos, there is a mitzvah of *oneg,* and not specifically of eating. One fulfills the mitzvah of *oneg* through eating only if he derives pleasure from his food. If one gets pleasure out of fasting, he can instead fulfill this mitzvah by fasting. However, it is written that there is no *simchah* on Yom Tov without food (*Mo'ed Kattan* 9a). Even if one does not have meat or wine, he still needs to eat and drink, and even if he enjoys fasting, it is forbidden on Yom Tov.

However, unlike on Shabbos, on Yom Tov, the food is not required to bring a person pleasure. Even if he does not have pleasure from the food, he has fulfilled the mitzvah of eating on Yom Tov. Because of this difference, it is not obvious that one should refrain from eating on Erev Yom Tov as on Erev Shabbos. Therefore, the Rambam writes (*Hilchos Yom Tov* 6:16; *Shulchan Aruch, Orach Chaim* 529) that it is forbidden to eat on Erev Yom Tov from the time of Minchah, similar to the halachah on Erev Shabbos. (The Rambam uses the word "*similar*" to show us that it is more definite that one may not eat on Erev Shabbos than on Erev Yom Tov.)   (*She'eilos Uteshuvos Chasam Sofer, Orach Chaim* 168)

The Magen Avraham writes in the name of the Levush, regarding partaking of a *seudas* mitzvah such as a *bris* or *pidyon haben* on Erev Shabbos:

Even if one feels that if he takes part in the seudas mitzvah *he will no longer be able to eat the Friday night* seudah, *he should still partake of the* seudas mitzvah. *This is because if the mitzvah is before him, he does not need to think about what will happen later. [If he indeed cannot eat the Friday night meal,] he should then eat three* seudos *on Shabbos day, as explained in* Shulchan Aruch (Siman 274).

Although this is what the Levush writes, the Magen Avraham rules that in practice we do not follow this ruling, because eating *seudas Shabbos* is obligatory while a *seudas bris* or *pidyon haben* is a mitzvah, but not halachically mandatory.

Therefore, the Magen Avraham rules that if one thinks that by eating a *seudas mitzvah* he will not be able to eat the Friday night *seudah* at all, he should refrain from partaking in the *seudas mitzvah*. (*Biur Halacha* 249:2, s.v. *muttar*)

Thursday Night L'chaim

Followers of Reb Yerachmiel Moshe of Kozhnitz, would gather together every Thursday night to discuss the greatness of various *tzaddikim*. Reb Yerachmiel would distribute whiskey and cake to each person present. They called this evening, "*Seudas Chuppah*."

(*Sifran Shel Tzaddikim*, chapter on Reb Yerachmiel Moshe of Kozhnitz, 18)

In a letter to his close circle of acquaintances, the Rebbe of Karlin wrote the following:

You should study Ohr Hachaim *together every Thursday night. You should then relate stories of* tzaddikim *and drink* l'chaim *with true feelings of love for one another. Enclosed is money for you to buy wine for the* l'chaim. *This is an appropriate preparation to greet the approaching Shabbos.*

(*Kisvei Kodesh, Michtavei Kodesh*, p. 83)

The Ribnitzer Rebbe, Reb Chaim Zanvil, would drink *l'chaim* every Thursday night and say, "In the merit of Reb Shalom of Prubisht."

Reb Shalom of Prubisht, the father of the Ruzhiner Rebbe, had instructed his chassidim to come together every Thursday night and discuss his manner of serving Hashem. He would add, "Whoever wants to merit a joyous Shabbos should talk about my tables and benches." This meant that if they had nothing to relate about his deeds, then at least they should speak of his tables and benches.

Harav Pinchas Brandwein of Yerushalayim added that he heard the following explanation of Reb Shalom's words, in the name of the Ruzhiner Rebbe:

What did Reb Shalom of Prubisht mean by telling his chassidim to speak of his tables and benches? He was referring to the wooden splinters which would come from his table. Those splinters were put into water that was used as a remedy for various ailments. Thus, "tables" was actually alluding to the wonders Reb Shalom was able to perform. Regarding the benches, the Rebbe was using a play on words on the word *benk*, which is "bench" in Yiddish, but can also mean "longing." The Rebbe was hinting to his intense longing for Hashem.

After drinking *l'chaim*, the Ribnitzer Rebbe would wish a *refuah sheleimah* to all the sick people of Klal Yisrael in the merit of Yisrael ben Perel, the Maggid of Kozhnitz. He explained that there is a *kabbalah* in the name of Reb Meir of Premishlan that if someone in the house is sick, one should drink *l'chaim* on Thursday night and say, "In the merit of Yisrael ben Perel, the Maggid of Kozhnitz, this sick person and all the sick people among Klal Yisrael should have a complete recovery."

The Ribnitzer Rebbe also instructed those who came to him for salvation to learn the entire Thursday night, without interruption, until dawn. They should then drink *l'chaim* and say the name "Yisrael ben Perel" together with their request. He said that this is a very powerful *segulah*.

(*Bilshon Chassidim Tiskadesh, Beis Hamaggid* 3:57)

Eating a Seudah on Erev Shabbos

There is a tradition handed down from those well-versed in Kabbalah, in the name of the Maggid of Kozhnitz, that just like on Motza'ei Shabbos there is an obligation to eat *seudas melaveh malkah*, on Erev Shabbos one should welcome the Shabbos with a small *seudah*. (*Pe'er Yisrael*, p. 206)

The *minhag* of eating a *seudah* on Erev Shabbos was of utmost importance to the first Munkatcher Rebbe. He instructed his wife not to give the leftover challah from that *seudah* to anyone, but rather to bake a kugel for Shabbos with it.

(Darchei Chaim V'shalom, Seder Erev Shabbos, p. 103)

The Ba'al Chakal Yitzchak of Spinka would eat borscht (a fermented beet drink) with potatoes and chicken at his Erev Shabbos *seudah*. *(Zemiros Shabbos Shabbason, Seder Erev Shabbos 9)*

In Western Europe, they washed on two loaves of bread on Erev Shabbos. The Alesker Rav added that his father-in-law, Reb Shalom of Belz, would make *Hamotzi* over two challos at every *seudas mitzvah*.

(Otzar Yad Hachaim 344, in the name of the Sefer Hamanhig)

Harav Itzikel of Pshevorsk related that he was not accustomed to washing for bread on Erev Shabbos. Then the Rebbe of Kalashitz told him that in Shiniva and Belz they ate a full *seudah* on Erev Shabbos which even contained meat. Upon hearing that, he felt obligated to wash for bread every Erev Shabbos. *(Siach Yitzchak, p. 41)*

Tearing Apart the Challah

It is said in the name of Reb Pinchas of Koritz that on Erev Shabbos one should not cut bread with a knife (see "Tearing Apart the Challah" below). The reason for this idea is hinted in the *pasuk* in *Tehillim* (145:16): *Posei'ach es yadecha*—"You open Your hand." The last letters of those three words—*chaf*, *saf*, *chaf*—spell the word "*chasoch*," which means to cut. The *pasuk* continues with, *umasbia l'chol chai*—"and You satisfy every living thing." Since on Erev Shabbos one shouldn't eat enough to be completely satisfied, he shouldn't fulfill the first part of the *pasuk* either, by cutting the bread on Erev Shabbos. Since Shabbos is the source of all blessing and sustenance in our lives, on Shabbos one should specifically fulfill the first part of the *pasuk* and use an especially sharp and smooth knife to cut the challah.

It is possible that this custom led to the Hungarian *minhag* to eat thin pitas (which don't have to be cut and are easily broken) on Erev Shabbos. *(Likutei Maharich, Hisnahagus Erev Shabbos)*

Another reason for tearing apart the challah is to differentiate between the challos eaten on Erev Shabbos and those eaten on Shabbos.

Additionally, Friday alludes to Yosef Hatzaddik, about whom it is written, *bashever asher heim shovrim*—"in payment for the provisions that they purchased" *(Bereishis 47:14)*, which refers to the Egyptians purchasing grain from Yosef. Since the words *shever* and *shovrim* come from the root word "break," we "break" apart the challah on Friday, which is the day that is connected to Yosef. *(Likutei Maharich, vol. 2, p. 3)*

Similarly, the Torah writes about Yosef, *V'Yosef...hu hamashbir*—"And Yosef...was the one who sold" *(Bereishis 42:6)*. The literal translation refers to the grains that the Egyptians purchased from Yosef. Again, since the word *mashbir* is associated with the *shoresh* "to break," this is another reason for breaking apart the challah on Erev Shabbos.

(Zemiros Ateres Yehoshua, p. 17)

The Erev Shabbos *seudah* is reminiscent of the meat that the angels roasted for Adam Harishon prior to his sin. Therefore, on Friday one should not wash past the tenth hour of the day, which was when the sin took place. Rather, the Erev Shabbos *seudah* should take place at the same time that the angels prepared the meat (i.e. earlier in the day). Since, at that point, Adam was going to live forever, this *seudah* symbolizes life, and therefore one should not use a knife, which can symbolize death.
(Shabbos Shalom Ma'amar HaShabbos; Mitzvos Asei, mitzvah 248, p. 137)

Another reason mentioned in the *Sefer Sivuv Rebbe Pesachyah* is that the *Kera'im* forbade using a knife on Shabbos, claiming that it violates the *melachah* of *mechatech*,

cutting. Therefore, on Erev Shabbos, the *Kera'im* would cut enough bread to last throughout Shabbos. Thus, the custom was *not* to use a knife on Erev Shabbos, in order to oppose the *Kera'im*.
(*Minhag Yisrael Torah*, vol. 1, 249:3)

Reb Moshe Melamed of Lutzk related that the elderly chassidim of Lutzk often repeated that on Erev Shabbos they did not use a knife, because the angels were guarding the knife to be used for cutting the kugel on Shabbos.
(*Kovetz Beis Aharon V'Yisrael* 103)

It is written in the *Shulchan Aruch* (*Siman* 250) that one should sharpen his knife on Erev Shabbos. Since the knife was given in to be sharpened, there was no knife in the house and they had to tear apart the bread with their hands.
(*Pisgamin Kaddishin, Parshas Vayakhel* 5768)

There is a dictum that a *minhag* breaks a *din*. The literal meaning of this expression is that there are times that a *minhag* overrides halachah. It can also mean that a *minhag* breaks the *middah* of *din* and turns Hashem's strict justice to compassion. Since tasting the food on Erev Shabbos is a *minhag*, we break apart the challah to allude that this *minhag* should break apart the *middas hadin*.
(*Zemiros L'Shabbos Kodesh Buhush, Hanhagos Kodesh* 10)

The Maharil had the *minhag* to bake a pita using very fine flour every Erev Shabbos and Yom Tov. Since the pita was very thin, there was no need to cut it. Instead, he placed his eight fingers on top of the pita and his two thumbs underneath it and recited the *brachah Hamotzi*. He then broke apart the pita, ate a *kezayis*, and distributed a *kezayis* to each person present.
(*Maharil Hilchos Seudah*)

For his noontime meal on Erev Shabbos, the Munkatcher Rebbe ate borscht or *russil* and a small slice of meat. The Rebbe would cut into a challah partially and then break it apart with his hands.
(*Darchei Chaim V'shalom, Seder Erev Shabbos*, p. 102)

The Spinka Rebbe's Erev Shabbos *seudah* consisted of borscht with potatoes and chicken. He did not use a knife to cut the challah; he tore it apart with his hands.

(*Minhagei Spinka*)

A follower of the Shiniver Rav once expressed his surprise at those who are accustomed to tearing apart the challah on Erev Shabbos rather than cutting it with a knife, as he felt that it appeared gluttonous.

The Shiniver Rav answered him with the following story:

In the times of Harav Nassan Adler, a large seudah *took place to which all the* gedolim *of Germany were invited. Although Harav Nassan was young in age, due to his stature they prepared a special couch in the front row for him. When Harav Nassan entered, most of the crowd was already assembled, and they all stood up in his honor and made room for him to pass to his seat in the front row. When Harav Nassan saw that the couch that had been prepared for him was made of silk and wool, which can be a question of* shatnez, *he instructed that they bring him another couch made of wood.*

One gadol *who sat near him could not contain himself and asked him, "Does this not appear to be haughty?"*

Harav Nassan answered him, "I don't know why the world is constantly afraid of appearing haughty but not afraid of haughtiness itself."

The Shiniver Rav concluded to his follower that he, too, was afraid of *appearing* gluttonous but was not as worried about gluttony itself.

(*Derech Hanesher*, p. 19)

In Belz, as well as in some other places, chassidim would tear apart the challos they ate on Erev Shabbos so that the knives remained sharp for Shabbos.

(*Sichos Kodesh* of the Ba'al Vayageid Yaakov of Pupa, p. 43)

The Ropshitzer Rav was extremely careful to hide his service of Hashem and pious deeds from the public. He therefore hired simpletons as his *gabba'im*, who were not able to understand his conduct. The Rebbe's followers once prevailed upon one of the Rebbe's *gabba'im* to reveal one of the Rebbe's customs.

He replied, "He takes a small fresh challah, tears it apart, and fills it with butter. Then he rolls in the snow." The *gabbai* did not realize that the Rebbe was practicing the lofty self-affliction of rolling in the snow.

This proves that the Ropshitzer Rebbe also did not use a knife on Erev Shabbos. (*Niflaim Ma'asecha*, vol. 1, p. 407)

Eating Dairy on Erev Shabbos

The Ropshitzer Rav would eat dairy foods on Erev Shabbos. He used to say in jest that eating dairy is similar to fasting (since one is refraining from eating meat). Since the *Shulchan Aruch* (*Orach Chaim,* section 249) states that righteous people would fast on Erev Shabbos (in order to have an appetite for the Shabbos meals), the Ropshitzer Rav ate only dairy in order to be able to eat meat on Shabbos with an appetite.

Conversely, the Stretiner Rebbe would specifically eat roasted meat on Erev Shabbos according to the *takanos* of Ezra (*Bava Kamma* 82).

Both of these paths are holy and proper.
(*Hadras Kodesh*, p. 22, section 100)

Some have the *minhag* not to eat dairy foods during the Erev Shabbos *seudah*. (*Zemiros Ateres Yehoshua*, p. 18)

The Sanzer Rav had a *minhag* not to eat cheese products on Thursday night or Erev Shabbos. (*Darchei Chaim* 52)

The *Sefer Hamatamim* explains that it is possible that on a short Friday a person will eat aged cheese which requires six hours of waiting time before eating meat, and he will then be unable to eat the Shabbos *seudah*. Or, he may forget that he ate the cheese and eat the Shabbos *seudah* without waiting, thus transgressing halachah. Therefore, a restriction was established that one should not eat cheese, even on the long Friday afternoons. It is possible that in Ropshitz they were only careful about not eating cheese, but they did eat other dairy products. *(Nezer Hakodesh, Nitzotzei Hakodesh, p. 84)*

Reb Shlomo of Bobov once asked his grandfather, the Sanzer Rav, to explain why he did not eat cheese on Thursday night and Erev Shabbos. The Sanzer Rav replied that he learned this from the Ropshitzer Rav. Reb Shlomo then asked his grandfather why Reb Shalom of Kaminka specifically ate cheese on Erev Shabbos. The Sanzer Rav replied that the Kaminka Rebbe also learned this from the Ropshitzer Rav.

When Reb Shlomo asked how the Ropshitzer Rav followed two opposing views, the Sanzer Rav explained that they were both together at the home of the Ropshitzer Rav at the time that he spoke about cheese on Erev Shabbos. He related that the Christians had a custom not to eat meat on Friday, and that some had the custom to specifically eat cheese on Friday (see *Magen Avraham* 551:128, where he writes that the gentiles did not eat meat on the sixth and seventh days of the week). The Ropshitzer Rav concluded by stating that this matter needed to be rectified.

The Sanzer Rav understood this to mean that one must rectify this matter by refraining from eating cheese on Friday; the Kaminka Rebbe interpreted it to mean that it needs to be rectified specifically by eating cheese. *(Magen Avos, p. 47)*

The descendants of the Sanzer Rav refrain from eating cheese on Friday, but the Sanzer chassidim generally do not keep this *minhag*. On Shavuos, when there is a *minhag* to eat dairy products *(Orach Chaim 494:2)*, the Sanzer descendants eat cheese even if it is Friday. *(Magen Avos, ibid.)*

Harav Yissachar Ber of Rodishitz was also accustomed to refraining from eating cheese on Erev Shabbos. It is told that he instructed many people who were suffering from toothaches to take upon themselves not to eat cheese on Erev Shabbos and this helped their pain disappear.

(Nifla'os Hasaba Kaddisha, vol. 1, p. 44b; vol. 2, p. 22b)

There are those who are accustomed to eating cheese on Thursday night and Friday because the Kaminka Rebbe said that he heard from his Rebbe, the Ropshitzer Rav, that eating cheese then is a *segulah* to be spared from toothaches.

(Oheiv Shalom, p. 27)

The Kalashitzer Rebbe used to repeat from the Ropshitzer Rav that bread with butter is not in the same category as cheese, and one is permitted to eat it on Erev Shabbos, even in large amounts. *(Divrei Chanah* vol. 1, *Halichos and Halachos,* p. 9)

Eating Meat on Erev Shabbos

Many *tzaddikim* had the *minhag* to eat meat products on Erev Shabbos so that their bodies should become accustomed to eating meat, and the change in diet should not cause them discomfort on Shabbos. *(Ohr Haner* 5)

Although it is written in the *Siddur Rabbi Shabsi* that one should not eat a *seudah* consisting of wine or meat on Erev Shabbos, in Poland they were accustomed to specifically eating meat on Erev Shabbos.

The reason for this this was that there was extreme poverty in Poland and people did not eat meat all week. Therefore, they ate meat on Erev Shabbos so that their bodies became accustomed to the change in diet, and they did not suffer any discomfort on Shabbos. However, even when following this *minhag*, one should be careful not to eat a lot of meat on Friday. *(Likutei Maharich, Seder Hisnahagus Erev Shabbos)*

The Kaminka Rebbes had the *minhag* to eat roasted meat with garlic on Erev Shabbos.

(*Magen Avos*, p. 50; See *Oheiv Shalom*, vol. 1, p. 77)

The Shiniver Rav and the Ropshitzer Rav were accustomed to eating roasted meat on Erev Shabbos. It is told that the Rebbe, Reb Elimelech, was also accustomed to doing so.

(*Magen Avos*, p. 50; *Hadras Kodesh*, p. 22, sec. 100)

The Gemara in *Chullin* (84a) states that a person should be careful not to eat more food than he can afford. Reb Elazar ben Azariah said that one who has one *manah* (currency used in the time of the Gemara), should buy a liter of vegetables to fill his pot. One who has 10 *manah* should buy a liter of fish to fill his pot, and one who has 50 *manah* should buy a liter of meat. One who has 100 *manah* should cook food every day. The Gemara asks, when should all the other people cook and eat their food if not every day? The Gemara answers, every Erev Shabbos, meaning, [for] every Friday night.

The literal meaning of this Gemara is that one should cook the best food he can afford on Erev Shabbos in honor of Shabbos, and the rest of the week he should eat cheaper food. But, since the Gemara uses the words, "Erev Shabbos," this proves that one should eat meat on Erev Shabbos.

(*She'eilos Uteshuvos Mor Va'ahalos; Ohel Brachos V'hoda'os* 39)

The Mishmeres Shalom writes that it was his father's *minhag* not to eat dairy products on Erev Shabbos, only meat. He did not eat as much as usual and was particular to eat garlic during the Erev Shabbos *seudah*.

It seems that this was in order to honor the Shabbos, since our Sages forbade us to enter Shabbos while fasting. One should greet the Shabbos with a clear mind, calmly, and happily (*Mishnah Ta'anis*). Therefore, an Erev Rosh Chodesh fast or *ta'anis bechorim* that should be held on Friday is pushed back and is held on Thursday.

Thus, it is appropriate to eat a tasty piece of meat on Erev Shabbos since meat contributes to a clear mind, as the Gemara cites the following incident: *Rava questioned Rav Nachman one night about a certain halachah. Rav Nachman answered him, but in the morning, he went back and told him the opposite. Rava explained that the night before he did not eat meat, and therefore did not have the clarity of mind to answer the question properly.*

Chazal quote the *pasuk* in *Mishlei* (15:15), *All the days of a poor man are difficult.* The Gemara asks, how can we say that all days of a poor man are difficult if he also gets pleasure from the Shabbos and Yom Tov food? We answer according to Shmuel that a change in diet can cause digestive problems, so even on Shabbos and Yom Tov, a poor man may suffer from the food that he is not accustomed to eating. Therefore, a poor person should eat some meat on Erev Shabbos so that the Shabbos food should not harm him and he should be able to fulfill *oneg Shabbos*.

Chazal say that one who keeps Shabbos is forgiven for his sins. We learn this from the phrase *(Yeshayah* 56:2): *Shomer Shabbos meichalelo*—"one who keeps the Shabbos from being desecrated." *Chazal* explain that we should not read it *meichalelo*, from being desecrated, but rather as *machol lo*—he is forgiven. In this way, Shabbos is comparable to Yom Kippur. Since on Erev Yom Kippur it is a mitzvah to eat meat *seudos*, it is appropriate to eat meat on Erev Shabbos.

(Mishmeres Shalom 24:9)

The Kedushas Tzion of Bobov would partake of a dish they called *knizhel*, cooked meat with garlic covered with dough, every Erev Shabbos. He then distributed some to his close followers. (Magen Avos, p. 50)

It is a praiseworthy *minhag* not to eat meat on Thursday night and Friday in order to honor the Shabbos by having an appetite for the meat. However, one should eat a *kezayis* of meat on Friday after his *seudah* (not as a main dish, but just a small amount after he has finished eating). This is to oppose the custom of the Christians who did not eat meat on Friday.

(Minhag Tov 46; *Magen Avos,* p. 47)

Drinking Mead

From when he was young, Reb Pinchas of Koritz was very careful not to drink mead (a drink of fermented honey and water) after immersing in the *mikvah* for Shabbos. He stated in the name of the Mezritcher Maggid that this *minhag* protects a person from fire and that this helped the community of Barshad during the fire that occurred there. *(Imrei Pinchas* 3:179)

The Karliner Rebbe would honor Reb Tzvi, the son of the Ba'al Shem Tov, with a drink of mead every Erev Shabbos after he immersed in the *mikvah*.

The Lechivitcher Rebbe sometimes gave Reb Michele a few glasses of mead on Erev Shabbos before *davening* so that he would be able to withstand the holiness of Shabbos.

(Sippurim Yekarim Maharam Midner; Kovetz Beis Aharon V'Yisrael)

Drinking Wine on Erev Shabbos

Rav Ovadiah of Bartenura writes in his *sefer, Darkei Tzion*, that while traveling to Yerushalayim he witnessed how on Erev Shabbos people would drink a bit of wine so that they welcomed Shabbos in a happy frame of mind. They then went to the *batei midrash* and sang and praised Hashem with joy. The Bartenura praised this *minhag*.

The Yerushalmi *(Brachos)* states that there was a *minhag* to drink wine on Erev Shabbos after *chatzos*.

(Otzar Yad Hachaim 874)

Russil

Russil is a dish of chicken and garlic that is roasted for a long time. In Belz they ate *russil* every Erev Shabbos and were extremely careful to uphold this *minhag*, to the extent that Reb Yissachar Dov of Belz expressed it as being in the category of a Torah commandment, meaning it was of utmost importance.

The Belzer chassidim washed for this *seudah* since they were careful only to eat meat within a *seudah*. This idea is taken from the words of Rashi on the words, *basar le'echol*, "meat to eat" (*Shemos* 16:18). Rashi states that meat is *le'echol*, for us to eat, but not to be satiated from it; one should not eat meat to the point of satiety. Therefore, chassidim only eat it within a *seudah* so that the bread and other foods satiate them and not the meat. (*Teil Talpios*, p. 384)

Chassidim were wont to say, "One who does not eat *russil* on Erev Shabbos eats a weekday meal on Friday night." This can be explained to mean that if a person eats meat on Erev Shabbos, by eating another *seudah* containing meat on Friday night he shows that he is eating solely in the honor of Shabbos, since a person does not usually eat meat twice in one day.

The well-known reason for this *minhag* is to fulfill that which is cited by the *poskim* (*Orach Chaim* 280), that one should eat garlic on Erev Shabbos, and *russil* contains garlic.

Another reason is that poor people who eat only dry bread all week can suffer discomfort from the change of diet on Shabbos, so there is a *minhag* to eat meat on Erev Shabbos to prevent this pain (*Bava Basra* 146; *Rashbam* ibid.).

An additional explanation is repeated from the Belzer Rebbe, Reb Yissachar Dov. During the time that Bnei Yisrael were in the *midbar*, they only ate meat that had been sacrificed as a *korban*. Therefore, every Erev Shabbos they sacrificed a *Korban Shelamim* in order to have meat for Shabbos. A *Shelamim* was eaten for two days and the night in between, and it was forbidden to leave over from it. Therefore, a person who brought a *Korban Shelamim* would eat more *seudos* than usual so that the *korban* would be consumed in time. In commemoration of this, we eat *seudos* containing meat on Erev Shabbos, Friday night and Shabbos day, which correspond to the three times that the *Korban Shelamim* was eaten.

In Belz, they were therefore accustomed to eating dairy during *melaveh malkah,* since Motza'ei Shabbos was a time that Jews did not eat meat because the *Korban Shelamim* was no longer allowed to be eaten and a new *korban* had not yet been sacrificed. (*Ha'ari Shebachaburah*, section 2)

It is a mitzvah to refrain from eating a *seudah* from the ninth hour of the day on Erev Shabbos. Righteous people refrain from eating a meal that is as large as one is generally accustomed to eating even earlier in the day. They would eat much less on Friday, such as a small amount of bread with radish. The *Siddur Reb Shabsi* states that one should not eat a meal of cooked food on Erev Shabbos. Perhaps, this is the reason that some do not eat any cooked food on Erev Shabbos except *russil*, so that they should eat less than during the week. (Those who eat *russil* do not eat fish, meat, or side dishes along with it. On Erev Shabbos, *russil* is the entire *seudah*, which is less food than usual.) (*Minchas Shabbos* 72:39)

Tasting the Shabbos Food

It is a mitzvah to taste the food on Erev Shabbos, since one should not enter Shabbos feeling hungry.
(*Magen Avraham, Orach Chaim* 250)

Righteous people are accustomed to tasting the Shabbos food on Erev Shabbos to be able to improve the taste of the food, if necessary. The Yerushalmi explains the phrase *To'ameha chaim zachu* (*Mussaf Shemoneh Esrei* of Shabbos) to mean that those who taste the Shabbos food will merit long life.
(*Kaf Hachaim* 250: 5)

The two reasons given above for tasting food before Shabbos differ in that if one cooks food for Shabbos on Thursday and tastes then, according to the first reason he has fulfilled the *minhag* of tasting the food for Shabbos and does not need to taste it again on Friday. However, according to the second opinion, the actual tasting on Erev Shabbos is a mitzvah, and one would need to taste the food again on Friday.

We rely on the women to taste the food they cook and ensure that it is tasty. However, it is the *minhag* of the righteous [men] to taste the food themselves on Friday, since aside from the stated reasons, there are concealed reasons as well.

(Likutei Maharich, vol. 2, p. 4b)

One who tastes the food on Erev Shabbos merits a long life. The *Yerushalmi* states that this is because it increases peace in the home by ensuring that one does not get angry on Shabbos over food that doesn't taste good. (*Chazal* obviously placed a great emphasis on peace in the home on Shabbos, since that is also the reason that we light candles.) (*Machzor Vitri*, vol. 1, p. 174, section 191)

On the sixth day, they gathered lechem mishneh, *two omers for each person* (*Shemos* 16:22). Rashi explains that *lechem mishneh* means *lechem meshunah*—different bread. The two *omers* of *mann* gathered on Friday were superior in taste and fragrance than the *mann* they received on the other days of the week, since it already had the taste of Shabbos. To commemorate this, we partake of some Shabbos food on Erev Shabbos.

(Chayei Chanoch, Beshalach)

We taste the Shabbos food prior to Shabbos so that we come to *Kabbalas Shabbos* with the merit of the Shabbos food. This is because the fervor of *Lechah Dodi* is drawn from the holiness of the Shabbos food.

(Avraham Bichiro, p. 16)

Tasting Each Dish or Specific Dishes

It is appropriate for a person to taste each dish cooked on Erev Shabbos. This can be compared to someone who is preparing a meal for an honored guest and tastes the food to

see if it is tasty. If not, he can add flavoring or even cook fresh food. All this is done in order to express to his guest his great happiness at hosting him by serving him in the best possible manner. So too, we want to express our great happiness at hosting the Shabbos.
(*Sha'ar Hakavanos Derushei HaShabbos*, p. 62; *Magen Avraham* 250:101)

Not all *tzaddikim* tasted each dish on Erev Shabbos; some chose just one dish to taste. (*Nemukei Orach Chaim* 250:1)

One should taste the cholent on Erev Shabbos. This is comparable to a person who is preparing a meal for a king and tastes the food to see whether it is good or if it is lacking anything, so that he can either correct it or prepare new food if necessary. (*Yosef Ometz Minhagei Frankfurt*, section 576)

Before lighting the candles, one should fulfill the *minhag* of *to'ameha*, tasting the Shabbos food, by tasting the *farfel* and fish. (*Zechor L'Avraham*, vol. 1, p. 287)

Reb Yissachar Dov of Belz explained that since Erev Shabbos is a time of *teshuvah*, we eat *farfel*, which comes from the word *farfalen* (fell away) in Yiddish, to hint that all our sins fell away and were nullified. (*Ish Chassid*, p. 43)

Tasting the Fish

We taste the fish on Erev Shabbos in our eagerness for the mitzvah of eating fish. (*She'eilos Uteshuvos Chavos Yair* 109)

One who eats a small, whole fish on Erev Shabbos says a *brachah rishonah* before eating it, but does not say a *brachah acharonah* afterward since it is not a *kezayis*. There is an opinion that one recites a *brachah acharonah* after eating a whole food even if it is less than a *kezayis*, but a part of the fish is generally removed so it is no longer whole. If one is unsure if he ate a *kezayis* he should not recite a *brachah acharonah*. (*Minchas Shabbos* 72:39)

The *tzaddikim* fulfilled the mitzvah of tasting the Shabbos food by eating fish, and made a *brachah* upon it before Shabbos because *tzaddikim* are *megulgal* (their souls are reincarnated) as fish. We eat fish as a preparation for Shabbos so that the merit of the *tzaddikim* should help us keep Shabbos properly.

Another explanation is that people would invest much effort in acquiring fish for Shabbos. During a *seudah*, one does not make a separate *brachah* on the fish. Therefore, it should be tasted before Shabbos so that he can make a *Shehakol* on it.

(*Dvar Tzvi Osiyos*, see *Divrei Torah* 43: 9)

Rebbe Yerachmiel Moshe of Kozhnitz wrote in his personal writings: *I once stood near the Karliner Rebbe when he ate fish on Erev Shabbos. After candle lighting, before he went to daven Minchah, he sat on his chair, and they brought him a slice of fish on a plate with a silver spoon. He said, "Eating fish on Friday right before Shabbos is obligatory."*

(*Kovetz Beis Aharon V'Yisrael*, year 18, issue 1, p. 134)

The Koidinover Rebbe relates that his father and grandfather would taste the fish after going to the *mikvah* every Erev Shabbos. Before tasting it, they said, *"To'ameha chaim zachu."*

(*Mishmeres Shalom* 25:64)

The Rebbe of Nassiod learned from the Divrei Chaim of Sanz that one should not eat fish on Erev Shabbos or Erev Yom Tov so that he will have an appetite for it on Friday night. However, one should still taste the fish on Erev Shabbos to fulfill the mitzvah of *to'ameha*, as stated in the *Shulchan Orach*.

(*Tehillos Chaim*, p. 305)

Harav Moshe Aryeh Freund would eat the onion that was cooked together with the fish during his Erev Shabbos *seudah*, because he attached great significance to it.

(*Zemiros Ateres Yehoshua*, p. 18)

Chapter 6
Seudas Shabbos

Eating Three Seudos

The Gemara points out (*Shabbos*, ch. 16) that the word *hayom*, today, is written three times in the *pasuk* (*Shemos* 16:25): *And Moshe said, "Eat it **today**, for **today** is Shabbos to Hashem; **today** you will not find it in the field."* Rashi states that the word "*today*," which appears three times, corresponds to the three *seudos* of Shabbos. It seems from his words that eating three *seudos* on Shabbos is an actual *mitzvas asei*, and if one fails to eat one of the *seudos*, his punishment is great.

(*Chareidim*, ch.14, *Mitzvos Asei Min HaTorah Hatluyos B'veishet*)

The *poskim* delved deeply into the Gemara and *Rishonim* to determine if the mitzvah of eating on Shabbos is *d'Oraisa* or *d'Rabbanan*. Those who hold that it is *d'Oraisa* bring proof from the fact that *Chazal* say that the three times it says the word "*hayom*" in the *pasuk* (*Shemos* 16:25), *Ichluhu hayom ki Shabbos hayom laHashem, hayom lo simtza'uhu basadeh*— "And Moshe said, 'Eat [the *mann*] today, for today is Shabbos for Hashem; today you will not find it [*mann*] in the field,'" refers to the three *seudos* of Shabbos. Those who disagree with this ruling hold that it is only an *esmachta*; the *pasuk* supports this mitzvah, but does not command it outright.

(*She'eilos Uteshuvos Nishal Dovid*, sec. 24)

The word "*hayom*" is written three times to refer to the three *seudos* of Shabbos. The Maharsha asks why the *pasuk* uses the word "*hayom*" to demonstrate this.

Suffering is referred to as night and redemption as day. Since one who eats three *seudos* on Shabbos is spared from three evil happenings, the *pasuk* uses the word *"hayom"* to allude to redemption from suffering. (*Maharsha, Shabbos,* 117)

Rabbi Shimon says: If one eats three *seudos* on Shabbos, a Heavenly voice announces, *He will delight in Hashem* (with the *Shechinah* in *Olam Haba*). One is required to take pleasure in all the *seudos* and to rejoice in every one of them. The *seudos* demonstrate *emunah*, which is why Shabbos is honored more than any other Yom Tov, since all the blessings are contained in it. Rabbi Abba would rejoice at each of the Shabbos *seudos*. When he finished eating the *seudos* he would say, "The *seudos* that proclaim *emunah* are finished."

(From the *Zohar* recited on Friday night)

The word *Bereishis* is an acronym for *ratzon Hashem* (spelled with two *yuds*) *tochal b'Shabbos shalosh achilos*—"It is the will of Hashem that one should eat three meals on Shabbos."

(*Agra D'kallah, Tzirufei Bereishis,* sec. 71)

The Raya Mihemna states that the secret of the three *seudos* is alluded to in the *pasuk, V'nahar yotzei mei'Eden lihashkos es hagan*—"And a river flowed out of Eden to water the garden." The word *oneg* is an acronym for *eden, nahar,* and *gan*. These three parts of Gan Eden allude to the three Shabbos *seudos*.

(*Pri Tzaddik, Kuntris Ameilah Shel Torah,* sec. 6)

Mekubalim write that Shabbos brings blessing and bounty to all the days of the week. The first *seudah* brings blessing to the first days of the week, the second *seudah* to the two middle days of the week, and *shalosh seudos* brings blessing to the last days of the week.

The three Shabbos *seudos* are derived from the three times that the word "today" (*hayom*) is written in the *pasuk, And Moshe said, Eat it today, for today is Shabbos for Hashem, today you will not find it in the field. Chazal* state that if you leave the Torah for a day, it will leave you for two. So too, if a person skips one *"day,"* i.e. one *seudah,* it will take away blessing from two days of the week.

(Avodas Hakodesh, sec. 4, *Etzba Ketanah)*

The Bartenura states that one is required to give a fifth of his earnings to *tzedakah (Pe'ah* 1:1). According to this, we can explain why we are specifically commanded to eat three *seudos* on Shabbos. Shabbos food is entirely holy, even if one does not have in mind to honor the Shabbos when eating it, and it has the power to elevate a person's food of the entire week, even if he did not eat it with the proper intentions. Therefore, we eat three *seudos* on Shabbos, which is a fifth of a week's meals: two meals every weekday totals twelve, plus the three Shabbos meals is fifteen, of which three is one-fifth.

(Ach Pri Tevuah; Mattan Shabbos 3:15)

Every food contains physical and spiritual components. Food is essentially physical, but its kosher status and the blessing recited on it give it a spiritual dimension. When eating a *seudas mitzvah,* the spiritual components are increased and outweigh the physical aspects, so that even the physical aspects are purified.

During the first *seudah* of Shabbos, the physical components of the food still outweigh the spiritual; by the second *seudah* the spiritual outweighs the physical, and by *shalosh seudos* the food is entirely spiritual, comparable to the *mann.*

(Lechem Rav, sec. 1821)

Three Meals Are Compared to...

The three *seudos* of Shabbos correspond to many different concepts:

- The first Shabbos of creation, the Shabbos of *Mattan Torah,* and the *Yom Shekulo Shabbos,* which refers to the days of Mashiach.
- The three *Avos*: Avraham, Yitzchak, and Yaakov.

- The three letters of the word *chessed*. One who does not eat three *seudos* withholds *chessed* from himself.
- The three parts of Gan Eden: *eden*, *nahar* and *gan*.
- The words *kadosh, kadosh, kadosh,* which symbolize the three levels of holiness that exist on Shabbos.
- The first, second, and third Batei Mikdash. When the Beis Hamikdash stood, there was tranquility for Hashem and the Jews, which was similar to tranquility on Shabbos.
- The letters *yud*, *heh*, and *vav*, which spell the Name of Hashem.
- The three concepts of *kesser*, *chachmah*, and *binah*.
- The three *middos* of *chessed*, *gevurah*, and *tiferes*.
- The three concepts of *nefesh*, *ruach*, and *neshamah*. Shabbos is like the *neshamah* of the six days of the week.

(*Mateh Moshe* 487)

The Arizal states the night *seudah* invokes the merit of Yitzchak Avinu and spares one from the birth pangs of Mashiach. The day *seudah* arouses the merit of Avraham Avinu and saves one from Gehinnom, since it says that Avraham Avinu stands at the entrance to Gehinnom to save his children who had a *bris milah*. The third *seudah* corresponds to Yaakov Avinu and spares one from the war of Gog and Magog. One should eat *melaveh malkah* to arouse the merit of Dovid Hamelech and be spared from torment in the grave.

(*Asarah Ma'amoros, Ma'amar Chikur Din* 1:23)

There was once a chassid of the Dzikover Rebbe who was appointed by the king to collect taxes on candles and meat. He was extremely harsh toward the townspeople and caused them much suffering. The townspeople went to the Dzikover Rebbe and described the situation to him.

The next time the chassid came to the Dzikover Rebbe, he gave him the following rebuke: The three Shabbos *seudos* correspond to Avraham, Yitzchak, and Yaakov. The Friday night *seudah* is the *seudah* of Avraham Avinu, during which we eat meat and have candles lit. During the second *seudah*, which corresponds to Yitzchak, we eat meat but do not light candles. During the third *seudah*, which is the *seudah* of Yaakov, we do not eat meat or light candles.

Avraham Avinu had two children, Yitzchak and Yishmael. Avraham told Yitzchak, "You should make sure to light candles and eat meat on Shabbos so that Yishmael will also have pleasure from Shabbos." How? The children of Yishmael will appoint a tax collector to collect tax on the candles and meat, and they will have pleasure from Shabbos through this income. Similarly, Yitzchak told Yaakov to eat meat so that the children of Eisav should have pleasure from the tax on the meat. But Yaakov Avinu, whose children were all *tzaddikim*, told his children not to light candles or eat meat, but just to rejoice with the Shabbos. (*Chemdah Genuzah*, vol. 2, p. 156)

The Friday night *seudah* corresponds to Yitzchak Avinu, and brings with it the blessing of children. The day *seudah* corresponds to Avraham Avinu, and brings with it the blessing of long years, and *shalosh seudos* corresponds to Yaakov Avinu, and brings with it the blessing of livelihood. Thus, by eating all three *seudos* one effects the three blessings of children, life, and livelihood. (*Chakal Yitzchak*)

Requirements for the Seudos

One is required to drink wine at each of the three *seudos*, since eating meat and drinking wine bring pleasure to a person, thus fulfilling the mitzvah of *oneg Shabbos*.

(*Rambam, Hilchos Shabbos* 30:9; *Shulchan Aruch, Orach Chaim* 250)

Aside from reciting Kiddush, which is a *mitzvas asei* at the first two *seudos*, one is required to drink wine during all three *seudos* in order to fulfill *oneg Shabbos*.

(*She'eilos Uteshuvos Maharam Alshaker* 106; See *Tur, Beis Yosef* 291)

One should serve as many tasty cooked foods as possible at every Shabbos *seudah*. One should partake of fine bread, fish, meat, and wine. At the very least, he should serve two cooked dishes at every *seudah*. (Beis Menuchah, p. 58)

One should prepare more delicacies for the Friday night *seudah* than for the day *seudah*. Each *seudah* should be less elaborate than the one preceding it, with *melaveh malkah* being the least elaborate. The *Midrash Rabbah* (Bamidbar 21:25) states that we learn this idea from the *korbanos* that were sacrificed on Sukkos. On the first day of Sukkos, 13 oxen were sacrificed and on each subsequent day fewer oxen were sacrificed. On the eighth day, only one ox was sacrificed. Similarly, if one has a guest, on the first day he should serve chicken, the second day he should serve meat, the third day he should give fish, and on the fourth he should serve vegetables, and then he should serve only grains.

Conversely, the Maharshal (4:58a) states that one should honor Shabbos day more than Shabbos night. Therefore, one should eat fish only during the day *seudah* and not at night, so that even if one prepares more delicacies for the Friday night *seudah* than for the day *seudah*, the day *seudah* still remains more special since it contains fish.
(Nefesh Yeseirah, Ma'areches 300, section 129)

All Shabbos foods have a connection to Shabbos. An incredible allusion to this is that all the Shabbos foods amount to the number seven. The *mispar kattan* of *yayin* (wine) is 7, meaning the sum of all the first digits of the letters of the word *yayin* add up to 7 (*yud*=1, another *yud*= 1, and *nun*=5, totaling 7). The numerical value of challah is 43, which in *mispar kattan* equals 7 (4+3=7). Fish, *dag*, has a numerical value of 7, and its *mispar kattan* is also 7, to demonstrate that fish is associated only with Shabbos. *Marak* (soup) also equals seven in *mispar kattan* (*mem*= 4, *reish* =2, and *kuf* =1). Meat, *basar*, in *mispar kattan* is 7 (*beis*=2, *sin*=3, and *reish*=2);

sheichar, beer, is 7 (*shin*=3, *chaf*=2, and *reish*=2), *paraparas*, dessert, is also 7 in *mispar kattan* (*peh*=8, *reish*=2, *peh*=8, *reish*=2, *aleph*=1, and *saf*=4); onions have seven layers; kugel in *mispar kattan* is seven (*kuf*=1, *gimmel*=3, and *lamed*=3), and the word *tavshil*, a cooked dish, is comprised of the same letters as *l'Shabbos*, for Shabbos.

(Kuntris V'Yosef Avraham, Derech Tzaddikim, p. 13b)

One should ensure that he has *basar*, *yayin*, and *dag*, (meat, wine, and fish) at each of the three *seudos Shabbos*. The first letters of each of these words (*beis*, *yud*, *dalet*) total seven in *mispar kattan*, and the middle and last letters also total seven.

(Shelah Hakadosh, Maseches Shabbos, Perek Ner Mitzvah)

In the *Tikkunei Shabbos* it is written that if a person delights in the Shabbos and increases his menu, he will merit two rewards which the letter *zayin* alludes to: *mazon*, sustenance, and protection from *klei zayin*, weapons, as we find in *Chazal* that he will be spared from the war of Gog and Magog. Indeed, the shape of a *zayin* is similar to both a sword and a sheaf of wheat, which symbolizes sustenance.

If one increases his menu on Shabbos, his *neshamah yeseirah* and *ruach hakodesh* will be increased.

(Tikkunei Shabbos)

The Ba'al Hatanya once stated that one should eat 24 kinds of foods on Shabbos, to correspond to the 24 verses in the prayer of *Hodu LaHashem* that is recited on Shabbos morning. One of those present questioned the Ba'al Hatanya by stating that there are actually 26 verses of Hodu LaHashem. The Ba'al Hatanya replied that conquering Sichon and Og were sudden occurrences and not included in the count.

(Shmuos V'sippurim, vol. 2, p. 156)

Belzer chassidim were careful not to add any additional dishes to the accepted menu of their Shabbos *seudos*.

(Ish Chassid, p. 43)

The Shiniver Rav said that one who knows the deep secrets of Shabbos understands that on Shabbos night the essential part of the *seudah* is the meat and fish, on Shabbos day it is the meat, and at *shalosh seudos* it is the fish.

(*Divrei Torah*, Cheshvan 5771, p. 41)

Extra Food on Shabbos

The *Zohar* states that every aspect of Shabbos needs to surpass that which is usually done during the week, including food. If a person is accustomed to eating bread and wine during the week, on Shabbos he should also eat meat. If he is accustomed to eating two cooked dishes during the week, on Shabbos he should eat three. If he is accustomed to eating three cooked dishes during the week, then on Shabbos he should eat four, etc.

During the week, a person is obligated to serve less food than the usual fare, or to leave one setting empty, to remember the *Churban*. On Shabbos, this is forbidden, since it detracts from the honor of Shabbos.

(*Kaf Hachaim* 242:9)

The *Midrash Rabbah* (*Eichah* 3:6) states that Reb Chiya Rabba went to Reb Yehoshua ben Levi and was served 24 cooked dishes during the week. Reb Chiya asked him what he serves on Shabbos. Reb Yehoshua replied that he serves double that amount.

We can interpret this to mean that Reb Yehoshua ben Levi cooked the same 24 dishes for Shabbos as he did during the week, but on Shabbos he ate double the usual amount from each dish.

Although most people commemorate the *mann* on Shabbos with *lechem mishneh*, there were *tzaddikim* who would eat double of each Shabbos food. Indeed, the Munkatcher Rebbe, the Ba'al Darchei Teshuvah, would be served two plates of each course and would partake of each one.

(*Chiddushei Maharya, Nedarim* 50b)

The reason why some *tzaddikim* eat double the amount of food on Shabbos can be understood from the following:

The Tosafos cites the *Midrash Shochar Tov* that the *Korban Mussaf* of Shabbos was the smallest of all the *mussafim* throughout the year; it consisted of only two sheep. Shabbos came before Hashem and complained that such a small *korban* was sacrificed on its day. Hashem replied that this *Korban Mussaf* is appropriate for Shabbos because Shabbos always contains double: The song on Shabbos contains two terms of praise, *mizmor* and *shir;* the mitzvah of *oneg* on Shabbos is written as *oneg* and *kavod;* punishment on Shabbos is double, as it says *michalileha mos yumas,* one who desecrates the Shabbos will surely be killed; bread is double, as it says *laktu lechem mishneh*, they gathered double bread. Thus, it is appropriate for the *Korban Mussaf* of Shabbos to contain two sheep.

This can be compared to a king who instructed his servants to prepare a meal for his children. The servants prepared two dishes. After they ate, the king instructed his servants to prepare a meal for him. When the servants asked him what they should prepare, the king asked, "What did you prepare for my children?" They responded by telling him what they prepared. The king then said, "Do not prepare for me more than you did for my children."

Similarly, just as Hashem instructed us to have *lechem mishnah,* two breads, on Shabbos, He instructed us to sacrifice for Him two sheep.

From the above, it seems that whatever one serves on Shabbos should be not only different from what is served during the week, but it should also be double—one should prepare two types of fish, meat, etc.

(*Darchei Chaim V'shalom* 394, p. 119)

The *Sefer Divrei Shalom* explains why everything on Shabbos is doubled: The two *keruvim* in the Beis Hamikdash demonstrate that nothing is one except Hashem. Shabbos, too, demonstrates the oneness of Hashem. Therefore, we double everything to show that every being has a partner, but only Hashem is one. *(Dvar Tzvi, Parshas Hamann*, sec. 23)

Reb Yosef of Rashkuv would instruct that double the amount of Shabbos food should be prepared each week. He would then eat twice from each dish. He explained that the first time, he ate to satisfy his hunger, but the second time he ate in honor of Shabbos. (*Mizekeinim Esbonan*, vol. 1; *Inyanei Shabbos*, p. 179)

Eating Shabbos Food with One's Hands

It is the *minhag* of many chassidim to eat fish with their hands, without any cutlery. The *Sefer Darkei Chaim V'shalom*, written by the Munkatcher Rebbe, connects this to the *pasuk* in *Bereishis* (9:2) *...and upon all the fish of the sea, [for] they have been given into your hand*. This alludes to the fact that fish should be eaten with one's hands.

(*Darkei Chaim V'shalom* sec. 395)

Korbanos were required to be brought with bare hands without any *chatzitzah* (foreign object) in the way (see *Pesachim* 57a). Since the table at which one eats is compared to a *Mizbe'ach*, perhaps this is the reason for eating Shabbos food with one's hands. (Ibid; *Minhagei Mahari Veil*, sec. 237)

There is a source in the Gemara for eating with one's hands. The Gemara in *Nedarim* (49b) states that Rabbah bar Rav Huna saw Rav Huna eating porridge with his fingers and asked him for an explanation. Rav Huna replied that porridge eaten with one's hands has a good taste. This demonstrates that even in the times of *Chazal* there were those who ate with their hands.

(*Vayevarech Dovid*, Reb Baruch Dovid, son of the Hornesteipler Rebbe)

Rabbeinu Chananal writes that it was the custom of the Greeks to eat with a two-pronged fork. They would hold the meat with this fork and then cut it and eat it. They would not touch the meat because it was not considered hygienic (*Bava Metzia* 25b). This seems to imply that eating with a fork and a knife is the way of the Greeks. (Ibid.)

Shabbos, specifically Friday night, is an auspicious time to bring down the holiness of the Torah. The *seudah* eaten on Friday night is called the *seudah* of Avraham Avinu. Regarding Avraham, it is written, *V'heyeih brachah* (*Bereishis* 12:2), and the *midrash* states that the power of giving *brachos* was given in the *hands* of Avraham. Therefore, one should eat the Shabbos food with his hands. (*Minchas Yehudah, Terumah*)

Some *tzaddikim* were accustomed to eating every solid Shabbos food with their hands. (*Darkei Hayashar V'hatov*, p. 23)

Sadigur chassidim were accustomed to eating all the Shabbos foods, except the kugel, with their hands, similar to the *kohen gadol* who performed the *avodah* with his hands. The Apter Rav was also accustomed to eating with his hands, but the Husiatyner chassidim ate only with forks.
(*Zemiros L'Shabbos, Minhagei Apta*)

The Ateres Tzvi of Ziditchov once ate the Shabbos *seudah* with the Yismach Moshe of Uhel. The Yismach Moshe picked up a fork, about to eat the meat. The Ateres Tzvi told him, "Is there not more holiness resting on your ten fingers than on this piece of metal?" Immediately, the Uheler Rav set down the fork and ate with his hands. (*Darchei Hayashar V'hatov*)

The Ateres Tzvi of Ziditchov was once at the *seudah* of the Maharam Ash. When the meat was served, the Maharam Ash ate it with a fork, whereas the Ateres Tzvi ate it with his hands. The Ateres Tzvi explained, "My hands were created by Hashem and perform many mitzvos, including laying *tefillin* and giving *tzedakah*. Before eating, I washed my hands and recited a *brachah*.

"A fork was created by a coarse gentile, and aside from *tevilah*, no other mitzvah was performed with it. And if it was among other vessels when it was immersed, the *brachah* does not even rest specifically on the fork. Therefore, I prefer to eat with my hands rather than with a fork."

Immediately, the Maharam Ash put down his fork and finished the meat with his hands. From that day on, the Maharam Ash did not use a fork for the Shabbos food. If the food was too hot, he waited until it cooled down.

(Shefa Tov, p. 38)

The Gemara in *Nedarim* (49b) says that one should not eat with his hands, since it is unhygienic because of the dirt that collects under the fingernails.

Reb Itzikel used to say that since chassidim are meticulous to cut their nails short every Erev Shabbos, there is no room for grime to collect, and they can eat with their hands.

(Ro'eh Even Yisrael, p. 192b)

Chapter 7
Friday Night—Beginning the Meal and Kiddush

Seeing the Shabbos Food

The midrash brings the *pasuk*: *We remember the fish that we ate in Egypt free of charge...* (*Bamidbar* 11:5) and then states that we learn from this *pasuk* to light candles for Shabbos.

Rav Eliezer de Avila explains the connection. The Jews in the *midbar* complained that they had no fish, even though the *mann* gave them the ability to experience the taste of any food they wished, because seeing food is an essential part of experiencing its pleasure. Since the Jews were not able to actually see the fish, they did not feel like they were eating it. Therefore, we light candles on Friday night so that we can see the food we eat and have complete *oneg Shabbos*.

(*Chomas Anach, Parshas Beha'aloscha* 6)

Not Eating before the Meal

It is a mitzvah to eat the Shabbos *seudah* with an appetite. Since bread is the essential part of the *seudah*, a person should not eat anything prior to the *seudah*, so that he will be able to eat the challah with an appetite. (*Darchei Moshe* 249: 4)

It is a mitzvah to refrain from eating anything on Shabbos after nightfall or after one has accepted Shabbos, and even after Kiddush before he has washed, so that he will eat the challah with an appetite. (*Otzar Halachos* 249: 18)

The Imrei Noam (*Parshas Emor*) writes that the words, *Zachor es yom haShabbos l'kadsho* (*Shemos* 20:8) begin with the same letters as, *Zeh hashulchan asher lifnei Hashem*—"this is the table that is before Hashem" (*Yechezkel* 41:22). We learn from this that the mitzvah of Kiddush, which is derived from, *Zachor es yom haShabbos l'kadsho,* should take place when the table is already set and one is ready to eat the *seudah*.

(*Birchas Avraham,* chap. 18)

Sending Away the Angels

The Sanzer Rav explains that we send away the *malachim* that accompany us home from shul, telling them, *Tzeischem l'shalom*, because angels can't eat. Since they can't join us as our guests, we tell them to leave. (*Mekor Chaim*, sec. 72)

Hastening to Recite Kiddush

The *Shulchan Aruch* states that when one arrives home he should eat right away. We learn this from *Zachor es yom haShabbos l'kadsho* which, *Chazal* explain, means to remember the Shabbos with wine immediately upon its arrival.

Commentaries on the *Shulchan Aruch* explain that the term, *he should hasten to eat right away* does not refer to the actual eating but to the recitation of Kiddush, because there can be no meal without Kiddush beforehand, and one must begin his meal immediately after Kiddush. However, there is no need to rush to finish the meal. On the contrary, if someone begins Shabbos before nightfall, it is actually better to end the meal after nightfall and eat at least one *kezayis* of bread after nightfall. (*Tur* and *Shulchan Aruch, Orach Chaim* 271:1)

Reciting Kiddush on Wine

One who recites Kiddush on wine on Friday night will live long in This World, and his *Olam Haba* will be increased.

(*Pirkei D'Rabbi Eliezer,* chap. 18)

Kiddush is recited over wine because wine brings joy to a person, as the *pasuk* in *Tehillim* (104:15) states: *And wine gladdens the heart of a person.* In addition, reciting Kiddush has the effect of reversing Divine justice to mercy, thus bringing joy.

(Sidduro Shel Shabbos 3:2:1)

We recite Kiddush on wine because, according to one opinion, the *Eitz Hada'as* was a grapevine.

Adam Harishon sinned on the tenth hour of Erev Shabbos, which is close to the beginning of Shabbos. (Indeed, it is from the tenth hour of the day that one may accept Shabbos.) This sin caused the *Shechinah* to recede to the Heavens. Therefore, we recite Kiddush on wine with the arrival of Shabbos to rectify Adam's sin that was done at that time, because when a Jew recites Kiddush, the *Shechinah* descends and rests at his Shabbos table.

(Ben Ish Chai, year 2, *Bereishis)*

The Bnei Yissaschar explains why we recite Kiddush on wine. Every *brachah* that *Chazal* established on specific foods, such as *Ha'adamah* on vegetables or *Ha'eitz* on fruits, is only applicable when the food is in its original form. If the food is no longer recognizable, it loses its status and its *brachah* becomes *Shehakol*. However, wheat and grapes are exceptions. When wheat becomes bread and grapes become wine, their status is enhanced and we recite the special blessings of *Hamotzi* and *Hagafen* over them.

This concept alludes to *teshuvah* done out of love, which changes sins into merits. Since Kiddush is an auspicious time for one to do *teshuvah*, we recite it over wine.

(Bnei Yissaschar, Tishrei 10:20)

When Shabbos arrives, we proclaim its holiness over wine, because wine satisfies and gladdens the heart. If one does not have wine, he can recite Kiddush on bread, since bread also satisfies and gladdens a person.

When Shabbos leaves, we are similarly obligated to proclaim the holiness of the day and its distinction from the days of the week over a cup of wine by reciting Havdalah. However, one may not recite Havdalah over bread. This is because on Motza'ei Shabbos, a person is probably already satiated from the *seudos* and will not be gladdened by eating bread.

(Shelah Hakadosh, Parshas Yisro, Torah Ohr 2)

Hashem commanded us to wear *tzitzis* and to wrap ourselves with them. This demonstrates that even one's body needs to be cloaked in a garment of Torah, and teaches that the physical aspects of life should be used to serve Hashem.

Similarly, Hashem commanded us to remember the Shabbos by reciting Kiddush on wine. Wine is a physical pleasure, and we are obligated to remember Shabbos with the physical pleasures of This World as well, and elevate them to a state of holiness.

With this we can explain the midrash on the *pasuk* (Bamidbar 15:39): *Do not follow after your hearts and your eyes that you are straying after them, so that you should remember, and perform all of My mitzvos.*

Do not stray after your hearts and your eyes means that one should not follow his desires, since doing so strengthens the power of the *yetzer hara*. But, the *pasuk* continues, *you should remember and perform all My mitzvos*. The midrash explains that "*all My mitzvos*" refers to Shabbos, which is equivalent to the entire Torah. This refers to Shabbos, to teach us that on Shabbos one is permitted fulfill his desires, because fulfilling one's desires on Shabbos is a mitzvah.

The *Chovos Halevavos* writes that all actions can be divided into three categories. A mitzvah, something which is compulsory; an *aveirah*, something that is forbidden; and *reshus*, that which is neither a mitzvah nor an *aveirah*, but

Shabbos Secrets • *Friday Night—Beginning the Meal*

permitted. However, if one's goal in performing a *reshus* is to serve Hashem, then the *reshus* also becomes holy.

This is why the *pasuk* uses the words, *l'ma'an tizkiru*—"so that you should remember." One should be sure to remember the lesson of Shabbos—elevate the mundane to holiness and be inspired to do so every day of your life. *(Maharam Schick)*

Another reason why Kiddush is specifically recited on wine and not on any other beverage is because the branches of a grapevine cannot grow unless they are supported by poles. The poles themselves produce no fruit, but without them the grapevine will perish. On Shabbos, we don't work and earn money, but Shabbos is the source of all blessings, and through Shabbos all of our endeavors during the week are blessed. Wine therefore symbolizes that just as the grapevine is fruitful only when supported by barren poles, the days of the week are fruitful only when supported by Shabbos.

(Beis Yisrael Hashaleim, Parshas Yisro, s.v. Zachor)

Another reason can be explained according to the *Zohar*: Jews are compared to a grapevine. Just as a grapevine does not accept any graft, the Jews do not accept any authority over them other than Hashem. This is the basis of Shabbos—it is a bond between Hashem and *Knesses Yisrael*. *Knesses Yisrael* is regarded as being wed to the *Shechinah* and consequently, does not submit to any other authority. Therefore, we remember the Shabbos with wine to remind us of our similarity to the grapevine—that Hashem is the only Power over us.

(Yishrei Lev, p. 14a)

The Shem Shlomo explains why we recite Kiddush over wine at the start of Shabbos. Wine that is touched by a non-Jew is *yayin nesech* and one may not drink it. We learn from this that Jews need to be separate from the nations. Thus, we recite Kiddush on wine to remind us to remain separate from the gentiles in every area of our lives.

(Drashos Dvar Tzvi, Parshas Shemini 5698)

The *brachah* of *Hagafen* is recited ceremoniously on many occasions, such as *bris milah*, *pidyon haben*, *chuppah*, and Shabbasos and Yamim Tovim. It is recited first, before the specific blessing that is designated for these mitzvos. Would it not be more fitting to start Shabbos and Yom Tov and other mitzvos with learning Torah or *tefillah*?

According to one opinion in the Gemara, the *Eitz Hada'as* was a grapevine from which Adam Harishon made wine. All holy acts and holy days of the year are to rectify this first sin. Therefore, *Chazal* have instituted that every holy act and time should begin with the *brachah* of *Hagafen*.

However, this holds true only according to the opinion that the tree that Adam ate from was a grapevine. Another reason can be learned from the following midrash:

Why are the Jews compared to a grapevine? Just as a grapevine is supported by poles made from old branches, Bnei Yisrael exists only in the merit of our forefathers.

The most significant part of everything is its beginning. Thus, at the beginning of every holy act, we start by reciting the *brachah* on the wine in order to connect our actions to those of our forefathers and to arouse their merit to help us fulfill the mitzvah properly. During *bris milah*, which is the first mitzvah performed with a newborn baby, we first make a *brachah* on the wine to instill in the child that he should follow the ways of our forefathers.   (*Dvar Tzvi, Shabbos* 65:1)

The Gemara in *Sanhedrin* (38b) states that Adam Harishon was created on Erev Shabbos. Rabbi Yochanan bar Chanina explains what transpired during the 12 hours of the first Friday of creation. During the first hour, Hashem gathered a pile of earth; during the second, He made a form, etc. During the ninth hour, Hashem commanded Adam Harishon not to eat from the *Eitz Hada'as*, and during the tenth hour Adam sinned by eating from the *Eitz Hada'as*, which was a grapevine, without making a *brachah*. During the eleventh he was judged, and in the twelfth he was banished from Gan Eden.

The twelfth hour is the time when Shabbos arrives and one recites Kiddush. The Maharsha writes that when Adam Harishon sinned he brought impurity to the world and this caused the *Shechinah* to ascend from the world. The *brachah* of *Borei Pri Hagafen* blesses Hashem for creating a grapevine to teach us that this *brachah* is regarded as a rectification (*tikkun*) for Adam Harishon's sin of eating from a grapevine without reciting a *brachah*, as mentioned in *Sefer Asarah Ma'amaros*. At the time that one recites Kiddush, the *Shechinah* descends and rests at a person's Shabbos table, thus proving that Adam's sin has been rectified.

(*Haggadah Chalukah D'Rabbanan, Kesones Pasim*, p. 30)

The Chida writes in the name of *Chazal* that a person should arouse himself to *teshuvah* before reciting Kiddush. *Vayechulu* is a testimony that Hashem created the world and rested on Shabbos. A wicked person cannot be a valid witness. Thus, a person should do *teshuvah* before Kiddush so that he can be a kosher witness.

The *sefarim* write that the mitzvos that a person does while he is still tainted with sin give strength to the Satan. Therefore, a person should be extremely careful to do *teshuvah* prior to performing any mitzvah. Accordingly, we can suggest that we recite Kiddush on wine on Shabbasos and Yamim Tovim to awaken the merit of our forefathers (see above) to assist us in doing *teshuvah* at the start of Shabbos. (*Dvar Tzvi Shabbos* 65:6)

The physical pleasures of *Olam Hazeh* prevent a person from recognizing that there is a Creator Who runs the world. Wine symbolizes ultimate physical pleasures and it inebriates a person so that he cannot see the spiritual light. On Shabbos, a person needs to recite Kiddush on wine in order to elevate physical pleasures and compel him to recognize that there is a Creator. This will infuse spiritual light into all his actions of the week and elevate them as well, so that they are only for the sake of Hashem. *(Haggadah, Bais Yaakov)*

Shabbos is the day that was given for Torah learning. We see in the Gemara that wine and its pleasant aroma help a person acquire Torah wisdom.

Another reason for reciting Kiddush on wine is that Shabbos is compared to the Beis Hamikdash, where they performed *nisuch hayayin*, the pouring of the wine on the *Mizbe'ach*. Nowadays, when there is no Beis Hamikdash, *Chazal* tell us that *nisuch hayayin* can be performed by *"pouring wine into the throats of* talmidei chachamim" (i.e. donating wine for *talmidei chachamim* to drink). *Talmidei chachamim* drink the wine in holiness and thereby elevate it, just as the *Mizbe'ach* sanctified the *korbanos* and their accompanying wine. Shabbos also has the power to sanctify and elevate the physical, and thus, the wine we drink at Kiddush is also similar to *nisuch hayayin*.
(Mesilas Yesharim; To'ameha Chaim Zachu)

The *Zohar* states that usually wine arouses the *yetzer hara*, except for on Shabbos and Yom Tov, when it becomes elevated. Therefore, there is a mitzvah to recite Kiddush on wine.
(Rabbi Dovid Meisels)

Kiddush is recited over wine as a reminder that one should learn the trait of *tznius* from the grapevine. The *Zohar* writes on the *pasuk* in *Tehillim* (128:3), *Eshticha k'gefen poriyah*— "Your wife is like a fruitful grapevine," that a woman who stays in her house and does not go outside is a *tzanuah* who will merit good children. Such a woman is like a grapevine. Just as a grapevine cannot be grafted with other plants, this woman doesn't mingle in public. *(Zohar, vol. 2, p. 115)*

Shabbos is equivalent to the entire Torah, and one who keeps Shabbos will merit to drink from the *yayin hameshumar*, the wine that is reserved since Creation. We drink wine on Shabbos to allude to this. *(Noam HaShabbos p. 41)*

The Gemara (*Sanhedrin* 38a) states that Yehudah and Chizkiyah, the children of Reb Chiya, sat together at a *seudah* near Rebbi and did not speak. Rebbi told them that he would give them wine so that they would speak.

The Ohr Lashamayim explains that a *tzaddik* is small in his own eyes and does not want to speak because he thinks he is not great enough. However, the bounty that Hashem sends comes through the *tzaddik* and requires that he speak of the good of Bnei Yisrael. Therefore, a *tzaddik* needs to drink wine to cause him to speak well of other Jews.

Therefore, we all need to make Kiddush on wine, to cause us to speak well of others. (*Rabbi Dovid Meisels*)

The Gaon of Selish says that one glass of wine in honor of Shabbos is greater than a thousand fasts, as is written in the midrash, *The honor of Shabbos is greater than a thousand fasts* (*Midrash Tanchuma, Bereishis* 83). (*Noam Siach Salka*, 145)

In *Yom Zeh Mechubad* we say *b'yeino yekadeish*—"with wine he will recite Kiddush." *Emunah* is like a secret, because one person does not know the level of *emunah* that exists in the heart of his friend. Wine has the same numerical value as the word *sod*, secret. This is what the *zemer* (song) is alluding to. Every person *b'yeino*, with his wine (i.e. with his secret, the amount of *emunah* he possesses), *yekadeish*, he will sanctify; according to the depth of his *emunah,* he will sanctify himself for Hashem. (*Imrei Pinchas, Rosh Hashanah*, 504)

Wine Brings Healing

The Gemara states that if one walks with large strides it takes away 1/500th of his eyesight. The Gemara concludes that one can restore his eyesight during Kiddush on Friday night. Rashi explains that this Gemara refers to drinking the Kiddush wine.

(*Maharsha Brachos* 43b, *Chiddushei Aggados*, s.v. *Lihadar leih*)

Rav Nitronai asks why we recite Kiddush in the *beis haknesses* even though we do not eat there and Kiddush needs to be recited again at the place where one eats the *seudah*. Kiddush wine brings healing, as the Gemara states that walking in large strides diminishes a person's eyesight by 1/500th and Kiddush restores it. Therefore, Kiddush is recited in shul in order to be able to distribute the wine for people to put on their eyes to effect healing.

(*Tur, Orach Chaim* 269; *Magen Avraham* 271:23)

The Gemara states that walking in large strides diminishes 1/500th of a person's eyesight and Kiddush restores it. The end letters of the words *Vayevarech Elokim es yom hashvi'i*—"And Hashem blessed the seventh day" (*Bereishis* 2:3), which refer to Kiddush, have a numerical value of 500, thus alluding to the fact that Kiddush restores 1/500th of a person's eyesight.

The *minhag* in Bavel and Narvona was that after Kiddush they added water to the Kiddush wine and then rinsed their faces with it, so as to benefit from this *segulah*.

(*Rokeach, Seder Kiddush Leil Shabbos*)

Since Kiddush wine is a remedy, during Kiddush all the fountains of healing are opened (i.e. Kiddush is an auspicious time for healing) (*Bava Basra* 58b).

(*Imrei Emes, Parshas Naso*, 5627, s.v. *B'zemiros*)

We can learn the healing power of wine from the story of a man who once had a chronic nosebleed and was losing a large amount of blood. He became increasingly ill until the doctors gave up hope on him. The man was already close to death and the entire household was weeping. Someone who saw how dire the situation was quickly ran to the wine cellar. He took a glass of strong, good wine and instructed the ill person to drink without letup. As soon as the ill man drank the wine, the bleeding stopped. The doctors were astonished and they blessed Hashem Who created many different remedies and cures in the world.

When this story reached Reb Pinchas of Koritz, he showed them where this remedy is alluded to in the Torah. The Torah states *(Bereishis* 49:11), *Uv'dam anavim susoh*—"and his robe in the blood of grapes." *Dam anavim* refers to wine, and *susoh* is from the same root as *asvisa* (healing) *(Shabbos* 110a).

Reb Pinchas of Koritz concluded that all types of remedies and cures are alluded to in the Torah, so that a person should know that all cures are in the hands of Hashem and he should beseech Hashem to heal him. *(Sifsei Tzaddikim, Dinov)*

A Full Glass

Chazal said that there are 10 requirements for a *kos shel brachah*, among them that the glass should be completely full. Rabbi Yochanan said that one who recites a *brachah* on a full *kos shel brachah* will be given an unlimited reward *(Brachos* 51a), as it says in *Tzur Mishelo*: *Al kos yayin malei... birchas Hashem*—"On a full glass of wine...the blessing of Hashem," which can be understood to mean that those who recite Kiddush on a full glass of wine will merit the blessings of Hashem. This is alluded to by the fact that *kos yayin malei* has the same numerical value as *brachah*.

The requirement for a full glass is not only when reciting the *brachah*, but also at the time of drinking the wine. Therefore, if some wine spilled during Kiddush and the cup is no longer full, it is proper to refill it before drinking.

(Tur, Orach Chaim 183; *Zemiros Divrei Yoel*, p. 64)

The Kiddush Cup

One should use a fine goblet for Kiddush. It is even more appropriate if one can enhance this mitzvah by using a silver goblet in order to honor the *Shechinah*, as it says: *This is my G-d and I will adorn him (Shemos* 15:2). *(Siddur Rabbi Shabsi* 63:2)

Some say that the source for calling the goblet which is used for Kiddush a *"becher"* is because *becher* is the same letters as the root of the word *brachah*.

The letters of the *aleph-beis* are divided into units, tens, and hundreds. The Maharal explains that the letters *beis*, *reish*, and *chaf* represent an increase, because each of them is the first of the plural of their unit. *Beis* has the numerical value of two, which is the first plural number. *Chaf's* numerical value is 20, the first plural number in the tens. *Reish*, whose numerical value is 200, is the first plural number in the hundreds. Thus, the word *becher* symbolizes an increase, and the goblet used for a *kos shel brachah* is called *becher* because it is a *segulah* for an increase in wealth and blessings.

(*Yiddish, Hasafah Hakedoshah,* p. 13)

There are those who are particular that the Kiddush cup should not have a rim. One reason for this is because, according to halachah, the cup should not be damaged in any way, even slightly, and if a cup has a rim it is difficult to be careful with this (since the rim is delicate). Another reason is that many are accustomed to using their Kiddush cups on Pesach, and in order to do so they first have to be kashered by immersing them in boiling water, which is easier if the cup has no rim. A third reason for using a cup without a rim is that, ideally, the cup should be completely full, and if there is a rim on the cup it is not considered entirely full. (*Halichos Hatzaddikim,* p. 165)

Rinsing the Cup

Rabbi Mordechai of Nadvorna would rinse the Kiddush cup himself. He would say that the Kiddush cup symbolizes the *neshamah,* and one needs to rinse his *neshamah* himself.

(*Oros Mordechai,* p. 115)

Borei Pri Hagafen

During the Friday night Kiddush, chassidim are accustomed to reciting the *brachah* of *Mekadeish HaShabbos* immediately after the *brachah* of *Borei Pri Hagafen* without pausing. This is to demonstrate that through Kiddush, we rectify the sin of Adam Harishon, which occurred through a grapevine.

(*Shulchan Menachem, Parshas Bereishis*)

Sitting While Drinking

It is proper for one to sit while drinking the Kiddush wine, as the Magen Avraham writes in regard to Havdalah: *One should only drink while he is sitting, as Chazal say: It is improper for a* talmid chacham *to eat and drink while standing* (Gittin 70a; Derech Eretz Zutah, chap. 5). *It is appropriate for every person to act like a* talmid chacham *in this regard.* (Kaf Hachaim 271:64)

Furthermore, the Rambam is of the opinion that for health purposes one should always sit while eating, as it says: *One should always sit or lean on his left side, and not walk around while eating.* (Rambam, Hilchos Dei'os 4:3)

Drinking Kiddush Wine

Ideally, one who makes Kiddush needs to drink *melo lugmav*, a cheekful, which for the average person is equivalent to more than half of a *revi'is*. One does not need to drink more than that. A very large person should drink more, but it need not be more than a *revi'is*. It is preferable for all the participants to also sip from the wine, although it does not have to be a specific amount. (Shulchan Aruch 271:13; Taz 17)

The person who recites Kiddush is required to drink from the Kiddush wine so that it should not appear as if he is degrading the mitzvah. (Maharam Chalavah, Pesachim 105b)

The one who recites Kiddush is required to drink *melo lugmav*, enough to fill his cheek, of the Kiddush wine. It is insufficient to just take a sip, as is customary with all other *kosos shel brachah*. This is because Kiddush needs to be drunk with pleasure, as the *pasuk* in *Yeshayah* (58:13) states, *V'karasa laShabbos oneg*—"and you should call the Shabbos oneg." *V'karasa laShabbos* refers to reciting Kiddush, and the word *"oneg"* proves that one must have pleasure from the Kiddush. He is therefore required to drink an amount that is substantial enough to provide pleasure.

(Higayon HaShabbos, p. 333)

In Ropshitz, they were accustomed to drinking only a small amount of the Kiddush and not most of a *revi'is*. This is in accordance to the Beis Yosef who quotes the *Rishon*, Reb Mordche Yashan, that the expression *melo lugmav* is not to be taken literally, but rather, it means enough to wet his throat. It is referred to as *melo lugmav* because it also wets one's cheeks. *(Beis Yosef* 271:14)

One is required to drink *melo lugmav* in one gulp without stopping. Ideally, this should not take more than the amount of time that it takes to drink a *revi'is* (ten seconds). One should be sure that it does not take longer than *kedei achilas pras* (the time that it takes to eat half a loaf of bread in the times of the Gemara; 2-9 minutes). *(Mishnah Berurah* 271:68)

After one drinks from the Kiddush wine, the remaining wine is considered defective *(pagum)*. This defect can be repaired by pouring a small amount of wine from the bottle into the cup. The wine can now be poured slowly back into the bottle, but it should not be done all at once.
(Bach 182, s.v. *V'Haram MiRottenberg)*

Preferably, one should distribute the remaining Kiddush wine to all the participants so that they should all drink from it out of respect for the Kiddush.
(Shulchan Aruch, Orach Chaim 271:14, *Darchei Moshe* 182)

Leaving Over Kiddush

The Gemara states that one who recites Havdalah on wine on Motza'ei Shabbos merits *Olam Haba*. The Gemara further explains that this refers to one who leaves over from the Kiddush wine to use for Havdalah. *(Pesachim* 113a)

The Arizal would leave over a small amount of wine in the Kiddush cup until the morning *seudah* so that the blessing from the Kiddush should remain. *(Pri Eitz Chaim)*

Chapter 8
Hamotzi on Friday Night

Challah

Loaves of bread are often called *"challah,"* as we find many times in the Torah (e.g. *challos matzos, challos lechem chametz*). Rashi explains that *"challah"* is a term used for special bread, as it says in the laws of *hafrashas challah: The first portion of your dough, you shall separate a loaf* [challah] *for a gift* (*Bamidbar* 15:20). There are those who say that the name challah has its source from the word *"chali"* which in Aramaic means sweet, since challah is generally sweeter and of better quality than regular bread. (*V'lechem Levav Enosh Yisad*, p. 28)

The *sefarim* state that it is forbidden to *daven* for one's livelihood on Shabbos. Therefore, we call the bread that is baked in honor of Shabbos "challah" which is an acronym of the phrase from *Mishlei* (30:8): *Hatrifeini lechem chuki*—"Give me sustenance of bread."

In Hungary, they called challah, *"barches,"* taken from the word *brachah*, as a *remez* that Hashem should bless all our efforts. (*Beis Yisrael Hashaleim* 72:6)

Reb Aharon of Belz would say that challah is called *"barches"* because it stems from the word *brachos,* and Shabbos brings *brachos* for the entire week. (*Betzila Dimheimenusa*)

The reason why some call challah *"barches"* is because it is pronounced *"bar ches,"* which means "eight days old." Challah corresponds to the loaves of *Lechem Hapanim* which were eight days old when the *kohanim* ate them.
(*Rabbi Dovid Meisels*, heard in the name of elderly chassidim)

Challah is an acronym for *chazarah l'derech hatovah*, returning to the proper path, or *chazarah l'derech Hashem*, returning to the ways of Hashem. (*Yismach Libi, Mishlei* 27:18)

Challah is an acronym for *cheilek l'Olam Haba*; through performing *hafrashas challah* one merits *Olam Haba*.
(*Yalkut Yitzchak*, Mitzvah 386; *Zecher Dovid*, p. 30)

Challah is an acronym for *chanun hamarbeh l'slo'ach*, Hashem is compassionate and always forgiving.
(In the name of *tzaddikim*)

It is possible that it is called challah to remind the woman when she bakes the bread that she should not forget to separate challah. (*Eishel Avraham* 260)

The midrash states: *Reb Yochanan asked why the mitzvah of challah is written next to the prohibition of* avodah zarah (*idol worship*). *The reason is to compare these two concepts. Whoever fulfills the mitzvah of challah it is as if he abolished* avodah zarah. *Conversely, whoever neglects the mitzvah of challah, it is as if he worships* avodah zarah.

Similarly, according to the Gemara (*Shabbos* 118b), whoever observes the Shabbos meticulously is forgiven for his sins, even if he worships *avodah zarah* like the generation of Enosh.

This demonstrates the connection between the mitzvah of challah and the mitzvah of Shabbos; both challah and Shabbos are the antitheses of *avodah zarah*. (*Rabbi Dovid Meisels*)

The long loaves of bread that are used on Shabbos are customarily called *koilish*. The source for this can be found in *Rashi* on *Pesachim* 48b. The Gemara there distinguishes between round loaves and long narrow ones. The long ones are termed by the Gemara as *chechin*, which Rashi translates into old French as *koilish*. (*Pesachim* 48b)

Lechem Mishneh

According to the Magen Avraham, there is no obligation *mid'Oraisa* to eat bread on Shabbos and Yom Tov. *Lechem mishnah* is eaten only because reciting Kiddush is contingent upon eating a *seudah*. *(Magen Avraham 168:9)*

There are differing opinions as to whether *lechem mishneh* is required by Torah law *(d'Oraisa)*. The Taz writes that if one does not have enough money to purchase both wine for Kiddush and challos, *lechem mishneh* takes precedence over wine because it is *d'Oraisa*, whereas reciting Kiddush on wine is only *d'Rabbanan* (Rabbinical law). *(Taz, Hilchos Chanukah 678:2)*

A person is required to recite *Hamotzi* on two loaves of bread on Shabbos, as it says in *Shemos* (16:22) with regard to the *mann*: *They gathered a double portion of bread*, and *lechem mishneh* is in commemoration of the *mann*.
(Brachos 39b; Shabbos 117b)

We recite *Hamotzi* over two loaves of bread to commemorate the *mann* of which a double portion fell on Friday for Shabbos. We should also contemplate the miracles of the *mann*. The *pasuk* in *Tehillim* (111:4) states: *He commemorated His wonders; Hashem is gracious and merciful.* The Metzudas Dovid explains that this commemoration refers to the *mann*, as Hashem commanded the Jews to put away a jug of *mann* to be preserved for generations.

The Metzudas Dovid further explains that because Hashem is gracious and merciful, He told us to commemorate the miracles of the *mann*. Thinking about the miracles that Hashem performed for us will lead us to be grateful to Him, which will earn us a reward. *(Rabbi Dovid Meisels)*

The two loaves of *lechem mishnah* correspond to the *Lechem Hapanim* that were baked on Erev Shabbos, placed on the *Shulchan* in two columns, and eaten the following Shabbos in the Beis Hamikdash. *(Pardes Hamelech)*

Shabbos is the day during which we strengthen our *emunah*. There are two aspects of *emunah*: One, which was handed down to us through *mesorah*, is *emunah* in *Yetzias Mitzrayim*. The other aspect of *emunah* is belief in the creation of the world, which can be recognized through reasoning and contemplating the wonders of Hashem. *Lechem mishneh* alludes to the fact that we should strengthen ourselves in both aspects of *emunah*. (Menachem Tzion, Bo)

In *Birchas Rosh Chodesh*, we *daven* that *Hashem* should send us *parnassah* and *chalkalah*, livelihood and sustenance. *Parnassah* refers to a person's own livelihood; *chalkalah* refers to his ability to give to others. Every person should *daven* for livelihood for himself and his family, and also that Hashem should provide him with enough that he should be able to sustain others, including impoverished *talmidei chachamim*.

Even if one's own sustenance is minimal, he is still required to give a part of what he has to the poor. The *pasuk* in *Yeshayah* (58:7) states, *Break your bread for the hungry*. This means that even if your bread is meager, you should still break off some and give it to the poor.

It is well known that Shabbos provides sustenance. It is said in the name for Reb Yaakov of Dinov that *kavod Shabbos* is an acronym for *kol birchain dileiala v'sata b'yuma shviah talyin*—"All *brachos* from the upper and lower worlds are dependent on Shabbos." Therefore, we recite *Hamotzi* on two whole loaves of bread. One loaf represents the livelihood that one should be blessed with in order to provide for his own needs, and the other represents the livelihood from which he will be able to give to others. The loaves are whole, alluding to the fact that we should have enough for ourselves, and not need to break off a piece of what we need for ourselves in order to give to others.

Another reason we recite *Hamotzi* on *lechem mishneh* is that during the week, we eat in order to have strength to serve

Hashem. On Shabbos, we also need to have in mind to fulfill the mitzvah of eating *seudas Shabbos*. *(Sova Semachos, Tazria)*

Shabbos was given for learning Torah. On Shabbos, a person is obligated to learn more Torah than he does during the week because on this day he has no work obligations. Bread can allude to Torah, as the *pasuk* says: Come, partake of my bread (*Mishlei* 9:5); the word "bread" refers to Torah. The two loaves of bread used for *lechem mishneh* teach us that on Shabbos, one needs to learn double the amount that he learns during the week. *(Mekor Chaim 274:1)*

The word *mishneh* is comprised of the same letters as *neshamah* (soul). By eating Shabbos food, one elevates his *neshamah*. *Tzaddikim* had the ability to elevate all the *neshamos* that were *megulgal* in their food.
(Gedulas Mordechai, Shabbos, p. 279)

We recite *Hamotzi* on two loaves of bread to symbolize that Shabbos contains a double blessing. This concept can be explained by understanding the partnership between Yissachar and Zevulun. Zevulun used to support Yissachar so that he could learn Torah. Yissachar then received a double blessing—one for himself and one that was transferred back to Zevulun. Similarly, the blessing of Shabbos is twofold. It receives a blessing for itself and it also influences the other days of the week. *(Sfas Emes, Vayechi 5653, s.v. B'inyan)*

Shape of the Challos

There are those, including the chassidim of Sanz, Kaminka, and Belz, who are accustomed to eating braided challos only at the day *seudah*. At the night *seudah*, they eat plain loaves that are not braided. *(Magen Avos, p. 202; Ish Chassid, p. 43)*

Harav Moshe Aryeh Freund, the Rav of Yerushalayim, would use a plain challah, which had no form and was not braided, for the Friday night *seudah*. For the day *seudah* he used a braided challah, and for *shalosh seudos* he used a challah that was comprised of 12 small challos baked together.

At night, he used the challah that was prepared for the day to complete the *lechem mishneh*. At the day meal, he used the challah that was prepared for *shalosh seudos* to complete his *lechem mishneh*. (*Zemiros Ateres Yehoshua*, p. 89)

At the night *seudah*, some recite *Hamotzi* on a plain challah, and during the day they use a braided challah. On Yom Tov, no distinction is made between the challos eaten at night and during the day. Although there are other deeper reasons for this, following is a halachic explanation:

The *Shulchan Aruch* (*Orach Chaim* 274:1) states that one should recite *Hamotzi* on two whole loaves of bread. For Kabbalistic reasons, on Friday night one should cut the bottom loaf, but on Shabbos day or Yom Tov night, he should cut the top loaf.

The Bach finds this difficult to understand, because by cutting the bottom challah on Friday night, it seems as if one is passing over a mitzvah, and if a mitzvah comes to a person he is not allowed to let it pass. Since the top challah is closer, one would think that he is required to cut the top challah and not pass it over in favor of the bottom one.

It seems that reciting *Hamotzi* over a braided and plain challah together resolves this difficulty. Generally, the better dishes are reserved for the day *seudah* since the honor of Shabbos day is greater than that of the night. Therefore, if a person puts the braided challah on top and has in mind to reserve it for the day *seudah*, it is not considered passing over a mitzvah if he uses the bottom challah.

On Yom Tov, the reason to use the bottom challah does not apply. We recite *Hamotzi* on the top challah and do not differentiate between the challos.

(*She'eilos Uteshuvos Kapei Aharon*, sec. 22)

The *Zohar* states that the three *seudos* correspond to the three *Avos*. On Sukkos, although there is an *ushpiza* for every day, Avraham is represented on all the days. So too, although the night *seudah* corresponds to Avraham Avinu and the day *seudos* correspond to Yitzchak and Yaakov respectively, Avraham Avinu is represented at all three *seudos*. Since the Friday night *seudah* corresponds only to Avraham Avinu, we recite *Hamotzi* on a plain loaf. At the day *seudos,* we use a braided loaf, comprised of a few strands, to hint that Avraham Avinu is also included.

(Ul'asher Amar, Hanispach Sefer Otzar HaShabbos)

One of the chassidim of the Yitev Lev married off a daughter. On Friday night, he told his new son-in-law that that they are accustomed to reciting *Hamotzi* on a plain challah on Friday night and a braided challah at the day *seudah*. The son-in-law replied that they should do the opposite. The chassid repeated his *minhag,* but again the son-in-law insisted that they do the opposite.

When the chassid repeated the incident to his Rebbe, the Yitev Lev advised him that since the son-in-law was deriding a *minhag,* his daughter should divorce him, as he will end up leaving Judaism. The chassid followed the Rebbe's advice and they divorced. Indeed, the young man ended up converting to a different religion. *(Siach Zekeinim, vol. 6, p. 40)*

It is a *minhag* to bake braided challos, each comprised of six strands, so that the two challos together total 12 strands, corresponding to the 12 *Lechem Hapanim*. *(Ketzei Hamateh)*

In Poland, Bohemia, and Moravia, they would bake braided challos. It seems that the reason for this was that they baked meat in the same oven together with the challos, rendering the bread *fleishig*. One is not allowed to use bread that is *fleishig* unless he changes its shape to make it recognizable, so they would braid the challos as a *siman*. *(Mekor Chaim, sec. 274)*

Some *tzaddikim* have a *minhag* to use challos that are each comprised of six small challos joined together, totaling 12 small challos. This *minhag* is based on the words of the Raya Mihemna that *lechem mishneh* alludes to the two *luchos* that were given on Shabbos. The *pasuk* states (*Shemos* 32:15), **mizeh umizeh heim Kesuvim**, and the word *zeh* has the numerical value of 12.

Also, the *luchos* themselves consisted of 12 parts—two tablets that had 10 commandments written on them.

(*Dvar Tzvi Shabbos*, sec. 125)

Preferably, the challos should be long, shaped like the letter *vav*, to complete the Name of Hashem of *yud*, *keh*, *vav*, *keh* known as the *Shem Havayah*. The cut in the challah is in the form of the letter *yud*, the five fingers in each hand that hold the bread are the two *hehs*, and the challah itself is in the shape of a *vav*, thus the Name of Hashem is formed when one cuts the challah.

The *Shem Havayah* symbolizes compassion, while Rosh Hashanah and Yom Kippur are times of *din*, justice. It seems that we eat round challos instead of long ones on Rosh Hashanah and Erev Yom Kippur because it is not the proper time to allude to Hashem's attribute of compassion.

(*Elyah Rabbah* 167; *Divrei Tzaddikim* 8:8)

It is said in the name of the Ropshitzer Rav that after the *Churban*, the *Anshei Knesses Hagedolah* instituted that one should bake two challos for Shabbos in the form of *vavs*, which have the numerical value of six. This alludes to the mystical secrets of the *Lechem Hapanim*, which were two sets of six challos. Even if one does not understand these secrets, if he bakes two challos in the form of *vavs*, it is as if he had them in mind.

This may reflect the meaning of the words in the song, *Azamer B'shvachin*: *Shechinta tistatar beshis nahamei listar,* when the Beis Hamikdash stood there were six challos on each side; *b'vavin tiskatar*, but after the *Churban* we have two challos, each in the form of a *vav*.

(*Chemdah Genuzah*, vol. 2, p. 26; *Magen Avos*, p. 201)

On the *pasuk, challah tarumu laHashem* (*Bamidbar* 15:20), Rashi defines challah as *tortel*, a round, appealing bread.

(See *She'eilos Uteshuvos Maharshal*, sec. 58)

Some opinions hold, as the Even Ezra explains, that the root of the word "challah" can mean round (*Vayikra* 2:4). Therefore, some Sephardim have the custom to bake round challos for every Shabbos. (*Yafeh L'lev*, vol. 2 242:2)

Aside from on Rosh Hashanah, when round challos are baked, challos used on Shabbos and Yom Tov are not round. The *pasuk* describes the *mann* as *k'zera gad*, and Rashi explains this to mean that the *mann* was round. It is interesting that we do not find that one should bake round challos in commemoration of the shape of the *mann*. (*Toras Shabbos* 274:2)

The *pasuk* (*Shemos* 16:5) says about the *mann* on Erev Shabbos, *v'hayah mishneh*—"and it was double." The Mechilta defines this phrase as *lechem meshunah*, different bread, because on every day of the week one *omer* fell, but on Friday a larger portion of *mann* consisting of two *omer* fell. Every day the *mann* had a good fragrance, but on Shabbos it was even better. Every day of the week the *mann* shone like gold, but on Shabbos it shone even more (*Mechilta, Parshas Vayisa, parshah* 2).

This Mechilta is the source for the *minhag* that the challos for Shabbos are baked with a special form and should have a special taste. It is possible that originally a different form was used for all Yamim Tovim, so that the challos on Shabbos would have a unique form, but over time round challos came to be used only for the Yamim Nora'im, and there is no special form used for the other Yamim Tovim.

(*She'eilos Uteshuvos Chemdas Tzvi*, vol. 3, 10:2)

The Elyah Rabbah states that there are those who bake three challos in three different sizes. At the night *seudah* they eat the medium challah, at the day *seudah* they eat the large one, and at *shalosh seudos* they eat the small one. However, the Kaf Hachaim states that he has not seen this *minhag* mentioned in the words of the Arizal, nor seen anyone who follows this *minhag*. *(Elyah Rabbah* 242:10; *Kaf Hachaim* 242:28)

Twelve Challos

The Ba'al Degel Machaneh Ephraim had a manuscript written by the Ba'al Shem Tov in which he wrote at length about using 12 challos on Shabbos. One of the reasons written was that the 12 challos correspond to the 12 *nevi'im* of the *Trei Asar*. Other *nevi'im* have their names immortalized by the name of their *sefer* (e.g. *Yechezkel, Yirmiyah*), but the 12 *nevi'im* of *Trei Asar* have no complete *sefarim* bearing their names. Therefore, to ensure that their names are mentioned, we take 12 challos, corresponding to their 12 names. Indeed, the Arizal would call the 12 challos by the names of the *Trei Asar*.

(Peninim V'avnei Cheifetz, Beshalach, p. 67)

There are those who bake a *"shtreimel* challah," a challah comprised of 13 small challos, the same number as the parts of a *shtreimel*. (*Shtreimlach* used to be made of 13 pieces of fur.)

(Sefer Kehillah)

The Lelover Rebbe was accustomed to using a challah that consisted of 12 small challos. The Rebbe instructed that the small challos be placed in six rows. In the first row, there was one challah, in the second row two challos, and in the third row three challos. The fourth row also contained three challos, the fifth row had two challos, and the sixth row one challah. A strand of dough was placed over the entire challah. Thus, the challos formed the shape of two triangles or two *segols* (one of the Hebrew vowels). The significance of two *segols* is mentioned in the *Zohar*. *(Zemiros Minhagei Lelov, Seder Leil Shabbos)*

Rabbi Elimelech of Tosh said that as soon as he began using 12 challos at his Shabbos *seudah,* no inhabitant of his city was lacking bread; as soon he began reciting Kiddush on whiskey on Shabbos day, there were no fires in the city; and when he began donning a white *bekeshe,* no son died during the lifetime of his father. *(Siach Zekeinim,* vol. 7, p. 346)

Loaves of Equal Size

The two loaves of challah used for *lechem mishneh* should be large in honor of Shabbos and similar in size. Those who are accustomed to using 12 challos should also bake them equal in size, specifically the challos that are used for *lechem mishneh.* This is because, according to the Arizal, one should hold the two challah loaves together while reciting *Hamotzi* so that they appear to be like one loaf of bread with two "faces," like the *Lechem Hapanim.* The challos can only appear like one loaf if they are the same size.

Another reason for baking the challos equal in size is that *Lechem mishneh* commemorates the *mann,* and the two portions that came down in the *midbar* on Erev Shabbos were equal. *(Pesach Hadvir* 274:6:4)

Different Types of Bread

The Kaf Hachaim states that Reb Eliyahu Chazzan advised him that one should eat various types of breads at the Shabbos *seudos.* At the Friday night *seudah,* a type of bread known as pitas are eaten. By Shabbos day, one should use wide loaves called *panis*, and at *shalosh seudos* a third type of bread called *subados* should be used. At *melaveh malkah,* biscuits *(rishas* or *ruskas)* are eaten, upon which one recites *Mezonos.* This is an old custom that was instituted so that all types of bread should become blessed with the holiness of Shabbos, and thus effect plentiful sustenance during the week. *(Kaf Hachaim* 36:45)

Topping the Challah

Belzer chassidim were careful not to sprinkle the challah with poppy seeds. It seems that the reason for this was because they suspected that the seeds might be infested with worms.

(Peninei Minhag)

Appealing, Tasty Challos

The *Yerushalmi* asks: If, for a *korban,* one has a choice between a fat animal and an animal with a nice appearance, which one should he use? It is better to use the fat animal because taste takes precedence over appearance. Similarly, one recites a *brachah* on bread that is baked with fine flour even if one has a roll that is made from coarse flour that is whole or has a nicer appearance.

Generally, there is an obligation to enhance the appearance of a mitzvah. However, the Bnei Yissaschar writes that regarding food that is consumed for a mitzvah, there is no advantage in enhancing its appearance. This is because food provides our bodies with pleasure, and if one enhances the appearance of a mitzvah food, it will seem like he is enhancing it for his physical pleasure, rather than for the sake of the mitzvah. Therefore, one should concern himself more with the taste of the challah than its appearance.

(Nimukei Orach Chaim 795:5)

The Rebbe of Zvolin would say, "A nice challah for Shabbos is equally important to me as a beautiful *esrog* on Sukkos." His son, the Ba'al Divrei Yisrael, added, "A *kezayis* of challah on Shabbos is as dear to me as a *kezayis* of matzah on Pesach night." *(Ma'amar Yechezkel, Kuzmir, vol. 2, p. 182)*

Setting the Challos on the Table

Some have the custom to place the challos on the table horizontally; others place them vertically, so that the challos appear like two *vavs*. Though there are several opinions, in practice, one should place them vertically.

The Arizal states that the bottoms of the challos should be placed against each other so that it appears to be like one challah with two "faces," similar to the *Lechem Hapanim*. This only holds true if the challos are placed on the table vertically. (*Likutei Maharich*, vol. 2, p. 36)

Some place the challos with their "faces" facing each other. This is because the challos correspond to the two *luchos*, and the *pasuk* states that at *Kabbalas HaTorah* Hashem spoke to the Jews face-to-face, so to speak. (*Mekor Chaim* 274)

If using 12 challos, one should place them on the table in the following manner: The two large challos in the middle—the braided challah on the right and the plain one on the left. Under each of these he should place a small round challah. He should put two small round challos to the right of the braided challah and two small round challos to the left of the plain challah. On each of the four round challos he should place a small long challah. (*Magen Avos*, p. 201)

Reb Aharon of Belz instructed his attendant to place the challos on the table as follows: First, the four large challos should be placed on the table. The challah which is being used for the night *seudah* should be at the right of the person reciting *Hamotzi,,* and the braided challah which will be used for the day *seudah* should be on his left. The challah which will be used for *shalosh seudos* should be beside the braided challah that will be used for the day *seudah*. The second challah which will be used for *lechem mishneh* for *shalosh seudos* should be placed to the right of the challah that will be used at night. This totals four challos. Afterwards, two more challos should be placed next to each of these four challos, totaling 12 challos. (*Kuntris Dibburei Kodesh*)

Covering the Challos

The *Tur* cites three reasons for covering the challos: The first is because the challah should be brought to the table after the Shabbos has been sanctified by reciting Kiddush. Uncovering challos after Kiddush has the same effect as bringing them later. Another reason is so that the bread should not be offended that we recite the *brachah* on the wine first, although we usually recite the *brachah* on bread first. Lastly, it is a remembrance of the *mann*, which was covered with dew above and below it. *(Tur 271)*

Reb Aharon of Belz said that one should use a special cover for the challos that is specifically designated for this purpose, and it should be used each Shabbos.

(Kuntris Dibburei Kodesh, p. 54)

Marking the Challah

Those who are scrupulous mark the challah by making a small cut with the knife prior to reciting *Hamotzi*. This is done in order to decrease the amount of time that elapses between reciting *Hamotzi* and eating the challah, because once the bread is marked, one does not need to spend time finding the right spot at which to cut it.

(Magen Avraham 274:1; Machatzis Hashekel)

Marking the challah prior to cutting it has deep mystical reasons; one should not deviate from this *minhag*. *(Yad Yosef)*

There are those who do not mark the challah prior to reciting *Hamotzi*. The basis is for this is a *Yerushalmi* *(Brachos 39b)* which states that one should not cut the bread until after he recites *Hamotzi*, because the halachah states that if one cuts bread prior to reciting a *brachah* then the *brachah* rests only on the piece that was cut. If that piece is lost, a new *brachah* is necessary. According to some opinions, in order not to enter into unnecessary complications, one should not mark the challah at all. *(Tzlach, Brachos 39a)*

The Shulchan Harav does not mention marking the challah. However, the general *minhag* is to mark the challah prior to reciting *Hamotzi*.

The Tzemach Tzedek once discussed a certain topic about which he felt it was unnecessary for one to be stringent. He remarked that being stringent with the topic under discussion when it is unnecessary is similar to one who searches for the mark he etched into the challah. The chassidim understood this to mean that even if one makes a mark on the challah, if he does not see it immediately after reciting the *brachah*, he does not need to search for it in order to cut at that specific spot. *(Ketzos Hashulchan 82:8)*

Prior to *Hamotzi* one should mark the challah in the third that is closest to him. One should mark it from left to right, diagonally towards oneself. One should also mark the bottom of the challah. *(Magen Avos, p. 205)*

The Gemara states that one should mark the bread to cut it at the spot where it is well baked, so that the *brachah* should be recited on the choicest spot of the bread. One should mark the bread from the bottom upwards.
(Shulchan Aruch 177:1; Rabbeinu Bacheye, Shulchan Shel Arba, p. 469)

In many areas, we find that we separate *reishis*, the first of something, for Hashem, such as *bikurim*, challah, and *terumah*. So too, we designate for Hashem the first slice of challah that we cut, by reciting the *brachah* on it. Therefore, just as *bikurim* needs to be from the first-ripened fruit, the slice of challah that gets designated for Hashem should be cut from the spot of the challah that was baked first (i.e. the most well-baked spot). *(Toras Chaim Sanhedrin 102b, s.v. Amar leih)*

Holding the Challah

One should hold the challah in his hands prior to reciting the *brachah* in order to minimize the amount of time that elapses between reciting the *brachah* and eating the bread. Another reason is so that it should be apparent that he is reciting the *brachah* over the challah. (*Beis Yosef*, in the name of the Rokeach and the Levush)

One should hold the challah in his hands while reciting the *brachah*. When saying the word *Hamotzi*, he should raise the challos slightly. (*Sha'ar Hamitzvos L'Arizal, Parshas Eikev*, p.40a)

With Ten Fingers

One should hold the bread with all 10 fingers while reciting the *brachah*. The 10 fingers correspond to the 10 tithes that are separated for Hashem: *bikurim, leket, shichechah, pe'ah, terumah, ma'aser rishon, ma'aser ani, challas ha'ohr, challas hakohen*, and the slice upon which one recites *Hamotzi*, which is designated for the sake of a mitzvah for Hashem.

(*Toras Chaim Sanhedrin* 102b, s.v. *Amar leih*)

Ten fingers correspond to the 10 words in the *brachah* of *Hamotzi*. They also correspond to the 10 words in the following *pesukim* about Hashem providing sustenance:

Matzmiach chatzir labeheimah, v'eisev la'avodas ha'adam l'hotzi lechem min ha'aretz—"Hashem causes grass to sprout for the animals and vegetation for the work of man, to bring forth bread from the earth" (*Tehillim* 104:14).

Einei chol eilecha yisabeiru, v'Atah nosen lahem es achlam b'ito—"Everyone's eyes look to You [Hashem] with hope, and You give them their food in its time" (ibid. 145:15).

Eretz chitah use'orah v'gefen use'einah v'rimon, eretz zeis shemen udevash—"A land of wheat and barley, vines and figs and pomegranates, a land of oil-producing olives and honey" (*Devarim* 8:8).

V'yiten lecha haElokim mital hashamayim umishmanei ha'aretz, v'rov dagan v'sirosh—"And may Hashem give you of the dew of the heavens and [of] the fatness of the earth and an abundance of grain and wine" *(Bereishis* 27:28).

The 10 fingers also correspond to the 10 steps of the process of creating a loaf of bread, from when the wheat is sown until it is baked: sowing, reaping, gathering, threshing, winnowing, selecting, grinding, sifting, kneading and baking.

(Rokeach, sec. 229; *Beis Menuchah*, p. 52b)

A Whole Loaf

The loaf of bread needs to be whole while reciting the *brachah*. This is because the table at which a person eats is compared to the *Mizbe'ach*, which symbolized completeness. All aspects of the *Mizbe'ach* were required to be complete and flawless. It was built with whole, uncut stones; the *korbanos* had no blemishes; and it was mandatory that the *kohen* himself have no defect. Since the bread eaten at the *seudos* on Shabbos is the main part of the *seudah* and comparable to the *korban*, the loaves upon which *Hamotzi* is recited need to be whole. Also, the knife should be smooth, similar to the knife used for a *korban*.

(Toras Chaim; Sanhedrin 102b, s.v. *Amar leih*; *Magen Avos*, p. 205)

Reciting the Brachah

The *pasuk* states: *The earth is Hashem's, and everything in it* (Tehillim 24:1). A different *pasuk* states: *The Heavens are for Hashem, but the earth was given to mankind* (ibid. 115:16). The Gemara in *Brachos* (35a) points out that there seems to be a contradiction in these two *pesukim*—does the world belong to Hashem or was it given to mankind?

The Gemara explains that the first *pasuk* is speaking of when a person has not yet recited a *brachah*. The second *pasuk* refers to after he has recited a *brachah*. The commentaries explain that by reciting a *brachah*, one acquires everything that is in the Heavens and earth from Hashem. If so, how can one recite *brachos* and eat on Shabbos if the act of acquiring is forbidden on Shabbos?

The halachah states that for the sake of a mitzvah, one is permitted to make an acquisition on Shabbos or Yom Tov (for example, one is allowed to take ownership of a *lulav* and *esrog* on Sukkos). Since eating and drinking on Shabbos is a mitzvah, acquiring the food is permissible.

Another reason that this is permitted is that there is a principle that when the fulfillment of a *mitzvas asei* requires transgressing a negative commandment, one may do so. In this case, the positive commandment of eating on Shabbos overrides the prohibition of making an acquisition on Shabbos. *(Nefesh Yeseirah, Ma'areches Shin, sec. 28)*

When one recites *Hamotzi*, he should take the two upper challos from the four middle ones and hold them together with both hands. The two bottoms of the challos should be connected so that it appears to be like one challah with two faces, one on the right and one on the left, similar to the *Lechem Hapanim* in the Beis Hamikdash.

(Sha'ar Hakavanos, Inyan Hashulchan)

The Arizal writes that when saying the word "*hamotzi*" one should stress the letter *heh* and pause between *ha* and *motzi*.

(Sha'ar Hamitzvos 54a, see there for further explanation)

Every food contains some spiritual components that give the food its existence. The Rambam writes that a person receives his sustenance from the spiritual components of the food, and an animal receives his sustenance from its physical components. This is alluded to in the *pasuk* in *Devarim* (8:3): *Lo al halechem livad yichyeh ha'adam*—"a person is not sustained by food itself"; *ki al kol motza pi Hashem yichyeh ha'adam*—"rather by the word of Hashem," i.e. the spiritual components of the food, that constantly give the food its existence.

Shabbos Secrets • *Hamotzi on Friday Night*

The Ba'al Shem Tov says that by reciting *Hamotzi*, one is *motzi*, he draws out, the spiritual components of the food from the *aretz*, its physical components.

(Kitzur Shulchan Aruch Im Sippurim Chassidi'im, p. 242)

When the Maggid of Mezritch would recite *Hamotzi* on Friday night, those present were able to see the fiery letters of the *brachah* emanate from his mouth. After the Maggid's passing, his chassidim traveled to many *tzaddikim* but did not witness this phenomenon anywhere else. When they visited the Chozeh of Lublin, the Chozeh sensed their mission, and after reciting *Hamotzi*, he exclaimed with wonder, "*Ososeinu lo ra'inu ein od navi*—'We did not see the signs, we have no *navi* left' *(Tehillim* 74:9)." This can be interpreted homiletically to mean: "Even if you don't see *ososeinu* (the letters—from the word *os*) [emanate from a *tzaddik*'s mouth], does that mean we have no *tzaddikim*?" *(Nifla'os HaRebbi M'Lublin*, sec. 188)

The Chozeh of Lublin once said, "A *brachah* of *Hamotzi* recited properly is better than a *bilkele* (roll)," meaning that a *brachah* of *Hamotzi* recited properly provides more pleasure than the food itself. *(Kedushas Tzion, Parshas Emor*, s.v. *V'hikravtem)*

Some are of the opinion that one can only fulfill the obligation of *lechem mishneh* through another person if he hears the *brachah* from him. He also needs to have in mind to fulfill his obligation [by hearing the other's recitation], and the person who recites the *brachah* needs to have in mind to exempt [the listener] from his obligation by saying the *brachah* for him]. One must also eat from the challah of the person who recited the *brachah*. *(Shulchan Aruch Harav* 274:4)

There are those who hold that even if one did not hear the *brachah* being recited, as long as one eats from the bread upon which *Hamotzi* was recited, he has fulfilled the requirement of *lechem mishneh*. This is because the obligation of *lechem mishneh* means to begin the *seudah* with *lechem mishneh*. When the host recites *Hamotzi*, that is the time that the *seudah*

begins for all those eating at his table, and the host acts as their emissary.
(*Eishel Avraham Butchatch; Likutei Maharich, Seder Seudas Leil Shabbos*)

One who eats in order to strengthen his body so that he is able to serve Hashem is performing a mitzvah by eating. This is hinted to in the letters of the word *ma'achal* (food), which are *mem, aleph, chaf,* and *lamed*, and are the same letters as in the word *malach* (angel). We can understand the meaning of the *brachah* of *Hamotzi* in this way: *Hamotzi lechem,* one can draw out the bread; *min ha'aretz,* from its physicality. By reciting the *brachah,* one can generate spirituality from the bread. By doing a mitzvah with a *ma'achal,* it becomes like a *malach*—entirely spiritual. (*Tzemach Tzedek*)

Lechem, bread, contains the same letters as the word *chamal,* compassion. If a Jew has compassion on another and gives him food, it arouses compassion in Heaven. This is the reason why Hashem created us with a need to eat—so that we should have the opportunity to give to others and bring Hashem's compassion upon ourselves.

This can be understood from the *brachah* of *Hamotzi*: *Hamotzi lechem*—Jews have the ability to draw out compassion, *min ha'aretz*—through our acts of kindness performed with physical, earthly food. (*Divrei Binah, Shiras HaShabbos,* p. 629)

Removing the Challah Cover

One should not remove the challah cover, but rather take out the challah from underneath it, similar to the *mann* that was removed from under the dew. This is done by *tzaddikim* and *gedolei Torah*. (*Likutei Maharich* vol. 2; *Darkei Chaim Sanz*)

Holding the Challah While Cutting It

The *Tur* states that a person should hold both challah loaves in his hands while cutting one of them (sec. 274). The Arizal seems to have a similar opinion. The Shulchan Aruch Harav, however, states that it is sufficient to hold both challos only during the recitation of *Hamotzi* and not while cutting.

(*Shulchan Aruch Harav* 274:2)

The Sanzer Rav would hold both challah loaves while cutting them. However, his son, the Shiniver Rav, did not follow this custom because, according to Rashi on the Gemara (*Shabbos* 117b), it seems that one is only required to hold both loaves in his hands during *Hamotzi*.

Some are of the opinion that if the two challos are touching each other there is no need to actually hold them while cutting. (*Darchei Chaim, Nimukei Orach Chaim* 274:1)

Cutting One or Both Challos

The Gemara relates that the *Amora* Rav Kahana held both challos in his hands while reciting *Hamotzi,* but then cut only one. He explained that we learn the obligation of *lechem mishneh* from what the *pasuk* (*Shemos* 16:22) states regarding the *mann*, that they gathered *lechem mishneh*. The root word *leket*, gathering, refers to gathering by hand, which teaches us that the challos used for *lechem mishneh* should also be held in one's hands. However, in the *pasuk* there is no allusion to *lechem mishneh* with regard to cutting the challah, so one does not need to cut both challos.

In practice, the *poskim* are divided in their opinions of whether a person is required to cut one or both challos. The Shulchan Aruch Harav holds that one only needs to cut one challah, and that it should be the one on his right side.

(*Shulchan Aruch Harav* 274:2; *Aruch Hashulchan* ibid.:3)

The *Shulchan Aruch* writes that one should recite *Hamotzi* on two whole challos. He should hold them both in his hands and cut open the bottom one. The Rema writes that this refers to Friday night, but on Shabbos day or Yom Tov one should cut the top challah. The reason for this is according to Kabbalah.

There are those recite *Hamotzi*, then take the top challah, put it beneath the other challah and cut it.
(Shulchan Aruch, Orach Chaim 274:1; Magen Avraham 274:1)

The *Shulchan Aruch* states that on Friday night, one should cut open the bottom challah. The *Sefer Darkei Chaim V'shalom* writes in the name of the Arizal that the Friday night *seudah* corresponds to Yitzchak Avinu. The Shabbos day *seudah* corresponds to Avraham Avinu. It is not fitting to place the challah of Yitzchak Avinu on top of the challah of Avraham Avinu, so on Friday night we cut the bottom challah.
(Kisvei Shir, p. 33)

There is a widespread custom for the person reciting *Hamotzi* to place the bottom challah closer to him. In this way, he avoids passing over a mitzvah when cutting the bottom challah. *(Taz ibid.:1; Elyah Rabbah 105)*

Slicing the Challah

After reciting Hamotzi, one should remove the challah cover from the challos and switch the left challah to his right hand and the right challah to his left hand. He should then cut the challah at the spot where it was marked, while the challos are touching each other and their two bottoms are connected.
(Magen Avos, p. 207)

Reb Avraham of Trisk would first cut into the bottom third of the challah at the Friday night *seudah*, he would begin cutting the top third of the challah at the day *seudah*, and at *shalosh seudos* he would begin cutting into the middle of the challah. *(Imrei Ya'i V'gadya Ya'i, p. 15)*

One should cut a large slice of challah that will be enough for him to eat throughout the entire *seudah*. Although during the week this would appear gluttonous, on Shabbos it is not. Since the person does not eat a large amount during the week, he demonstrates that he is doing so solely in the honor of Shabbos, out of love for the mitzvah.

(Tur and *Shulchan Aruch, Orach Chaim* 274)

According to Kabbalah, a man should cut a *kezayis* of challah for himself and a *kebeitzah* (a larger amount) for his wife.

The Gemara states that a person should always be careful with the honor of his wife because blessing is found in a person's home only in the merit of his wife *(Bava Metzia* 59a), as the *pasuk* in *Bereishis* (12:27) states regarding Avraham Avinu: *And he [Pharaoh] benefited Avram for her [Sarah's] sake.* With this we can understand the words of Rava who said that a person should honor his wife in order to become wealthy.

We also find in the words of the Rambam that one should honor his wife more than himself. Since bread is an important item, one should honor his wife with a large slice of challah.

(Yafeh L'lev 274:2)

There are those who cut a large slice of challah for themselves, but are not particular to do so for the members of their family, and there are those who cut larger slices of challah for the members of their family than for themselves.

The chassidim of Ropshitz used to cut a separate slice of challah for each person in the family, even if they were not present, and even after they got married.

(Zara Kaddisha Linsk, p. 233; *Magen Avos,* p. 213)

One should cut the slice of *Hamotzi* into several parts, corresponding to the number of people called up to the Torah on that day. On Shabbos, he should cut the slice into seven pieces; on Yom Tov, five pieces; on Rosh Chodesh and Chol Hamoed, four pieces; and during the week and on Shabbos by Minchah, it should be cut into three pieces.

(Elyah Rabbah, Orach Chaim 167:2)

One should cut the slice of *Hamotzi* into seven parts because the challah gives sustenance for the seven days of the week.
(Bikurei Tzion, p. 72)

The Kedushas Tzion of Bobov would put the slice of bread in his mouth but would not chew it until he cut a slice for his wife. His son, Reb Shlomo of Bobov, was at first accustomed to cutting a slice for his wife prior to eating his own slice. Later, he changed his custom and he would take a small amount of bread into his mouth and chew it and then cut a slice for his wife while the first bite of challah was still in his mouth, but he had not yet swallowed it. *(Magen Avos, pgs. 211–212)*

There are those who cut the challah for their family only after they eat a *kezayis*. *(Darchei Chaim V'shalom, sec. 393)*

Distributing the Challah

The one who recites *Hamotzi* should immediately eat a small amount of challah and then cut more slices and distribute challah to all those at the table. He should not pause between reciting the *brachah* and eating the challah.

The Arizal seems to be in agreement of this view *(Sha'ar Hakavanos)*. *(Taz 167:15; Magen Avraham 167:34)*

There are those who are accustomed to distributing the challah to their family prior to eating their own slice of challah. The Sanzer Rav remarked to his nephew, the Bobover Rebbe, that according to Kabbalah one should cut a slice of challah for his wife before partaking of his own challah.
(Siddur Ya'avetz; Siddur Kesser Nehora; Zemiros Divrei Yoel)

There are those who place a slice of challah on the table in front of each person. The host should not place the challah into people's hands, as that is the custom of mourners.
(Shulchan Aruch, Orach Chaim 167:18; Elyah Rabbah ibid.:24)

Many *talmidim* of the Ba'al Shem Tov did not follow this custom and did place challah into the hands of those present. This is because this *minhag* is only found from the time period of the Rambam and is not found in the words of *Chazal* or the Arizal. *(Nimukei Orach Chaim* 167:18)

One should not toss bread, even if it will not be ruined, as doing so degrades the bread and it appears as if he is rejecting the good that Hashem bestows upon the world.
(Shulchan Aruch, Orach Chaim 171:1; *Magen Avraham* 171:1)

However, many *gedolim* would toss the challah slices to reach those who sat too far, since they were particular not to place the challah into another person's hand (as it is stated in the *Shulchan Aruch* to be the custom of mourners—see above). They were of the opinion that in this case, tossing the bread is not degrading to the bread, since the Magen Avraham writes that if one tosses the bread for another person's benefit there is no concern of degrading food.

The Ksav Sofer was accustomed to tossing the challah to those sitting at his table. His son, Rabbi Shimon Sofer, was puzzled by this custom since the halachah states that one should not throw food, particularly bread.

However, Rabbi Shimon found support for his father's *minhag* in the words of the *Sefer Toras Chaim,* that one's table is comparable to the *Mizbe'ach* (*Sanhedrin* 102b, s.v. *Amar leih*). The *Sefer Hisorerus Teshuvah* writes that, accordingly, the food atones for our sins just like *korbanos*. The slice of *Hamotzi* corresponds to the fats of the *korban* that were designated for Hashem and burned on the *Mizbe'ach*. There was a mitzvah to toss these fats onto the *Mizbe'ach* (*Rambam, Hilchos Beis Habechirah* 2:13). Therefore, tossing the bread does not degrade it, but rather honors it since it is being treated like the fats of a *korban*.
(She'eilos Uteshuvos Hisorerus Teshuvah, vol. 1, 132)

One needs to clarify this matter, as the Magen Avraham states that tossing bread is forbidden (167:38).

(She'eilos Uteshuvos Mishnas Yaakov)

Dipping the Challah into Salt

It is a mitzvah to bring salt to the table prior to reciting *Hamotzi*. This is because the table at which one eats is compared to the *Mizbe'ach*, and the food he eats is like a *korban*. Since every *korban* was sacrificed with salt, we dip the challah into the salt. This protects a person from harm.

(Shulchan Aruch, Orach Chaim, Rema 167:5)

The Tosafos writes that Rabbi Menachem was extremely careful to bring salt to the table when eating a meal with bread (*Brachos* 40a).

The midrash states that since people are not performing any mitzvos while they are waiting for everyone to wash their hands for bread, the Satan can use the opportunity to speak out against them. However, the covenant of the salt, which is on the table, protects them.

(Brachos 40a, Tosafos, s.v. Havei melach)

The abovementioned midrash can be explained as follows: Salt symbolizes a covenant, an agreement between people, since it is always eaten with other foods and never alone. This shows unity. Similarly, when we wait for one another to wash, it demonstrates our unity. It is this unity that actually protects from the Satan.

(Imrei Shaul)

When Hashem separated the waters between Heaven and earth, the lower waters cried to Hashem that they wanted to remain close to Him. Therefore, they merited that the salt for *korbanos* was taken from them. The Oheiv Yisrael states that salt gives food a good taste because something which pleads to be close to Hashem brings good to the world.

(Yalkut Oheiv Yisrael, Achilah, p. 105)

The midrash states that the lower waters are called "Weeping Waters" because the lower waters started crying that they did not want to be distanced from Hashem. Hashem told them, "Since you cried for My honor, the upper waters cannot sing *shirah* until they receive permission from you."

Salt proves that the lower waters' intentions were for the sake of Heaven, since the salt that is derived from these waters is used for *korbanos*. *(Higyonei Haparshah, Vayikra)*

There were idols worshippers who were careful not to salt the meat that they sacrificed for their idols, so as not to draw out any of the meat's blood. This was because they believed in the power of the star *Madim*, which represents blood. Conversely, Hashem commanded us to salt meat in order to draw out the blood so that our actions will be unlike those of idol worshippers. We put salt on the table to demonstrate that, contrary to the idol worshippers, we *do* use salt.

(Divrei Tzaddikim 40:40; Rabbeinu Bacheye)

Chazal state that one who learns Torah needs *yiras Shamayim* in addition to his Torah learning *(Shabbos 31a)*, and explain this concept with a parable: If someone has wheat, he should mix into it soil that contains a large concentration of salt to keep it from becoming wormy. Torah is like the wheat and *yiras Shamayim* is like the salt. Just as salt preserves food, *yiras Shamayim* will provide a person with a long life through learning Torah.

That is why on Shabbos we dip the challah into salt, to demonstrate that a person needs to have Torah and *yiras Shamayim* together. (See *Sefer Vayidaber Moshe*, p. 93)

The *pasuk* states, *V'chol korban minchascha bamelach timlach*—"And you should salt every one of your meal offering sacrifices with salt" *(Vayikra 2:13)*. The word *"bamelach"* (with salt) contains the same letters as the word *"balechem"* (with bread). This hints to the Torah, which is sometimes referred to as bread.

The concept of a bris (covenant) is mentioned in connection to both salt and Torah. This teaches us that just as the world cannot exist without salt, it also cannot exist without Torah.

Salt alludes to sustenance for the soul, which is Torah. When *Chazal* state that one should not recite *Hamotzi* until the salt is brought to the table, it is to remind us that the most important thing is the "food" with which we sustain our souls—i.e. the Torah. If we are lacking in Torah, we are lacking in true sustenance.

(Sifsei Kohen, Vayikra 3:13)

A third of the world is desert, a third land, and a third water. The sea came before Hashem and said, "The Torah was given in the desert, the Beis Hamikdash was built on land, but what do I have?"

Hashem replied, "In the future, the Jews will sacrifice *korbanos* on the *Mizbe'ach* with salt."

Today, when there is no Beis Hamikdash, the table at which a person eats is compared to the *Mizbe'ach*. Therefore, we place salt on the table. This is why the *pasuk* states with all your *korbanos* you should offer salt, and not simply with every *korban* you should offer salt. It demonstrates that this refers to any table at which a person eats his meals.

(Sifsei Kohen, Parshas Vayikra 2:13)

After eating the first *kezayis* of bread, Reb Yehoshua Heschel, the Rav of Kapish, would take another slice of challah, dip it into salt, and say, "*Al kol korbancha takriv melach*—with all your *korbanos* you should offer salt *(Vayikra 1:13)*." He was accustomed to saying throughout the *seudah*, "*Zeh hashulchan asher lifnei Hashem*—this is the table that is before Hashem," several times. He would say that since the table at which one eats is compared to a *Mizbe'ach*, one should visualize himself as if he is bringing a *korban*.

(Zichron Yehoshua, Erech Seudah, p. 44b)

Besides the ideas already discussed above, placing salt on the table arouses a person to contemplate several lessons:

Salt can inspire a person to realize that he was created solely to thank Hashem. Rabbi Abba states that at the beginning of creation, Hashem was praised only by the water. If the praise of the water was so valued by Hashem, how much more so is the praise of a person who possesses the power of speech and for whom Hashem does so much kindness.

Salt demonstrates that Hashem gives reward and punishment. The water was rewarded for wanting to be close to Hashem by being the receptacle of salt, which is essential for the world's existence. Salt demonstrates that punishment exists, since the generations of the *mabul*, Enosh, and Sedom were punished with water (from which salt is derived).

By putting salt on the table a person is reminded that the people of Sedom, who did not do *chessed*, were punished with salt, and he will be inspired to increase his acts of *chessed*.

When a person is sitting at his table laden with food and surrounded by his family, he may become arrogant and rebel against Hashem. The waters were first in the Heaven, where they had the opportunity to praise Hashem. They were later sent down to this world as salt. This teaches us that a person should appreciate all that Hashem has granted him and recognize that it is a gift from Him.

Salt reminds a person to lament over his deficiencies in his service of Hashem, just as the lower waters cried over not being close to Hashem.

A person should have the courage to do what is right. He should learn from the water which had the courage to break through its boundaries in order to reach upwards and be close to Hashem.

Salt also reminds a person that Hashem forgives. Hashem forgave the water for breaking through its boundaries and rewarded it with the decree that salt would be used for *korbanos*. *Melach*, salt, contains the same letters as *machal*—Hashem forgave. (*Sifsei Kohen, Vayikra* 2:13)

Salt contains two opposite forces: water and fire. It comes from the sea but is formed through heat, which causes the water to evaporate. Water represents the trait of *rachamim*, compassion, and fire represents *din*, justice.

Hashem made a pact with the world that in order for it to exist it needs both compassion and justice. Salt has the power to preserve food and enhance its taste, but it can also destroy food because no produce can grow in salty earth. Since salt represents *rachamim* and *din* together, which give the world its existence, Hashem commanded us to sacrifice *korbanos* with salt. (*Rabbeinu Bacheye*; *Kli Yakar*)

A person is required to connect all his daily physical deeds to his service of Hashem. This can be accomplished by restricting physical pleasures. Salt represents restraint because the Yam Hamelach (literally the Salty Sea, also known as the Dead Sea) is at the border of Eretz Yisrael. We bring salt to the table to demonstrate that a Jew needs to have boundaries and restraint while eating and enjoying physical pleasures.

Reb Aharon of Belz explains a passage in the *Zohar* according to this idea. The *Zohar* states that the time of eating is a time of battle, *milchamah*, which has the same letters as *melach mah* (What does salt teach us?). While a person is eating, he needs to remember what the salt is there to teach him—that he should set boundaries and limit his physical pleasures.
(Reb Yissachar Dov of Belz, *Parshas Terumah*)

When the Beis Hamikdash stood, there was a *Mizbe'ach Hachitzonis*, outer *Mizbe'ach* and *Mizbe'ach Hapenimis*, inner *Mizbe'ach*. The inner *Mizbe'ach* alludes to the rectification of a person's soul, and the outer one alludes to the rectification of a person's body. Every day, the *avodah* took place on both of these *Mizebechos*. Today, when we no longer have a Beis Hamikdash, a person needs to ensure that he serves Hashem every day with his body and soul so that he rectifies them both.

Since a person is made up of body and soul, he is part of both the upper and lower worlds. There is no other creation that has a part of both worlds besides salt, since it comes from both upper and lower waters.

Therefore, it is a mitzvah to have salt at every *seudah* to allude to the fact that while eating, a person should serve Hashem with his body and soul together. Perhaps this is the reason that many salt holders have two parts to them; to remind one that he should rectify both his body and soul while eating. *(Binyan Tzvi Toras Belz, Vayikra)*

The table at which one eats is compared to a *Mizbe'ach*, and we dip the challah into salt to show that our food is like a *korban*—a person sacrificing from himself. How? If a person is eating and he is satisfied, and he restrains himself from eating more, it is as if he is fasting, and fasting atones for sins like a *korban*. *(Orach Ne'eman, Orach Chaim 167)*

Dipping the Challah Three Times

According to Kabbalah, one should dip the slice of challah in the salt three times and eat it immediately. One should not sprinkle the salt on the challah as that can cause poverty.
(Be'er Heitev, Shulchan Aruch 167:8; Tzelosa D'Avraham, p. 141)

According to Kabbalah, salt is associated with *middas hadin*, and bread with *middas harachamim*. When we dip the bread into salt, the bread is on top and the salt is on the bottom; this reinforces the concept of *middas harachamim* over *middas hadin*. *(Ohr Tzaddikim Derech Seudah, Maharam Paprish)*

Dip the bottom edge of the challah into salt three times.
(Magen Avos, p. 208)

When a person is satiated, it is possible that he will forget about Hashem, as it says in *Devarim* (8:12-14): *...and your silver and gold increase, and all that you have increases, and your heart grows haughty, and you forget Hashem, your G-d, Who has brought you out of the land of Egypt, out of the house of bondage.* Therefore, we dip the bread into salt three times to allude to the *mishneh* is *Pirkei Avos* (3:1): *Akavya ben Mehalalel says, contemplate these* **three things** *and you will not come to sin...*
(Beis Yisrael, Vayikra 2:13)

Sugar Instead of Salt

It is said in the name of the Chasam Sofer that if there is no salt on the table one may use sugar, because both of them improve the taste of food. *(Aleph Ksav, sec. 37)*

Although there are those who are of the opinion that one may dip the challah into sugar instead of salt, according to Kabbalah, one should dip the challah specifically into salt.
(See Kaf Hachaim 167:37, 38; Magen Avos, p. 209)

Not Dipping in Salt

The Chasam Sofer did not dip the challah into salt at the Friday night *seudah*. The reason for this is that it is supposed to remind us of the *korbanos* that were sacrificed with salt. However, there were no *korbanos* sacrificed on Friday night. (During the week, the fat and certain parts of the *korban* were burned on the *Mizbe'ach* each night, but on Shabbos this was forbidden, and the Shabbos *korbanos* were sacrificed during the day.) Also, dipping bread into salt protects a person from suffering, and Shabbos itself already protects. *(Minhagei Chasam Sofer 3:64)*

The Re'ah is of the opinion that one should dip the challah in salt on Friday night. He explains that not only did the part of the *korban* that was burned on the *Mizbe'ach* require salt, but also the other parts of the *korban*. Therefore, even on Friday night there were *korbanos* that were being eaten which required salt. (*Kovetz Kol HaTorah*, issue 59, p. 94)

The Ya'avetz writes that not dipping the challah into salt on Friday night is alluded to in *Brachos* 2b. The Gemara mentions eating bread with salt during the week with the phrase, *"from the time that a pauper eats his bread with salt each night."* However, regarding Friday night, the Gemara writes, *"from the time that people arrive home to eat their bread,"* and does not mention salt.

One reason that some do not dip the challah into salt is that challah is in commemoration of the *Lechem Hapanim,* which were eaten without salt.

Another reason is that every substance in this world can be separated into its components. Salt, even when separated into its most minute particles, will still be a mixture. All the days of the week have a partner besides for Shabbos. Since salt symbolizes fusion, it is not fitting to dip the challah into salt on Shabbos. (*Hilchasa Rabbasa L'Shabbasa*, p. 382)

Eating the Hamotzi

There are those who break off a piece of the challah that was dipped into the salt and then eat it. This is because the Shulchan Aruch states *(Orach Chaim* 170:67) that a person should not eat an entire *kebeitzah* at once, as this is considered gluttonous. The Taz and the Magen Avraham explain that, according to the *Shulchan Aruch*, if a person holds a *kebeitzah* of bread in his hand at once, even if he takes only a small bite of the bread, it is considered gluttonous.

(*Magen Avos*, p. 209; *Mishmeres Shalom* 27:5)

Conversely, many *tzaddikim* were accustomed to biting into the slice of challah upon which *Hamotzi* was recited in order to demonstrate their love for the mitzvah. Just as, on Shabbos, if one cuts a slice of challah large enough to last the entire *seudah* it is not considered gluttonous, if he bites into the *Hamotzi* piece, since it is clear that he is doing so because of his love for the mitzvah, it is permitted.

(Aruch Hashulchan 170:11; *Zemiros Ateres Yehoshua*, p. 91)

Some are of the opinion that a person should eat a *kezayis* of challah without interruption, but one may rely on the more lenient opinion for the *shiur* of a *kezayis* and eat a smaller amount. *(Magen Avos*, p. 209)

Reb Aharon of Belz would take a very large slice of challah and eat it without interruption. He did not eat it together with any other food or drink, or soak it in any liquid (during the week, Reb Aharon would soak his bread in liquid and then eat it, since he had difficulty eating). He pushed himself to eat it quickly, in the time of *kedei achilas pras,* without speaking during that time.

Reb Aharon would eat a very large *shiur*, two to three *kebeitzos,* to ensure that he had eaten a *kezayis* according to all opinions. At the very least, he was careful to eat one *kebeitzah*. After eating the first large slice of challah, Reb Aharon would take another slice of challah, dip it into the wine in his goblet and eat it. *(Halichos Tzaddikim*, p. 228)

Ideally, one should eat a bit more than a *kebeitzah* of challah, since a *kebeitzah* can be considered a *seudas arai*, a snack, and not a *seudas keva,* a proper meal. However, others are of the opinion that even a *kezayis* is sufficient.

(Magen Avraham 291:1, *Shulchan Aruch Harav* 274:6)

A person should eat the slice of challah that *Hamotzi* was recited upon before eating other bread, so that it is eaten with an appetite. This demonstrate one's love for the mitzvah.

(Rema 167:20; *Shelah, Sha'ar Ha'osiyos, Kedushas Ha'achilah)*

A person should eat the slice of challah that *Hamotzi* was recited upon before eating other bread.

This can be learned from the words of the Arizal that if one can have lofty thoughts in mind during the entire time that he eats, that is a great thing, but at the very least he should have them in mind while eating the *kezayis* upon which the *brachah* was recited. It would appear from the words of the Arizal that the *kezayis* upon which one recites the *brachah* should be eaten first.

However, the *Sefer Chassidim* writes that a person should leave over a small piece of the slice upon which *Hamotzi* was recited and eat it at the end of the *seudah*.

In practice, we follow the view of the Arizal and eat the entire slice of *Hamotzi* at the beginning of the *seudah*. If one wishes to follow the view of the *Sefer Chassidim*, he should leave over a piece from the loaf upon which *Hamotzi* was recited but not from the actual slice. *(Kaf Hachaim 167:137)*

One should not serve an animal or a gentile from the slice of *Hamotzi*, since doing so degrades the mitzvah.
(Magen Avraham, Orach Chaim, 167; Mishneh Berurah ibid.:97)

Crumbs of Hamotzi

The Chasam Sofer would eat the crumbs from *Hamotzi* as a *segulah* for a sharp memory.
(Minhagei Chasam Sofer 5:3; Tomer Devorah, Minhagim 5:3)

One should eat the crumbs from the *kezayis* of *Hamotzi*, as it is a *segulah* for wealth. *(Meishiv Devarim 32:38)*

One should be extremely careful with the crumbs from the slice upon which *Hamotzi* was recited, as they are compared to the organs of a *Korban Olah*. If an organ of the *Korban Olah* fell down, the *kohanim* were required to place it back on the *Mizbe'ach*. So too, one should be careful that the crumbs of the slice of challah upon which *Hamotzi* was recited do not land on the floor.

Crumbs on the floor can lead a person to poverty.

(*Kav Hayashar*, sec. 70)

One should be careful that the crumbs that fall from the bread while cutting the bread after reciting *Hamotzi* do not fall onto the floor but on the table or tablecloth. After one eats the *kezayis* of *Hamotzi* he should gather the crumbs and eat them. Since they are leftovers of a mitzvah, they have the power to prevent one from harm. (*Sefer Kasuv*, p. 24)

The Strelisker Rebbe would crumble the challah on Shabbos. He would say that the reason for this is because a child crumbles his food. This is difficult to understand, but it is possible that this demonstrates that we Jews are beloved by Hashem like children, and Hashem has pleasure from us like a father from his children. (*Imrei Kodesh Strelisk*, p. 62)

Some are accustomed to giving the challah crumbs to their children, as a *segulah* for them to have children who will find favor in the eyes of others. (Veitzener Rav, Reb Tzvi Hersh Meisels)

The *minhag* is to gather the crumbs from the challah onto a spoon. This may be an allusion to the *avodah* that was performed on Shabbos with the *Lechem Hapanim*. There were two spoons of *levonah* (frankincense, one of the ingredients of the *ketores*) on the *Shulchan* with the *Lechem Hapanim*, which were offered up on the *Mizbe'ach* before the *Lechem Hapanim* were eaten. Since the challah is commemorative of the *Lechem Hapanim*, we eat the crumbs with a spoon to allude to the *levonah*. (*Rabbi Dovid Meisels*)

The Power of Crumbs

There was a man from Eretz Yisrael who went off the *derech*. He ended up in India and one day entered a restaurant and ordered many different *treif* foods. The waiter first brought him bread and water to eat while his meal was being prepared. After a while, he came out with a large plate of pasta. The man protested that he had not ordered pasta.

"You are Jewish," said the waiter. "And this is what Jews eat."

The man was stunned. "Do I look Jewish?" he asked the waiter. "What makes you think I'm a Jew?"

"It's simple," answered the waiter. "I watched you while you were waiting for your food, and when I saw you gather up the crumbs from your bread and eat them, I knew you must be Jewish."

The man said, "Hashem, I grew up learning that You are in the whole world. I ran away to India to deny it, but I clearly see that You are even here, stopping me from eating *treif* food. I promise I will come back and do *teshuvah*."

He returned to Eretz Yisrael and indeed became a *ba'al teshuvah*. *(Rabbi Dovid Meisels)*

Dipping the Hamotzi into the Kiddush Wine

Reb Yehoshua of Belz said that dipping the slice of *Hamotzi* into the Kiddush wine and eating it on Friday night is a *segulah* to be saved from chest pains.
(Reb Yehoshua of Belz, *Hilchasa Rabbasa L'Shabbasa*, vol. 1, *Toldos*, p. 35)

There are differing opinions as to whether the *Eitz Hada'as* was a grapevine or a wheat stalk. There are those who dip the challah into the wine to rectify the sin of the *Eitz Hada'as* according to both views. *(Shulchan Menachem, Bereishis)*

Chazal say that until 40 years of age food is beneficial; after 40 years of age, drinking is beneficial *(Shabbos* 142b).

Reb Shmelke of Nikolsburg explained that until 40, the *yetzer hara* tries to persuade a person to enjoy his youth and indulge in food, convincing him that he will do *teshuvah* when he is older. A young person should take a lesson from bread which, when fresh, has a good taste, but when it becomes old, it loses its taste. After 40 years of age, the *yetzer hara* tells a person that he is too old and weak to do *teshuvah*. At that time, a person should be inspired by wine which only improves with age.

To allude to the above concept, we dip challah into wine. This reminds us that one should accomplish and learn as much as possible in his youth, but in his later years he should not claim that he is too old to learn. (*Rabbi Dovid Meisels*)

Delicious Taste of Challah

The challah that is eaten on Shabbos has a better taste, aroma, and appearance than bread eaten during the week. It seems that the source of this is found in the *Mechilta D'Rabbi Shimon Bar Yochai* (*Shemos* 16:5). In regard to gathering the *mann* on Erev Shabbos, the *pasuk* states, *v'hayah mishneh*—"and [the *mann*] was double." The *Mechilta* explains this to mean, *v'hayah meshuneh*, and it was different, meaning the *mann* gathered on Erev Shabbos was better. Each day of the week the *mann* had a pleasant aroma, and on Shabbos even more so. Each day of the week the *mann* was golden in its appearance, and on Shabbos even more so.

(*Kovetz Beis Aharon V'Yisrael*, year 10, issue 3, p. 115)

One Friday night, when Reb Meir Premishlaner was eating the challah, he sensed in it a taste of Gan Eden. He asked the Rebbetzin which ingredient she put into the challah that gave it such a special taste. The Rebbetzin replied that the Jewish maid had baked the challah that week. When they asked the maid what she had done differently, she replied that she had recited Hallel while baking the challah since she remembered from her youth that while kneading the dough for the matzos for Pesach they recited Hallel. She decided that, if so, she should also recite Hallel while baking challos. Reb Meir Premishlaner declared that this was the reason that there was a taste of Gan Eden in the challos. (*Gilyon V'shinantam*)

Challah as a Segulah

While eating the first bite of challah, a person should have in mind that he should not lack sustenance on Sunday. While eating the second bite he should have in mind that Hashem should provide him with sustenance for Monday, and so on for each day of the week.

(*Ateres Menachem*, sec. 197; *Divrei Menachem, Likutim*, p. 36)

It is a *segulah* to leave a piece of the Friday night challah on the table to bring *brachah* to the entire week. At the home of Rabbi Yosef Yozpa, the son of the Chasam Sofer, several times when a Shabbos candle fell onto the tablecloth he placed a piece of challah near it and the fire was extinguished. He learned this from his father, the Chasam Sofer. This demonstrates that the challah from Shabbos has the power to protect.

(*Shevet Mi'Yehudah, Beshalach*, s.v. *V'es kol*)

Eating Challah with Each Dish

Rabbi Meir was accustomed to eating more bread on Shabbos than during the week, because he ate bread with each dish.

(*Rashi, Kesubos* 64b, s.v. *Miskavnin l'hakal*)

Rabbi Meir states that it is normal for a person to eat bread together with every dish. During the week one only has a small amount of food, and so he only eats a small amount of bread throughout the meal. On Shabbos, he eats more foods and therefore eats a larger amount of bread.

(*Yerushalmi Eiruvin* 8:2, *Pnei Moshe*)

There were *tzaddikim* who ate a piece of bread together with the first bite of each dish served at the Shabbos *seudah*. Rashi and the Ba'al Hama'or were of the opinion that one should do so because food is only considered part of the *seudah* and does not need a separate *brachah* if eaten together with bread. Although this is not generally practiced, the Beis Yosef writes in the name of the Maharya that one should follow Rashi's opinion. (*Shulchan Rabboseinu*, p. 180; see *Zemiros Divrei Yoel*, p. 96)

Chapter 9
The Friday Night Seudah

Eating the Seudah in its Proper Order

The four different Shabbos foods that we eat at the *seudah* correspond to the four letters of the *Shem Havayah*—*yud, keh, vav, keh*. When writing a *sefer Torah*, it is not imperative that the letters of each word be written in order, except for the names of Hashem. If so, then the Shabbos food, which corresponds to the *Shem Havayah*, also needs to be eaten in order. If the *Shem Havayah* is written in order, it arouses compassion; if not, it arouses the attribute of justice, Heaven forbid. Thus, Reb Shalom of Belz states that the Shabbos *seudah* needs to be eaten in its correct order.

(*Ha'ari Shebachaburah*, p. 288; *Magen Avos*, p. 427)

The foods which Jews are accustomed to eating on Shabbos have holy sources, and a *minhag* that is accepted by Jews is equal to that which is written in the Torah. Our traditional Shabbos menu is based on the foods eaten by the Marranos in Spain, who recognized one another through their Shabbos foods. It is said in the name of *tzaddikim* that the Shabbos foods we eat have a particular order, and there are lofty reasons for each food. (*Matamim*)

The mishnah states that a *korban* which is holier is sacrificed first. For example, a *Korban Chatas* is sacrificed before a *Korban Asham*. The holier *korban* is also eaten first (*Zevachim* 89a).

At our Shabbos table, the holiness of Shabbos rests upon our food just like it rests upon the *korbanos*. Therefore, we need to eat the Shabbos foods in their order of importance. The foods for which we have a source should be eaten before other food. One should also eat the living things, such as fish, chicken, or meat before eating other foods, such as salads.

The Ye'aros Devash reinforces this concept, stating that Hashem accepted the *korban* of Hevel who offered an animal, and not the *korban* of Kayin who offered flax. A *korban* represents the person sacrificing it as if he is sacrificing himself, and therefore it is preferable that the food we eat should first should be from a living being. (*Rabbi Dovid Meisels*)

The Brisker Rav ate an extremely minimal amount of food each day. After moving to Yerushalayim, he was very weak, and the Rebbetzin began preparing chicken for him each day, in addition to his usual meal. However, her plan did not work. The Rav ate the chicken soup that was served first, and did not touch the chicken or the rest of the meal.

When the Rebbetzin once chanced upon the doctor of Yerushalayim, Reb Moshe Wallach, she expressed her concern that the Rav was not eating properly. The doctor advised her to serve the chicken as the first course so that the Rav would eat some chicken.

The following day, the Rebbetzin served the Rav the chicken as the first course. The Rav inspected the chicken and said, "The bone is curved, which means it was broken and then healed. According to halachah one may eat it, but I never ate chicken that was halachically questionable. Should I start to do so in my old age?"

The Brisker Rav did not partake of the entire meal for fear that it had touched the chicken or the soup.

Since this incident, the Yerushalmi Jews began eating the chicken at the beginning of the *seudah* and the soup at the end of the *seudah*. This way, if there is any question about the chicken, they will be aware of it and not partake of any of the other foods. *(Yerushalayim Shel Ma'alah)*

Friday Night Foods

In the Friday night song, *Azamer B'shvachin* we say, *l'apasha zinin,* one should have many different foods for the Shabbos *seudah*. *Zinin* is similar to the word *zayin*, seven. Thus, it alludes to eating seven types of food at the Shabbos *seudah*. *(Pri Tzaddik, Emor, sec. 6)*

These are the seven dishes: fish, soup, meat, compote, cooked carrots, *farfel*, and liver.

The *Sefer Mishnas Chassidim* states that the seven types of food and drinks of the Friday night *seudah* correspond to the seven *middos: chessed, gevurah, tiferes, netzach, hod, yesod,* and *malchus*. *(Mishnas Chassidim, Leil Shabbos 4:6)*

A person should prepare as many foods as he is able for the Friday night *seudah*. If he can, he should prepare ten dishes which correspond to the ten *sefiros*. At the very least, he should not prepare less than two cooked dishes, one dish more than during the week, meaning chicken soup and *tzimmes*.
(Shulchan Hatahor 242:2-3)

The Komarno Rebbe would eat the following ten dishes on Friday night: fish, filled fish, soup, chicken, meat, stuffed chicken neck, *lokshen* kugel, sweet carrots *(tzimmes)*, *farfel*, and compote. *(Minhagei Komarno, sec. 188)*

One should partake of at least two cooked dishes at the Friday night and Shabbos day *seudos*. We see that at the *seudas hamafsekes* eaten on Erev Tishah B'Av it is forbidden to eat two cooked dishes; this demonstrates that two cooked dishes have the status of a *seudah*.

At *shalosh seudos* it not necessary to eat two cooked dishes; according to the strict letter of the law one may even eat fruit for *shalosh seudos*.

(*Magen Avraham* 242:1, in the name of the *Zohar*, *Bereishis* 48b)

Hot Food

It is a mitzvah to keep the Shabbos food hot, since by eating hot food one honors and takes delight in the Shabbos.

(*Orach Chaim* 257, *Rema*)

The food should be eaten while still hot.

(*Siddur HaYa'avetz*, Beginning *Hanhagos Erev Shabbos*)

Many are careful that the hot dishes eaten on Shabbos are hot enough to give off steam. It is told in the name of Reb Shalom of Belz that this is because the steam rising from the food is a commemoration of the *Lechem Hapanim,* which emitted steam.

(*Minhagei Pri Eliezer*, p. 225)

The Me'or V'shemesh would relate many *divrei Torah* between each course of the Shabbos *seudah*. He would expound on each thought for a long time and in the meantime, the food turned cold. It was later revealed to him that this practice caused displeasure in Heaven.

There is a source for this in the words of one of the *Rishonim*, the Rokeach, who writes: *After eating a hot dish one should sing* zemiros Shabbos (54).

(*Darkei Chaim V'shalom*, sec. 404, *He'aros*)

Reb Yechiel of Aleksander was once served soup at the Shabbos *seudah*, which he immediately ate. His son, the Yismach Yisrael, then asked his father for *shirayim* from the soup. Reb Yechiel gave his son the soup but the Yismach Yisrael was unable to eat it because it was so hot. The Yismach Yisrael then asked his father in astonishment, "How were you able to eat such hot soup?"

His father replied, "This soup is not hot to a person who burns with love for his Creator." *(Emunas Moshe, Yisro 11)*

A plate of soup was once served at the Shabbos *seudah* to the Shiniver Rav, without a spoon. The Rav tried to decide on the proper course of action: if he would wait until the spoon was brought, the soup would cool off, and it is proper to eat it as hot as possible to fulfill *oneg Shabbos*. On the other hand, eating the soup without a spoon is a lack of good manners. Ultimately, he decided that the mitzvah of *oneg Shabbos* takes precedence and he should drink it straight from the bowl.

(Noam Siach, p. 153)

Reb Asher of Ropshitz would eat very hot food on Shabbos. Reb Asher once spent Shabbos in Tarna and he wanted to eat the *seudah* at his lodgings so that the food should not turn cold from being moved to a new place. However, there was already a very large crowd eating the *seudah* there, so he found another place nearby where he could eat the *seudah*. He wrapped the food very well, on all sides, so that it should not cool down.

After bringing over the food, he said, "If food, which has no eyes or ears, needs to be wrapped up so well in order for it not to cool down when taken outside, and even then, it still cools down, how much more so must a person, who has eyes and ears, be careful when walking in the street even a short distance that he should not 'cool off' [in his service of Hashem]." *(Temidim K'sidram, p. 1204)*

The Tosher Rebbe would say, in the name of his grandfather, that although during the week eating very hot foods can harm one's health, on Shabbos, the hotter the food the better. This is because on Shabbos, a special light spreads upon the world, and the heat of this light enters the Shabbos food.

(Avodas Avodah, p. 146)

On Shabbos one eats hot foods, on Erev Shabbos one bathes and immerses himself in hot water, and on Motza'ei Shabbos one eats and drinks hot things, and bathes in hot water (*Shabbos* 119b).

In order to prepare hot water, one needs to create peace between water and fire, because naturally, water extinguishes fire, and fire evaporates water. The Gemara (*Brachos* 56b) states that one who sees a pot in a dream should say, "Hashem should bring peace upon us," because the pot symbolizes peace between water and fire.

Shabbos is called *"Shabbos Shalom"* because it brings peace over the entire universe. To allude to this, we eat hot food on Shabbos, which can only come about when there is peace between water and fire. (*Zemiros Shabbos Shalom Umevorach*, p. 12)

Chapter 10
Not Just an Appetizer—
The Significance of Fish

Reasons for Eating Fish on Shabbos

The *Shulchan Aruch Harav* states an opinion that eating fish on Shabbos is a Torah obligation (*d'Oraisa*).

(*Shulchan Aruch Harav* 242, *Kuntris Acharon* 4)

One should make sure to eat fish at each of the *seudos*, because there are deep, mystical reasons for this *minhag*. Most *tzaddikim* are *megulgal* in fish and by eating fish on Shabbos, we rectify their souls. If a person who eats fish on Shabbos is also eventually *megulgal* in a fish, Hashem will arrange it so that he will be eaten by a pious Jew, measure for measure.

(*Kitzur HaShelah; Minchas Shabbos* 72:28)

The Ropshitzer Rav said that the word, "Shabbos" begins with the sound, "*sha*" to allude to the fact that mundane matters should not be discussed on Shabbos.

Perhaps this is one reason why we eat fish on Shabbos. Unlike any other kosher creature, fish are always silent. This demonstrates that one should remain silent on Shabbos [aside from speaking words of Torah and *tefillah*].

(*Ohr Yesha*, p. 10; *Imrei Yehudah Barzan, Parshas Shelach*)

The Gemara states that every place where there is desecration of Shabbos, there is a fire (*Shabbos* 119b). By observing Shabbos properly, one is saved from fire. The Gemara also states that desecrating the Shabbos causes wild animals to come (*Shabbos* 33a). These examples demonstrate that by observing the Shabbos properly, a person is spared from all evil, and spared also from the suffering of *galus*. Indeed, *Chazal* state that if the Jews would keep two Shabbasos properly, they would be redeemed.

All animals make noise when they are hurt, but fish cannot cry out, even when being harmed. If a person, Heaven forbid, desecrates the Shabbos, various forms of suffering will befall him and he will cry out in pain. However, if a person keeps Shabbos properly, the merit of Shabbos will protect him and he will have no need to cry out. Even if he did sin, he will not need to cry out in pain from the punishments, because one who keeps Shabbos properly, even if he worshipped *avodah zarah* like the generation of Enosh, will be forgiven for his sins.

Therefore, we eat fish on Shabbos to hint to the fact that by keeping Shabbos one will have no need to cry out from pain or suffering, just like a fish. (*Tiyul B'pardes, Dagim*)

Shabbos food has the taste of the *mann*. The *mann* in the *midbar* could taste like any food except fish. Hence, we eat fish on Shabbos so that we fulfill the mitzvah of *oneg Shabbos* with every possible taste. (*Oheiv Yisrael, Parshas Eikev*)

During the creation of the world, Hashem blessed the fish on Thursday, man on Friday, and on Shabbos, Hashem blessed the Shabbos. These three blessings are combined when a Jew, who is called man, eats fish on Shabbos. When one does so, he is blessed with a triple blessing. Three times the word *brachah*, with the addition of the letters *yud, keh,* and *vav* (the Name of Hashem which is the source of *brachah*) has the same numerical value as the word Shabbos.

(*Bnei Yissaschar, Shabbos* sec. 11, *Ma'amar* 3:16)

The *pasuk* in *Bereishis* (1:22) states regarding the fish: *And Hashem blessed them, saying, "Be fruitful and multiply, and fill the waters of the seas..."* The Ohr Hachaim states that fish required a special blessing since they are a cold-blooded species and, naturally, they would be unable to reproduce.

(Igra D'kallah, Bereishis 24:73)

Eretz Yisrael is a place of *kedushah,* and if one is there, he has a *tzelem Elokim,* the image of Hashem, which Adam possessed prior to his sin of eating from the *Eitz Hada'as*, and which departed after he sinned. Through the holiness of Shabbos, a person also merits a shining face, no matter where he is, as *Chazal* state that one cannot compare the countenance of a person on Shabbos to his countenance during the week. When a person conducts himself with holiness on Shabbos, this *tzelem* is returned and his face glows, since the holiness of Shabbos is comparable to Eretz Yisrael.

Fish have scales, which is their sign that they are kosher. When certain fish are removed from the water, which symbolizes purity, they shed their scales. However, as long as they had the scales when they were in the water they are still kosher.

So too, the Jews only have a *tzelem Elokim* in Eretz Yisrael, and when they are taken out of Eretz Yisrael they lose it. Outside of Eretz Yisrael, they only have the *tzelem Elokim* on Shabbos. Even so, they are still "kosher." Therefore, we eat fish on Shabbos to allude to these ideas.

(Avnei Hamakom, Avnei Shoham sec. 103)

Every creation has its roots in the upper worlds. Fish have a more elevated source than other animals. *(Divrei Tzaddikim)*

Before eating meat or poultry, one needs to perform several mitzvos, such as slaughtering and salting. Since fish do not have any of those mitzvos, we have a mitzvah to eat fish on Shabbos. *(B'tzila Demheimenusa,* p. 4)

This world is composed of four components: water, fire, air, and earth. Water is on the highest level and earth is on the lowest level. Fish come from water, which is on the highest level, as opposed to meat which comes from the earth, the lowest level. We eat fish on Shabbos since Shabbos also stems from an elevated spiritual realm.

(Ben Ish Chai, Halachos, Shanah Shniyah, Vayeira, sec. 18)

The Rebbe of Gastinin states that Shabbos is a day of *penimiyus*; it possesses an inner essence that is covered and not easily revealed, as the *Zohar* states that Shabbos is a day designated for the soul. Similarly, fish are always covered with water. The Ba'al Avnei Nezer adds that this concept is alluded to in the Gemara that states that a person should delight in the Shabbos with spinach and large fish *(Shabbos* 118b). For spinach, the Gemara uses the phrase *toch toch,* which hints to inner essence. We eat filled fish to allude to *penimiyus* even further.

(Avir Haroim, vol. 2, sec. 374)

The Significance of Fish

The holy souls of *tzaddikim* who sinned descend to this world and are *megulgal* in fish.   *(Ohr Hachaim, Bereishis 1:26)*

Why do we eat fish during all three *seudos* on Shabbos? The three *seudos* are parallel to the three *Avos* and their power to bring the blessings of children, life, and sustenance to this world. Avraham corresponds to children, as Hashem promised him that his children will be as numerous as the stars *(Bereishis* 15:5). Yitzchak alludes to wealth as it says: *And Yitzchak sowed in that land, and he found in that year a hundred-fold, and the Lord blessed him* (ibid. 26:12). Yaakov corresponds to life, as the *Zohar* states that one who sees Yaakov in a dream is blessed with a long life *(Zohar,* vol. 1, p. 168a).

Fish correspond to children, life, and sustenance. The *pasuk* states, *and may they multiply abundantly like fish...* *(Bereishis* 48:16). *Chazal* say that there are three species in the world that have more strength as they get older, and one of them is fish (*Shabbos* 77b). The story of *Yosef Moker Shabbos*, [a poor man who, by finding a gem inside of his Shabbos fish, was miraculously rewarded with a tremendous fortune because of his great dedication to honoring Shabbos], demonstrates that fish also allude to sustenance (ibid. 119a).

(Imrei Noam, Likutim Shabbos, section 2)

The Sanzer Rebbe was unsuccessful in acquiring fish for Shabbos one week, even after investing a large amount of effort. At the Shabbos *seudah*, at the time that the fish is usually eaten, the Rebbe said, "Who needs fish? Fish is the only species that eat one another alive although they did each other no harm."

The following Shabbos, when the fish was placed on the table, the Rebbe said, "What a special dish! Fish is the only species in the generation of the *Mabul* that did not sin. Hashem chose fish to be the species in which tzaddikim are *megulgal*. Although fish consume other fish, they do not chase them. If one splits open a fish, he can see that the head of the consumed fish entered first, because the small fish swam towards the larger fish and wanted to be consumed."

The chassidim who were present for both Shabbasos were astonished to witness how the Rebbe demeaned fish one Shabbos, and praised it highly the next.

The Rebbe explained, "This is the correct way for a Jew to live. He should always accept with love the path that Hashem, Who runs this world with goodness, designates for him. Last week it was decreed that we should not have fish for Shabbos, therefore I focused on the negative aspects of fish. Now that we merited having fish for Shabbos, I am praising it, to thank Hashem for it." *(Haparshah V'hasippur, Shoftim*, p. 240)

The fish species did not sin during the generation of the *Mabul*. Therefore, it is a food fit for kings.

(Siach Sarfei Kodesh, vol. 1, sec. 413)

Throughout the generations, *tzaddikim* went to great lengths to ensure that they had fish at every Shabbos and Yom Tov *seudah*. There are many elevated concepts regarding fish, and *tzaddikim* would have lofty thoughts while eating it.

(Sefarim Hakedoshim)

Tzaddikim like to eat fish because fish contain the *gilgulim* of *tzaddikim*. A fish, unlike other animals, does not have a neck; its body is attached directly to its head. This alludes to a *tzaddik* who is completely and directly attached to Hashem.

(Toras Moshe, Beha'aloscha, s.v. Sheish mei'os ragli)

The Chozeh of Lublin once asked the Yismach Moshe why we eat fish at every *seudas Shabbos* or *seudas mitzvah*, since there is no known source for this in Tanach. When Avraham Avinu served the angels, he gave them butter and meat, but we do not see any mention of fish. In *Parshas Yisro* as well (18:12), the *pasuk* states: *And Aharon came and all the elders of the Jews came to eat bread with Moshe's father-in-law—* there is no mention of fish.

The Yismach Moshe replied that the reason that Hashem permitted us to eat animals is so that the *neshamos* that are *megulgal* in them should be rectified by a Jew eating the animal with holiness and purity.

Every animal can have *kashrus* concerns except fish—a fish with the necessary *simanim* is always considered kosher. In previous generations, it was not necessary for *tzaddikim* to be *megulgal* because they perfected themselves while they were still alive. Today, however, even *tzaddikim* need to be *megulgal*, but they are *megulgal* in fish, which have no questions of *kashrus*. Therefore, we eat fish on Shabbos so that we can connect to the *tzaddikim* within them and rectify them.

(Beis Tzaddikim Ya'amod, vol. 3, p. 53)

The word *dag*, fish, is comprised of the letters *dalet* and *gimmel*, which have the numerical value of four and three. This alludes to the four *Imahos* and three *Avos*.

(*Matamim Hachadash*)

Shabbos is called "king." Just as a king provides for his servants, in the merit of Shabbos we have sustenance the entire week. There was a well-known saying in Southern Yemen that "Shabbos without fish is like a king without servants."

(*Michlul Hama'amarim V'hapisgamim*, Megillas Esther, p. 55)

Fish as the First Course

The Tiferes Shlomo writes that *lechem mishneh* on Shabbos alludes to Yosef Hatzaddik because twice the word *"lechem"* has the same numerical value as the word "Yosef." Observing Shabbos properly is a rectification for the *shevatim* selling Yosef, as it says in *Parshas Va'eschanan* (5:26), *And you should remember that you were a slave in Mitzrayim, and Hashem took you out of there, therefore I command you to keep the Shabbos*. The *Zohar* states that the word *"slave"* in this *pasuk* refers to Yosef Hatzaddik.

Fish also alludes to Yosef Hatzaddik, as Yaakov Avinu blessed the children of Yosef that they should multiply like the fish in the sea and the evil eye should have no control over them. The *minhag* is to eat fish after *lechem mishneh* because both allude to Yosef.

(*Noam HaShabbos*, p. 46)

The Yalkut Reuveini states that one should first consume foods that are easier for the body to digest before eating heavier foods, so fish is eaten before the meat since it is easier for the body to digest.

(*Kaf Hachaim* 157:38)

Fish were the first living beings to be created. Therefore, fish are closer to their source, and to the words of Hashem which created the world. The holiness of Shabbos is our source of life, so we begin our Shabbos *seudah* with fish.

Another reason for eating fish as the first course at the Shabbos *seudah* is because *ayin hara* (the evil eye) has no power over fish and we want to be blessed that no *ayin hara* should affect us.

Fish symbolize life since they were the first living beings to be created. When we eat fish, we *daven* that all those who are waiting to be blessed with children should have their *tefillos* answered.   (*Imrei Emes Lublin, Parshas Bo, Leil Shabbos* 5637)

The fish is eaten first so that the *neshamos* of the *tzaddikim* who were *megulgal* in fish should be rectified first.
(*Magen Avos*, p. 223)

Reb Yehoshua of Tamashov was once in Brod for Shabbos. That week there was no fish available in Brod, and soup was served for the first course. Reb Yehoshua asked why there was no fish and was informed that there was none to be had.

Reb Yehoshua related that the reason we eat the fish first is because there is a possibility that meat and chicken may be questionable in regard to *kashrus*. However, any fish that possesses *simanim* is definitely kosher. Therefore, one should start the *seudah* with fish so that, just like the fish is definitely kosher, all the foods should be entirely kosher.

Reb Yehoshua explained that since there was no fish, he could not assume that the rest of the food was kosher and could not eat anything from the *seudah*. Indeed, it was later discovered that there may have been a problem with the *kashrus* of the meat.   (*Kuntris Eit Shamein*)

One of the grandchildren of Reb Dovid Moshe of Chortkov once invited his grandfather to a *seudah* for an occasion. His grandfather asked him if he prepared fish for the *seudah*. When the grandchild answered that he did not, Reb Dovid Moshe replied that he would not attend. When his grandchild asked him for an explanation, he explained that fish is permissible to eat without any further preparation. Meat however, must be slaughtered, checked, and salted. Therefore, it is good to begin one's *seudah* with a dish that is permissible without any doubts, and then one can assume that the entire *seudah* will be kosher. (*Divrei Dovid*, sec. 59; *Ner Yisrael, Achilah*)

One should begin his *seudah* with fish, and end the Shabbos with fish at *shalosh seudos*. (*Shiras HaShabbos*, p. 223)

In earlier times, the *minhag* was to eat meat before the fish. This is the reason that it says in *zemiros, basar v'dagim v'chol matamim*—meat and fish and all delicacies, with meat listed first. (*Otzar Yad Hachaim* 116)

Segulos from Eating Fish

Dag has a gematria of seven. One who eats *dag* on the day of *dag* (i.e. Shabbos, the seventh day) is spared from *dag*, an acronym for *din Gehinnom*, the punishment of Gehinnom.
(*Shulchan Lechem Hapanim*, sec. 242, p. 3)

The Arizal writes that the numerical value of the words "Yitzchak" and "Rivkah" is the same as the word "*tefillah*." This demonstrates that through the power of their *tefillah*, Yitzchak and Rivkah had the ability to remove harsh judgments.

The word *dag* in its full form (the letters *dalet* and *gimmel* written out; *dalet* spelled out is *dalet, lamed* and *tav*; *gimmel* spelled out is *gimmel, yud, mem,* and *lamed*) also has the same numerical value as the words Yitzchak and Rivkah together.

This teaches us that a person who eats fish in honor of Shabbos will have the harsh judgments that were decreed on him reversed. (*Midbar Kadeish, Balak*)

There was once an epidemic in the city of Belz. At his Shabbos *seudah,* the Sar Shalom of Belz said, "I already remarked several times that if a Jew keeps Shabbos properly and takes pleasure in it, he will be protected from all harm.

There are those who are afraid to eat fish during an epidemic, even on Shabbos, but in truth, a small amount of fish eaten in honor of Shabbos will only protect a person."

(*Halichos Hatzaddikim*, p. 329)

There was once a gravely ill chassid whose days were numbered. He decided that he wished to die in the house of a *tzaddik* and instructed his family to carry him to the home of the Sanzer Rav so that his soul should depart from the Rebbe's holy home. His family obeyed his wishes. When the Sanzer Rav became aware of his presence, he took a piece of fish and gave it to him to eat. Although it was well-known that eating fish was deathly for this particular illness, the chassid did not doubt his Rebbe and ate the fish. As soon as he finished eating the fish, he felt a bit better. His condition continued to improve until he was completely well.

Perhaps the Sanzer Rav served the ill chassid fish and not a different dish because it is written that the word *dagim* is an acronym for *Yud Gimmel Michilin D'rachamin*, the Thirteen Attributes of Mercy (*Eikev*, p. 271b, 272a), so eating fish has the ability to evoke the Thirteen Attributes of Mercy.

(*Beis Hayayin*, p. 193)

The Yitev Lev would often travel to Reb Shalom of Belz. Once, the Belzer Rav handed him *shirayim* of a piece of fish. The Yitev Lev was uncertain whether he should eat it since he had a high fever. When the Belzer Rebbe saw his hesitation, he said to him, "Eat the fish, because the *shirayim* of my fish are a *segulah* against illness." Indeed, the Yitev Lev ate the *shirayim* and recovered.

(*Pe'er V'kavod Eirech Maran Maharash*, sec. 8)

A chassid once fell ill and was extremely weak. He came to Reb Aharon of Karlin on Shabbos, and when the Rebbe distributed *shirayim* of the fish to those present, he included the ill man. The chassidim remarked to the Rebbe that fish is harmful to those suffering from his illness.

The Rebbe replied, "Who is to say that fish doesn't agree with illness? Maybe illness doesn't agree with fish?"

The chassid ate the fish and his illness disappeared.

(*Pri Yesha Aharon Karlin*, p. 317)

The Gemara states that Rava would salt the fish himself. The Spinker Rebbe would salt the fish himself each Erev Shabbos and would say that the word, "Rava" has the same numerical value as *banei, cheiyei, umezonei* (children, health, and sustenance), which teaches us that fish on Shabbos can brings us these blessings. (*Pe'er Yosef, Hakdamah*)

We can say that fish is called *"fish"* in Yiddish based on the *pasuk* in *Bereishis* (1:22): *Pru urevu*—"be fruitful and multiply." Targum translates this *pasuk* as *pushu usegu*, they will multiply and proliferate. Indeed, *Chazal* state that the evil eye has no control over fish (*Brachos* 40a). Thus, the name fish itself (similar in spelling to the word *pushu*) hints to its ability to bring about the blessing of children. (*Halichos Tzaddikim*, p. 344)

The *sefarim* state that the Name of Hashem, *Shakai*—*shin, dalet, yud*, is the name that is designated for granting children. When Hashem blessed both Avraham Avinu and Yaakov Avinu with children, He appeared to them with the name *Shakai*. The numerical value of *pru urevu* is 500, the same as the value of the word *Shakai* written out in its full form (*Chida*, in the name of *Sefer Imrei Noam*).

Therefore, we drink whiskey immediately after eating fish to form Hashem's name of *Shakai*—the first letters of the words *dagim* (fish) and *yayin saraf* (whiskey) are *dalet, yud* and *sin*. (*Rabbi Dovid Meisels*)

There was once a city with a large Jewish population. Their *rav* was a *mohel* and he spent most of his time performing circumcisions.

Once, one of the king's ministers persuaded the king to grant him a monopoly over all the fish in the sea. The price of fish became prohibitive and people were unable to afford it, even in honor of Shabbos.

From then on, the *rav* noticed a steady decline in the number of births in the city. The elders of the city explained that this was due to the fact that people could not afford to purchase fish, even for Shabbos, and fish is a *segulah* for children.

The *rav* took a piece of earthenware upon which he wrote the Name of Hashem. He instructed his student to throw the vessel into the sea. From that day on, no fish would swim to the surface of the sea. The fishermen stood at the sea all day but were unsuccessful in catching even a single fish. The king soon noticed the absence of fish from his daily menu and personally went down to the sea to investigate. He too attempted to catch some fish but was unsuccessful. The king issued a decree that anyone who possesses information to explain this phenomenon should step forward. Two fishermen related how they saw a Jew place an object in the water after which the fish no longer rose to the surface.

The king gave the Jews three days to present the responsible party to him, threatening to banish them from the city if they did not comply. The *rav* presented himself to the king and explained, "Nature was created by Hashem so that the world should continue to exist. Shlomo Hamelech said that a person cannot stop the air from flowing, because air is necessary for the existence of the world, and as such, one cannot charge for it. So too, water, which is vital for our existence, is free of charge. One can charge for the service of transporting it, but not for the water itself. So too, one can charge for the service of catching fish, but not for the fish itself.

"I have been the *rav* and *mohel* here for tens of years and have always performed several *brissim* a day. Now, however, that number has been decreasing steadily, and several days can pass without me performing even one *bris milah*. The elders revealed to me that this is due to the lack of fish. Repeal your decree and fish will once again grace our tables."

The king heeded his words and together they went down to the sea. The *rav* recited *hataras nedarim*, and before he had even finished, the sea split apart and schools of fish appeared at the surface. The king was so overcome that he blessed the Name of Hashem. They escorted the *rav* home with a royal procession, song and dance.

(*Ahavas Chaim, Bo*, in the name of the *Pla'ei Hatzaddikim*)

The Biala-Bilitz Rebbe, Reb Aharon Halberstam, once suggested the following *segulah* to someone who wished to be exempted from the army: He should light a candle every Erev Shabbos for the merit of the *neshamah* of Rav Nachman bar Yitzchak, and he should buy large fish in honor of Shabbos.

Why did Reb Aharon suggest this? The Gemara states that Reb Nachman bar Yitzchak said that one who delights in the Shabbos will be spared from the oppression of the government. This Gemara continues by stating that one should delight in the Shabbos with large fish (*Shabbos* 118b). Therefore, Reb Aharon advised, eating fish on Shabbos in the merit of Reb Nachman Bar Yitzchak will be a *segulah* for being exempted from the army. (*Mibe'er HaShabbos*, p. 387)

Reb Gershon Chanoch Henoch of Radzin would say that one should carry with him the eye of a fish as a *segulah* to be spared from *ayin hara*. Chazal state that *ayin hara* does not have control over fish (*Brachos* 20a), so fish can ward off an evil eye, especially fish cooked in honor of Shabbos. Reb Gershon himself carried with him the eye of a fish and it was noticed several times that when he ate fish he put away the eye.

(*Dor Yesharim*, p. 74)

Varieties of Fish

Reb Aharon of Belz would say that it is interesting to note that there are so many types of fish in the world, some of them much higher quality, yet people use carp as their fish for Shabbos. When they brought him carp that was covered in scales so that it appeared golden, he appreciated it greatly.

(*Halichos Hatzaddikim*, p. 299)

It's important to eat fish every Shabbos, because fish come from a very lofty place, and the fish's open eyes are symbolic of Hashem always watching us. When the Torah says that one may eat all fish with scales, it means particularly the lox fish (salmon). This fish has an additional scale which other fish don't have, which shows that this is the best of all fish.

(*Me'or V'shemesh, Likutim, s.v. Masechta Chullin*)

The *hecht* fish, today known as pike, is considered to be the king of the fish and swims at the head of the fish.

(*Chashavah Latovah*, Aleksander Rebbe)

Tzaddikim say that they prefer to eat pike, since it possesses *bitachon*. It does not pursue fish for its meals but waits for the fish to come to it. (*Shabbos Shalom, Ma'amar Shiras HaShabbos*)

Reb Aharon of Belz attached much value to the pike fish. He said in the name of his father that the pike fish is the king of all fish. (*B'tzila Dimheimenusa*, p. 98; *Halichos Hatzaddikim*, p. 296)

Herring can help curtail a person's negative desires.

(*Sefer Chassidim*, sec. 390)

There are those who are accustomed to eating black bread dipped in olive oil with herring before eating other fish on Friday night. (*Minhagei Lelov*)

Many *tzaddikim* cooked the fish with sugar and were careful to only eat sweet fish on Shabbos, and not pickled fish.

The cook once prepared tasteless fish for Reb Aharon of Belz. He said in jest, "This fish is 'real' fish—without salt or sugar, just fish itself."

(*Divrei Chanah*, vol. 2, p. 364; *Halichos Hatzaddikim*, pp. 308, 310)

The Gemara in *Shabbos* (ibid.) states that even something small prepared in honor of Shabbos brings *oneg Shabbos*. The Gemara explains that this refers to small fish fried in their own oil with flour. This is the source for eating pickled fish, because those small fish were generally prepared with flour and vinegar.
(Vayageid Moshe, Shabbos Kodesh)

Reb Moshe of Dezh would eat herring at each Shabbos *seudah*. He would say in jest, "The Gemara states that Hashem salted the *livyasan* for the *tzaddikim* to eat when Mashiach comes. Does Hashem not have anything else to serve the *tzaddikim* besides fish that is thousands of years old? It must be that *tzaddikim* enjoy eating salted fish."
(Seudasa D'Malka, p. 32)

It is the *minhag* of Jews to eat ground fish on Friday night, called gefilte fish. This is made by taking out the flesh of the fish, grinding it, and then returning it to its place in the fish, under the skin, so that the fish still has its original appearance. This fulfills *minhag* of eating a filled food that is mentioned in the Gemara. There are also those who made a large loaf of ground fish, called gefilte fish, as well.

The Rema writes that in several locations they ate a dish which consisted of dough on the top and bottom, filled with meat. This was eaten on Friday night as a remembrance of the *mann,* that had dew above and below it. Kugel similarly fulfills this idea with its crust on the top and the bottom. Since on Friday night there are those who do not eat kugel, they eat gefilte fish which is surrounded by the skin (see above) to remember the *mann*. Since there are those who do not eat fish at the day *seudah* (they eat it before the *seudah* after Kiddush), they eat kugel. On Yom Tov, when fish and gefilte fish are eaten during the day, kugel is not eaten. *(Halichos Hatzaddikim, p. 306)*

There are those who place the ground fish in the skin of a cooked fish. One should chop the onions very finely so that

they are not recognizable. This is an important preparation for Shabbos, comparable to preparing the Shabbos candles.
(Nesiv Mitzvosecha, Shvil Emunah 6, sec. 5)

It is a *minhag* to eat filled fish to symbolize that the coming week should be filled with everything good.

Another reason for eating "gefilte" fish is to remind a person to "feel" the Shabbos in his heart.
(Minchas Shabbos, Oneg Shabbos ibid.)

Reb Yosef Dov of Brisk was careful to only eat gefilte fish on Shabbos since it does not have bones. When he was served other fish, he would chew the bones and suck them before discarding them, in order to avoid any prohibition of *borer*.
(Zichru Toras Moshe, sec. 20, *Kehillas Yom Tov, He'arah* 3)

Another reason for eating filled fish is so that one should not come to transgress the prohibitions of *borer* or *muktzeh* by either touching or picking out the bones.
(HaShabbos Noam Haneshamos, p. 67)

The Rebbe of Visket once gave *shirayim* of his fish to one of the people present at his table. The man replied that he does not eat gefilte fish. The Rebbe said, "A fool does not feel [the sanctity involved]."   *(Da'as Zekeinim, Pe'er Mikedoshim*, p. 19)

They would serve the Toldos Aharon Rebbe cooked fish and filled fish, with a small amount of carrots with sauce. He would first eat from the filled fish and then from the cooked fish. He ate the fish with challah.
(Zechor L'Avraham, Seder Leil Shabbos, p. 309)

The Sanzer Rebbe ate two types of fish each Shabbos. First, he ate pickled fish, then cooked fish.   *(Darchei Chaim*, sec. 58)

After the passing of the Sanzer Rav, the Minchas Elazar was at the Shabbos table of his son, the Shiniver Rav. When the fish was served, the Shiniver Rav first ate the cooked fish and then the pickled fish. His brother, the Gorlitzer Rebbe, asked him why his actions differ from those of his father, the Sanzer Rav, on the first Shabbos after his passing.

The Shiniver Rav replied, "When our father was Rav in Rudnick, fish was scarce. Father worried all week whether we would have fish for Shabbos. Therefore, at the beginning of each week, when there was fish available, he purchased it immediately and pickled it so that it should last until Shabbos. If there was fish available closer to Shabbos, he bought it and cooked it without vinegar. Since there is a principle that that which is constant comes first, when there were two types of fish in front of him, my father first ate that which he was accustomed to, the pickled fish that we usually had.

"When Father became Rav in Sanz, where there were fish available in abundance, he prepared the pickled fish on Erev Shabbos, as well. Since until then he ate the pickled fish first, he did not wish to change his custom, and continued doing so. I, however, never accepted this custom upon myself. Since I derive more pleasure from plain fish, I eat it first."

(*Sefer Darchei Chaim V'shalom*, sec. 394, p. 130)

The *pasuk* states, *Es Shabsosai tishmoru*—"My Shabbos you should keep," twice (*Shemos* 31:13; *Vayikra* 19:30). The Gemara states that all the fundamental aspects of Shabbos are double (*Midrash Shocher Tov* 92b), so there are those who eat two types of fish. (*Pnei Menachem, Amarim*)

The *Zohar* states that the food and drink, clothing, and every aspect of Shabbos should be more plentiful and better than that of during the week (*Eikev*, p. 271b, 272a), as the Gemara states that one should take pleasure in the Shabbos by eating large fish. This demonstrates that aside from increasing one's menu on Shabbos, each dish should be better and more than during the week, i.e. fatter or larger. Therefore, in Sanz they ate two types of fish each Shabbos—pickled and cooked.

(*Dvar Tzvi Kedushas Shabbos*, sec. 18)

We eat two types of fish on Shabbos because the words *yayin*, wine; *basar*, meat; and twice the word *dag*, fish, total the same numerical value as Yerushalayim, from where all blessing originates. A person should have this in mind while eating the fish and this will bring blessing to his sustenance the entire week.

(Zemiros Beis Sofrim, p. 103)

Large Fish

The Gemara states that one who takes pleasure in the Shabbos is granted his heart's desires. The Gemara then asks: *With what should a person take pleasure in the Shabbos? With a dish of spinach, large fish, and heads of garlic.*

(Shabbos 118b)

It is a mitzvah to eat large fish on Shabbos. Since they are big, they symbolize the higher worlds. The open eyes of fish allude to Hashem's watchful eyes over us within the higher worlds, about which it is written: *He does not slumber or sleep, the watchman of Yisrael* (Tehillim 121:4).

(Divrei Emes L'haRebbi M'Lublin, Mattos, s.v. Od l'pasuk)

It is said in the name of the Chiddushei Harim that the Shabbos itself desires large fish to be eaten.

(Or Pnei Yitzchak, p. 136)

In the song *Azamer B'shvachin*, written by the Arizal, we say the phrase *v'nunin im rachashin*. Reb Yaakov of Posen defines *nunin* as large fish, such as the one bought by Yosef Moker Shabbos, and *rachashin* as small fish eaten at *shalosh seudos*.

According to Kabbalah, one should serve one large fish and one small fish at every *seudas Shabbos*; one can be *mesakein* more *neshamos* through small fish.

(Yosef Ometz, sec. 550; Chemdas Hayamim 8:34)

In Poland, there was a fish called *plush*. When this fish was brought to Reb Yissachar Dov of Belz, he was very pleased.

He explained that the Gemara states that *oneg Shabbos* refers to eating large fish *(Shabbos* 118b). This is explained as "the largest of its kind." The *plush* fish was small in size and the largest of them was not bigger than any other average-size fish. Thus, with *plush* it was possible to eat the largest of them, whereas with other fish, the largest were so huge that it was not practical to obtain them for the Shabbos *seudos*.

(Halichos Tzaddikim, p. 298)

Placing Fish on the Reverse Side of the Plate

The Kapisher Rav once told his followers that he had heard from the Lisker Rebbe that one should eat the fish on the reverse side of the plate. The reason for this is that the *aleph-beis* in its correct order alludes to *rachamim*. The *aleph-beis* in backward order alludes to *din*. The word *dag*, fish, contains *aleph-beis* in its reverse order (first *dalet* and then *gimmel*). Therefore, we turn over the plate to demonstrate that we wish to reverse the *middas hadin* to *middas rachamim*.

The Kapisher Rav added that through charity and kindness one can also overturn harsh judgment. Therefore, *dag* is an acronym for *dalim gemol*, doing *chessed* with the poor.

(Ohr Hayashar V'hatov, p. 160)

When the fish was served to the guests at Reb Hershel Lisker's table, the Rebbe's attendant announced that all those present should turn over their plates and eat the fish on what is usually the underside of the plate. All the guests did so except for one person. The Rebbe, who had been immersed in holy thoughts, suddenly turned to this guest and said, "You wish your circumstances to be reversed, so turn over the plate."

From that point on the guest's fortune was overturned, and his livelihood took a turn for the better.

(Darchei Hayashar V'hatov, p. 299)

The Order of Eating the Fish

Tzaddikim were accustomed to placing the fish on the plate so that the head of the fish was to the right of the person eating it. They first ate the eye of the fish and then a bit from the fish on both side of the eyes and then underneath it. This formed the shape of the *nekudah segol* which corresponds to Bnei Yisrael who are referred to as the *Am Segulah* and are compared to fish. (*Pardes Hamelech*, p. 391)

Reb Shmuel Tzvi of Spink would first eat a *kebeitzah* of challah dipped into the sauce of the fish. Then he ate the head of the fish, took the eye, sucked it, and placed it in his pocket. Next, he took out some fish from the cheeks and then opened the head and searched for the brain.

After that, he ate the gefilte fish which was in the skin. He then dipped the challah into the fish sauce of the pickled fish twice and ate two bites. Then he dipped his challah into the sauce once. (See *Zemiros Tiferes Tzvi* for more reasons and insights)

One should begin eating the Shabbos fish by eating the eyes. (*Toras Avos, Shabbos* 77)

The Head of the Fish

There were *tzaddikim* who were accustomed to eating from the head of a fish on Friday night. (*Zemiros Divrei Yoel*, p. 85)

While eating the fish, Reb Aharon of Belz once pointed to a certain spot on the head of the fish. He remarked that his father, Reb Yissachar Dov of Belz, had told him that this piece is the choicest part of the fish. (*Halichos Hatzaddikim*, p. 337)

The Ba'al Avnei Nezer was accustomed to first eat the eyes or the brain of the fish. Once, as he began eating the head of the fish on Friday night, his face became aflame with holy excitement and he praised the taste of the fish several times. He then related a story of his father-in-law, the Kotzker Rebbe, who was once at the home of Reb Bunim of Peshischa. When Reb Bunim served the Kotzker Rebbe the head of the fish, Reb Bunim asked him, "Do you recognize this person?" [Reb Bunim was asking the Kotzker Rebbe if he recognized the *tzaddik* who had been reincarnated in that fish.]

(*Avir Haro'im*, vol. 2, sec. 373, 375)

The Eyes of the Fish

The reason for eating the eyes of a fish is because fish do not have eyelids and their eyes are constantly open. This alludes to the fact that Hashem's eyes are constantly upon those who fear Him, and He watches over them with tremendous compassion. (*Ta'amei Haminhagim*, sec. 306; *Minchas Yaakov*)

Reb Eliezer Yerucham, the son-in-law of the Divrei Chaim of Sanz, related that after the passing of the Divrei Chaim, they found many white balls in the pockets of his Shabbos clothing. These were the eyes of fish, particularly the *hecht* (pike) fish. The Divrei Chaim attached deep meaning to this custom.

(*Tehillos Chaim*, p. 286)

One of the chassidim of Reb Yaakov Tzvi of Parisov came to his Rebbe on Rosh Hashanah night and mentioned his daughter, who was blind. The Rebbe handed him the eye of the fish and said, "*Tov ayin hu yevorach*—'He who has a good eye will be blessed' (*Mishlei* 22:9)." He was hinting that blessing would come through this eye. He instructed the chassid to give the eye to his daughter to eat. He also told him to move to a different location in order to avoid an evil eye. The chassid followed the Rebbe's instructions and his daughter's sight was restored. (*Toras Rand*)

Reb Yosef of Yample, the son of Reb Yechiel Michel of Zlotchov, once ate the Shabbos *seudah* with his Rebbe, Reb Yisrael of Ruzhin. He noticed that the Rebbe began partaking of the fish by eating its eye. He tried to understand why the Rebbe did so.

Shabbos Secrets • *The Significance of Fish*

Chazal say that the fish remained alive by the *Mabul* because they did not sin. *Chazal* say that all sins begin with the eyes, since the eye sees, the heart desires, and then the hands commit the deed. Since the fish did not commit any sin (which originates from the eyes), Reb Yosef assumed that perhaps this was why the Rebbe began eating the fish with the eye.

The Ruzhiner Rebbe turned to him and said, "Your thoughts were indeed correct. Those are my intentions when eating the eye of the fish."

(*Tiferes Banim*, vol. 2, sec. 122; *Yismach Yisrael; Likutei Torah*)

The Rebbe of the Chemdas Hayamim would say the following while eating the eye of the fish (which refers to the eye of Hashem): *The open eye, the heavenly eye, the holy eye, the eye that observes, the eye that does not sleep or slumber, the eye that guards, the eye that is the source of all existence, should look upon on us with compassion.* (*Chemdas Hayamim* 8:34)

Not to Insult the Slices of Fish

If Reb Aharon of Belz wanted to reach a piece of fish, he would turn the plate around so that the piece was right in front of him. In this manner, he turned the fish plate many times while eating the fish. His intentions were not to pass over a slice of fish so as not to insult it. If the Rebbe was so careful not to embarrass a piece of fish, how much more so must one be careful with the honor of his friend.

(*Halichos Hatzaddikim*, p. 333; *Eidus Chayah*, p. 203)

Warm Fish

The Gemara (*Kiddushin* 25a) states that one of the elders of the city of Nezunia once asked Rav Hamnuna a question which he was unable to answer. The elders then asked Rav Hamnuna, "What is your name?"

He answered, "Rav Hamnuna."

They said to him, "It is not fitting to call you Hamnuna, but rather Karnuna."

Tosafos explains in the name of Rabbeinu Chananal that the elders intended to degrade Rav Hamnuna (ibid., s.v. *Hamnuna Karnuna*). Since Rav Hamnuna was unsuccessful in answering their question, it was not fitting to call him *"cham nuna,"* warm fish, which is a delectable, tasty dish, but rather *"kar nuna,"* which is cold, tasteless fish.

(*Chiddushei HaRitva, Kiddushin* 25a, s.v. *Lav Hamnuna*)

One should eat fish at night and not save it for the morning, since people like hot fish better than cold fish. Since it is not possible to eat hot fish on Shabbos day, one should eat fish at night. (*Aruch Hashulchan* 271)

Challah with Fish

Reb Mordechai of Lechovitch said that one should eat fish with challah, which is made of grains, since *dagan*, grains, and *dagim*, fish, have the same numerical value.

(*Ohr Yesharim*, p. 17)

Another reason for eating challah with the fish is that grain products have a tendency to warm the body and fish cools it down.

(*Levushei Machlul, Cheilek Michalalta Umilbashta, Kuntris Acharon*)

One of the Ropshitzer Chassidim would say when eating the fish, "Hashem, I am grateful to have challah and fish to eat. Hashem, please give me also a little bit of Shabbos with the challah [let me truly sense the Shabbos.]"

(*Mizekeinim Esbonan*, vol. 1, p. 179)

Weekday Bread with Fish

Many are accustomed to eating the fish on Friday night with bread that was baked for use during the week. The Shiniver Rav explains that this is because challos were once made with chicken fat (*Pri Megadim* 242), and fish and chicken cannot be eaten together.   (*Likutei Maharich, Seder Hisnahagus Erev Shabbos*)

The Satmar Rebbe, Reb Yoel Teitelbaum, added to the Shiniver Rav's words that, in truth, there are hidden reasons for this *minhag*, but the Shiniver Rav would conceal deep secrets in simple explanations.   (*Zemiros Divrei Yoel*, vol. 1, p. 314)

The Rebbe of Unsdorf gives another reason for this *minhag*. In earlier times, in addition to the challos, people would bake their entire week's supply of bread on Erev Shabbos. They ate some of this bread with the fish to demonstrate that this bread was also baked in honor of Shabbos and not solely for during the week.
(*Ta'amei Haminhagim*, sec. 247; *Beis Yisrael Kama, Mattersdorf*, p. 232)

Since Shabbos is the source of all blessing (see *Zohar*, Vol. 2, p. 88a), we eat weekday bread on Shabbos to bring blessing on our sustenance for the entire week.

We eat the bread specifically with the fish because the evil eye has no control over fish, and they multiply rapidly. Thus, fish symbolizes abundance and we wish to have abundant livelihood throughout the week.

This may be what *Chazal* are alluding to when they say, *Asei Shabbascha chol, v'al titztareich labriyos*. By eating a weekday food on Shabbos, one will have enough livelihood all week and not need to depend on others.   (*Magen Avos*, p. 227)

Weekday bread (which is made from grains other than wheat) complained to Hashem that it is not eaten on Shabbos or Yom Tov. The fish also complained that the mitzvos which are performed with animals, such as *shechitah,* are not performed with them. Therefore, we appease both the bread and the fish by eating a piece of weekday bread with the fish at the Shabbos *seudah*.   (*Brachah Shlomo Titchin*, p. 1)

Dipping Challah into Fish Sauce

One should eat a *kebeitzah* of challah at the beginning of the *seudah*, before the fish, in order not to forget to eat a *kebeitzah* in the timeframe of *kedei achilas pras*. We dip the slice of *Hamotzi* into the fish sauce prior to eating the fish to ensure that one is able to eat a *kebeitzah* in the proper amount of time, because that helps a person eat it faster.

(Minhagei Pri Eliezer, pp. 210, 222)

The Skulener Rebbe would dip his challah into the fish sauce so that it was easier for him to chew and eat in the time of *kedei achilas pras*. (<i>HaShabbos Noam Haneshamos</i>)

The Belzer Rebbes would dip the challah into the fish sauce. They would then have the plate removed from the table and not distribute *shirayim*. Only then did they begin eating the fish without the sauce. (<i>Halichos Hatzaddikim,</i> p. 328)

There are those who have the custom, after eating a *kezayis* of challah, to place seven pieces of the slice of *Hamotzi* into the fish sauce, and then eat them with the sauce before partaking of the fish. (<i>Piskei Teshuvos</i> 274:4)

The Kedushas Tzion of Bobov used a special bowl for the fish sauce. He dipped the challah into the fish sauce and only afterwards ate the actual fish. (<i>Magen Avos,</i> p. 224)

Reb Shlomo of Bobov once encountered a person who did not eat the fish sauce. Reb Shlomo told him, "All the Shabbos foods have an order and a reason," implying that one should not skip any dish. (Ibid.)

Dipping the challah into the fish sauce unifies the four levels of creation: *domeim*, *tzomei'ach*, *chai*, and *medaber*—inanimate objects, plants, animals, and human beings. These four categories correspond to the four letters in the Name of Hashem of *yud-keh-vav-keh*. The fish sauce is an inanimate object, the fish is a living being, the challah is derived from wheat which is a plant, and the person eating it is a human being. One who eats for the sake of Hashem in honor of Shabbos unifies all of the above and elevates it to its source, Hashem. *(Zemiros Noam Eliezer Skulen, p. 64)*

The Gemara in *Pesachim* states that the Jews at the Yam Suf, as they exited the sea on one side, were afraid that the Egyptians were exiting it on the other side. Hashem then commanded the sea to cast out the Egyptians so that the Jews could see them dead. The water obeyed this command, and when the Jews saw the dead Egyptians it reinforced their *emunah* in Hashem.

Fish sauce symbolizes the sea because it is the source of the fish. The sea caused the Jews to strengthen their *emunah* in Hashem by *Krias Yam Suf*, so we honor it by eating the fish first. *(Rabbi Dovid Meisels)*

Many are accustomed to eating the congealed sauce of the fish to allude to what the *pasuk* states in regard to *Krias Yam Suf*: *...the running water stood erect like a wall; the depths congealed in the heart of the sea (Shemos 15:8)*.

(As heard by author)

The *pasuk* in *Bereishis* states: *And the gathering of the waters, He called seas (Bereishis 1:10)*. Rashi explains that although it was one gathering, it was called seas, in the plural form, because each body of water is different. Because of this, the fish that come from different seas have different tastes, as Rashi states that one cannot compare the taste of fish that comes from the waters of Akko to the fish that comes from Aspamia. This demonstrates that the essence of the fish is the water from which it originates.

Fish sauce is the source of the cooked fish, and there is a *minhag* to dip the challah into it, to remind us that just as the taste of the fish comes from its source, everything in this world resembles its Source. *(Rabbi Dovid Meisels)*

Pepper in the Fish

Before eating the fish, the Skulener Rebbe would take a handful of pepper and sprinkle it on the fish, specifically the head. If there was no pepper on the table, he would request it and relate the following story:

The Berditchever Rav was once a guest at a certain Jew's home. While they were eating, the host asked the Berditchever Rav if he loved pepper. When the Berditchever Rav heard the question, he became filled with a tremendous fervor, and in his excitement, he jumped onto the table and exclaimed, "Do I love pepper? I love Hashem!"

The Skulener Rebbe would complete the story and say, "But in honor of Shabbos I allow myself to request a bit of pepper." It is assumed that the Rebbe had loftier reasons for doing so. The Rebbe would put so much pepper on his slice of fish that it appeared to be impossible to eat, but he ate it without any difficulty. *(HaShabbos Noam Haneshamos*, p. 64)

Reb Aharon of Belz once said in jest, "In the past, chassidim liked to put a lot of pepper in their fish, today's chassidim put a lot of sugar in their fish."

The Rebbe was alluding to the fact that although in the past generations one was able to accomplish much by being forceful, in our weak generation, after the Holocaust, one needs to act with pleasantness and softness.

The Paltishaner Rebbe related that Reb Aharon of Chernobyl was accustomed to cooking the fish with a large amount of pepper, and the fish was very spicy. When Reb Yissachar Dov of Belz ate at the home of his grandfather, Reb Aharon, it was very difficult for him to eat the fish since in Belz they cooked sweet fish and he was not accustomed to it. When Reb Aharon distributed *shirayim* of the fish, he gave Reb Yissachar Dov from the head of the fish, which did not have as much pepper. *(Halichos Hatzaddikim*, p. 311)

Eating Other Foods with Fish

There are those who eat radishes with the fish, and some eat them with the soup, because radish is a food that is reserved for Shabbos. The *Sefer Maggid Meisharim* writes that the angel who learned with the Beis Yosef once told him, "How did you want me to speak to you last night if you ate a large amount of radish? Do not eat it, except for a small amount on Shabbos."

(Maggid Meisharim, Bereishis, p. 8)

Reb Aharon of Karlin once traveled through Chernobyl. He went to visit Reb Aharon of Chernobyl, who requested that he stay with him for Shabbos. On Friday night, the Chernobyler Rebbe served fish with mustard. The Karliner Rebbe remarked, "For the Shabbos fish, mustard is not necessary." The Chernobyler Rebbe then instructed that the mustard be removed from the table. The next week, when the mustard was served, the Chernobyler Rebbe said, "Reb Aharon says that mustard is not necessary with Shabbos fish."

(Pri Yesha Aharon, p. 140)

Reb Aharon of Belz once said that there is no reason to put carrots on gefilte fish. He said that the fish vendors place carrots on the fish as a decoration, but it has no connection to fish. *(Halichos Hatzaddikim, p. 310)*

Many place carrots on gefilte fish because the evil eye has no control over fish and they are blessed with many offspring. Carrots in Yiddish are called *mehren*, which also means, "increasing" and hints to the blessing of many offspring.

Another reason for placing carrot slices on the fish is because sliced carrots resemble an eye, alluding to the eye of Hashem always watching us. (As heard from elderly chassidim)

The Gemara *(Nedarim* 54b) states that fish is hard on the eyes. Therefore, we eat carrots, which enhance eyesight, with the fish. *(Rabbi Dovid Meisels)*

Before eating the fish, there are those who are accustomed to eating the onions (*betzalim*) that were cooked with the fish, which alludes to the *tzeil*, shadow, of Hashem, as the *pasuk* (*Tehillim* 91:1) states, *b'tzeil Shakai yislonan*—"in the shadow of Hashem a person will shield himself." This demonstrates that we are sheltered in the shadow (i.e. protection) of Hashem at the *seudas Shabbos*. (*Minhagei Hayehudi Hakadosh of Peshischa*)

Separating Between Fish and Meat

One should wash his hands between eating the fish and the meat. He should also eat bread that is soaked in liquid, which fulfills both *kaniach* and *hadachah*, wiping and rinsing out one's mouth. Some are of the opinion that this is not necessary because one is permitted to eat fish and meat one after the other, as long as they are not cooked together (*Hagahos Mordechai*). Indeed, while some do have the custom to wash their hands between fish and meat, most do not, but one should eat and drink between the fish and the meat.

(*Shulchan Aruch, Yoreh De'ah* 116:3)

The *Tur* writes the following about rinsing one's mouth between milk and meat, but it can also be applied to rinsing one's mouth between fish and meat:

One needs to perform *kaniach*, wiping out one's mouth well—accomplished by eating; and *hadachah*, rinsing out one's mouth—accomplished by drinking. One can wipe out his mouth with any food that he wishes, except for flour, dates, and vegetables, which stick to a person's gums and do not wipe out the mouth properly. Afterwards, one should perform *hadachah* and rinse his mouth by drinking either wine or water.

There are those who soak the bread in the wine or water and then eat it so that they fulfill *kaniach* and *hadachah* at the same time. However, it is better to perform *kaniach* and *hadachah* separately. (*Tur, Yoreh De'ah*, sec. 89)

Shabbos Secrets • *The Significance of Fish*

The Tur writes the following words *(Orach Chaim 116)*: *My esteemed father was accustomed to washing his hands between meat and fish, according to the principle that one is required to be more careful with something which poses a danger than with that which is forbidden.*

It is also advisable to drink something between fish and meat so that the two don't get digested together, because the process of digestion resembles the process of cooking.
(*Shelah Hakadosh, Sha'ar Ha'osiyos; Emek Brachah*, sec. 5)

The Rosh was accustomed to washing his hands between the fish and meat. He soaked a piece of bread in wine and ate it between the fish and meat in order to fulfill both *kaniach* and *hadachah*. Therefore, after the fish, many are accustomed to dipping a piece of challah into the Kiddush wine.
(*Tur, Yoreh De'ah* 116, *Prishah*)

Before drinking whiskey after fish, one should dip a piece of challah into it and eat it. This is similar to what is mentioned in the *Rema*, that one should eat bread dipped into liquid so that he fulfills *kaniach* and *hadachah* between meat and fish. (*Rema, Yoreh De'ah*, 116:3; See *Be'er Heitev, Orach Chaim*, 174:8)

Drinking Whiskey after Fish

After eating the fish, one should drink whiskey. *Tzaddikim* have said that by doing so one alludes to the Name of Hashem of *Shakai*. The first letters of the words *dagim* (fish) and *yayin saraf* (whiskey) (*dalet, yud,* and *sin*) are the same letters as the word *Shakai*. Therefore, one should not wash his hands until after drinking the whiskey, so as not to form a break in the letters of *Shakai*. (*Darkei Chaim V'shalom*, sec. 396)

However, there were those (including the Satmar Rebbe) who did wash their hands after the fish before drinking the whiskey.
(*Zemiros Divrei Yoel*)

The *minhag* in Belz was to bring a cup of whiskey to the table after the fish and not place the bottle on the table. Once, when a bottle of whiskey was brought to the table, Reb Aharon of Belz exclaimed, "Am I a drunkard that you place an entire bottle on the table?" (*B'kedushaso Shel Aharon*, p. 441)

One should not drink water after eating the fish, as it is harmful. Perhaps that is why some have the custom of drinking whiskey instead.
(*Moed Katan* 11a, *Tosafos*, s.v. *Kavra*; *Digas Hayam*, p. 115)

Reb Shalom of Kaminka once asked the Sanzer Rav: If two types of fish are eaten, does that necessitate drinking whiskey twice?

It is said in the name of Reb Simchah Bunim of Peshischa that some are accustomed to eating herring at the beginning of the *seudah*, before the other fish. There are those who also drink some whiskey between the herring and the fish, and those who don't.

Reb Simchah Bunim said that this depends on one's custom with regard to *Pirkei Avos* on Shabbos. When reciting *Pirkei Avos*, we start with the phrase of *Kol Yisrael*...which affirms that every Jew has a portion in *Olam Haba*. After reciting *Pirkei Avos*, we say *Ratzah Hakadosh Baruch Hu l'zakos es Yisrael*, which states that Hashem wished to give us merit, and therefore He gave us the Torah and many mitzvos.

At the end of the summer, there are several Shabbasos during which two *perakim* of *Pirkei Avos* are recited. At those times, some recite these two *pesukim* between each *perek* and some only say them at the beginning and end of their entire recitation of *Pirkei Avos*.

This is how one knows whether he should drink whiskey between the herring and the fish. If one recites these *pesukim* between the two *perakim,* he should drink whiskey between the herring and the fish. If he does not recite these *pesukim*, then he does not need to drink whiskey between them.

Reb Eliyahu Yosef of Rozhvadov explains that fish cools down the body and whiskey warms it up. So too, *Pirkei Avos* a can cause a person to feel broken and discouraged when he realizes how much he needs to improve. Therefore, we say the pesukim of *Kol Yisrael* and *Ratzah Hakadosh Baruch Hu,* which give a person encouragement and joy.

One who feels discouraged when reciting *Pirkei Avos* and needs to "warm himself up" immediately between each *perek*, should also drink whiskey between the herring and the fish. One who does not feel that way need not drink the whiskey between the two.   (*Kol Mevaser* vol. 2, p. 254; *Derech Tzaddikim* 29b)

After the fish, the Lelover Rebbe would drink whiskey and then rub the remainder onto his palms and sniff it. Some say this was so that none of it should go to waste. Another reason is that since his *minhag* was not to wash his hands between fish and meat, he sniffed the whiskey to demonstrate that he placed it on his hands in order to wash them.   (*Minhagei Lelov*)

If there was *sheichar*, beer, on the table, the Munkatcher Rebbe was accustomed to drinking it after the whiskey. It was once heard from him that this is an allusion to the *Geulah*, as Hashem told Rachel Imeinu, *"Yesh sechar lepe'ulaseich, veshavu banim l'gevulam"* (*Yirmiyahu* 31:15). *Sechar* contains the same letters as *sheichar*.   (*Darkei Chaim V'shalom*, sec. 396)

Drinking Wine after the Fish

There are those who drink the remainder of the Kiddush wine after drinking the whiskey.   (*Minhagei Pri Eliezer*, p. 222)

Many are accustomed to drinking wine after the fish, since they do not consider whiskey to be a beverage that is drunk on Shabbos, but rather during the week on a *yahrtzeit*.

(*Mishmei D'Reb Tanchum*, sec. 18)

In the *pasuk, Zachor es yom haShabbos* (which is a reference to Kiddush), the word *zachor* has the same numerical value as the word *kavra* (fish, in Aramaic). This is a hint that one should drink wine after fish. *(Shem MiShimon, Yoreh De'ah, sec. 13)*

The Apter Rav writes that the *mann* had the ability to taste like anything in the world except fish (Eikev, *V'ya'ancha v'yeiravcha*). The Chasam Sofer writes that he heard that the *mann* did not have the taste of wine *(Parshas Devarim* [beginning], 5594). Since the Shabbos food tastes like the *mann*, perhaps we drink wine after the fish to complete *oneg Shabbos* with every taste. *(Rabbi Dovid Meisels)*

Chapter 11
Splendid Soup

Soup from Mashiach's Bowl

Reb Aharon of Belz related that the Chozeh of Lublin once instructed his attendant to take all the soup and give it to a person who was standing near the oven. The man ate all of the soup and did not leave any over. When the attendant returned to the Rebbe with the empty bowl, the Rebbe said, "This man is Mashiach, and he came specifically to eat the soup." The chassidim immediately went to find the man but he was no longer there. They then began calling the bowl from which he ate, "Mashiach's bowl." Reb Yehoshua of Belz bought this bowl for a large sum of money. *(Temidim K'sidram*, p. 1204)

Soup with Lokshen

The *minhag* on Friday night is that after the fish, we eat chicken soup in order to fulfill *oneg Shabbos*. This is based on the Gemara *(Brachos* 44a) which states that a *seudah* without soup is not considered a *seudah*.

Some eat two bowls of soup; one bowl of soup with noodles *(lokshen)*, and one bowl of soup with a type of pastry called *kezil*. The Darkei Teshuvah and Sanzer Rav had this custom.
(Darkei Chaim V'shalom, sec. 394)

There is a *minhag* to eat the soup with long and thin noodles, *lokshen,* which become tangled together. This symbolizes that Shabbos is a time of unity and harmony, as we say, "*Shabbos Shalom*." *(Imrei Pinchas*, vol. 1, *Sha'ar HaShabbos*, sec. 29)

Lokshen is similar to the words *"lo kashin,"* not difficult. Since *Chazal* say that earning a livelihood is difficult (*Pesachim* 118a), and all the blessings of the week are dependent on Shabbos, we eat *lokshen* to signify that our livelihood should be earned without difficulty.

(*Magen Avos,* p. 240; *Zemiros Nitei Aharon,* p. 115; *Tuv Ta'am*)

The root word of *lokshen* is an acronym for *"L'kavod* **Shabbos Kodesh.**" (*Zemiros Nitei Aharon,* ibid.)

Reb Pinchas of Koritz would say that the more elevated a person is, the more refined his eating habits. He would cite as proof that gentiles do not derive pleasure from eating soup with *lokshen*, but only from coarse foods.

(*Imrei Pinchas, Sha'ar Gimmel, Seder Hayom V'inyanei Tefillah*)

In Sanz, they would eat soup with long *lokshen* to correspond to the letter *vav* and chickpeas to correspond to the letter *yud* of the *Shem Havayah*. In Shiniva, they would eat small lokshen to correspond to the *yud,* and long beans to correspond to the *vav*. (*Yud Gimmel Oros*)

It is the custom of Jews to eat soup with *lokshen* on Friday night in order to abolish harsh decrees, since *lokshen* contains the words *"lo kashin,"* not difficult.

(*HaShabbos Noam Haneshamos,* p. 74)

Reb Mordechai of Nadvorna would say that one should eat *lokshen* (which in is the shape of threads) on Friday night to symbolize that a person is endowed with special grace from Hashem known as *chut shel chessed* (a thread of grace).

(*Chemdas Yamim,* p. 52)

Reb Elimelech of Lizhensk once lodged at an inn and heard the innkeeper complain to his wife, "How much longer will we need to eat kasha? We should be able to eat *lokshen* already."

The Ziditchover Rebbe gave the following explanation to this story. We shouldn't have *kashios* (questions) on Hashem.

Rather, it should be *lo kashin*; we should not have questions anymore.

This idea may be alluded to in the phrase, *Kashin mezonosav shel adam k'Krias Yam Suf*—"a person's sustenance is hard like the splitting of the Yam Suf" (Pesachim 118a). A person sometimes has difficulty understanding Hashem in regard to his livelihood and may ask questions. The answer to this is *Krias Yam Suf*. Just as at *Krias Yam Suf* even a maidservant was able to perceive Hashem's greatness, a person should constantly look to see the hand of Hashem in his life and in his quest to earn a living. *(Ayalah Shluchah, Yisro)*

Reb Yerachmiel Moshe of Kozhnitz would eat soup with *lokshen*. He once quoted the *pasuk* in *Ovadiah* (1:18), *Ubeis Eisav l'kash*, which he interpreted to mean that by eating *lokshen* in the soup, one negates the power of Eisav. During the week, he did not eat *lokshen* since it alludes to the lengthening of the *galus*.

(Sipran Shel Tzaddikim, Ma'areches Mem, Hanhagos, sec. 16)

Reb Yitzchak, the son of Reb Moshe of Rozhvadov, was going to be having surgery and was forbidden to eat on the Shabbos before the surgery. He requested that he be given, at the very least, "one noodle" in honor of Shabbos. His strong feelings about Shabbos food were evident.

(Mishmei D'Rabbi Tanchum, sec. 13)

There is a story told of a chassid who knocked on his neighbor's door to request a bit of *lokshen* on Friday night, as he did not have any. The neighbor replied that he only had raw *lokshen*. Undaunted, the chassid took some *lokshen* and ate it raw. *(Shulchan Menachem, Parshas Beshalach)*

Square Noodles

During the Yamim Nora'im we *daven* to Hashem to rule over all four corners of the earth. Therefore, there are those who have the custom of putting square noodles (which have four corners) into their soup during the month of Tishrei.

Another reason for this custom is so that one should not mention the word *din* (harsh decrees) by saying *"dinne lokshen"* (thin *lokshen*). *(Zemiros Tiferes Tzvi,* p. 109)

The Belzer chassidim have the *minhag* to put *farfel* in their soup, instead of *lokshen.* It is said in the name of the Rebbe of Maglintza that *lokshen,* since it is long, symbolizes the length of *galus.* (See *Sifran Shel Tzaddikim, Ma'areches Mem, Hanhagos,* sec. 16)

The Debreciner Rav was once a guest at the Shiniver Rav's home for Shabbos. The Shiniver Rav ate his soup with small square *lokshen* in it. He then explained to the Debreciner Rav, "Next week is my mother's *yahrtzeit.* My mother invested a lot of effort into our upbringing and was very particular that we should eat our food with proper manners. When we were young, she would constantly instruct us to eat the *lokshen* in a dignified manner. Finally, she decided to cook square noodles and it solved the problem. Therefore, this week I told my Rebbetzin that she should cook square *lokshen,* for the merit of my mother's soul." *(Gilyon Kerem Shlomo)*

Beans in the Soup

The Lisker Rebbe says that one who eats beans every Friday will not leave This World without repenting.

(Ohr Hayashar V'hatov, p. 161)

Some say that beans have the merit of being eaten on Shabbos because only kosher animals eat beans.

(Tiferes Avos, Minhagei Maharyav, p. 71)

The Satmar Rebbe added long *lokshen,* soup nuts, and beans to his soup. *(Zemiros Divrei Yoel,* vol. 1, p. 94)

It was heard from the Chozeh of Lublin that he ate beans in the soup because they are in the shape of the letter *yud,* and *lokshen* is in the shape of a *vav*, alluding to the *Shem Havayah*. *(Kedushas Naftali, p. 240)*

The Sanzer Rav was once served soup without beans. He explained that the beans are in the shape of a *yud*, the *lokshen* in the shape of the letter *vav*, and the plate and the soup are the two letter *hehs*. He requested that they bring beans from a neighbor. *(Zemiros Divrei Yoel, vol. 1, p. 94, He'arah sec. 3)*

The Sanzer Rav writes that it is questionable whether chickpeas require a *brachah* when eaten during a *seudah*. The Sanzer Rav would eat some challah with his first and last bites.

If one eats chickpeas during the *seudah* (i.e. not in the soup) most Shabbasos of the year, it is considered part of his *seudah* and he does not need to recite a *brachah*, although he should eat some bread at the beginning and the end. However, one who only eats chickpeas in the soup, and only occasionally eats them on their own during the *seudah* (such as at a *shalom zachar*), needs to recite a *brachah*.
(Os Shalom, Hilchos Milah 65:33, in the name of the Divrei Chaim)

Gur chassidim do not recite a *brachah* on beans that are eaten during the Shabbos *seudah*, since they consider them a regular food eaten at the Shabbos *seudah*. The Divrei Chaim holds differently, because beans weren't such an integral part of the *seudah* where he lived. *(Michtavei Torah, Gur, Michtav 37)*

The Toldos Aharon Rebbe ate soup with *lokshen* and beans on Friday night. He was careful that each spoonful contained at least one noodle and one bean.
(Zechor L'Avraham, Seder Leil Shabbos, sec. 35)

The *Midrash Aggadah* in *Vayigash* states that Yosef Hatzaddik sent his father Yaakov from *"the good of the land Mitzrayim,"* which refers to a certain type of bean which is soft, good for the elderly, and alleviates worries and troubles.

Once Yaakov would know that Yosef was alive, he would no longer have any reason to worry and the beans shouldn't have been necessary. Yosef realized, though, that since Yaakov was so accustomed to worrying, it had become part of his nature and he would need a remedy for it.

The *Yerushalmi* (*Yuma* 1:4) states that on Erev Yom Kippur, the *kohen gadol* was not allowed to eat this type of bean since it induces sleep, and he needed to be awake all night.

(*Divrei Negidim, Vayigash*)

According to the above midrash, it is a *minhag* to eat beans at a *shalom zachar* and many eat them every Friday night, since it relaxes a person and helps him sleep.

(*Amud Aish, Aish Das, Vayigash*)

Spices and Salt in the Soup

There are those who put spices in the soup.

(*Darkei Chaim,* Sanz, sec. 58)

Reb Tzvi Hersh of Liska testified that the Ruzhiner Rebbe ate an extremely minimal amount. He would eat three or four spoonfuls of soup. When the Lisker Rebbe once tasted the soup, it was so salty and spicy that it was almost inedible.

(*Ner Yisrael*, vol. 4, p. 179)

Reb Shlomo of Karlin was once a guest at the home of the Ba'al Hatanya. The Ba'al Hatanya's wife wanted to prepare the Shabbos food in honor of the special guest, but the usual cook claimed that since she cooked each week, she deserved to cook that week as well. The Ba'al Hatanya told his wife that if she just adds a bit of salt to the pot, she has fulfilled the mitzvah of serving a *talmid chacham*, so that is what she did.

Many people heard of this, and one by one they came, without each other's knowledge, and added some salt to the soup. When Shabbos arrived, and the soup was served, Reb Shlomo of Karliner could not eat it because it was so salty.

However, the Ba'al Hatanya ate the soup. When the Ba'al Hatanya noticed that Reb Shlomo was not eating, he thought that perhaps it was because the soup was missing salt. The Ba'al Hatanya added some more salt to the soup and returned it to Reb Shlomo.

Reb Shlomo then asked the Ba'al Hatanya if he did not taste how salty it was. The Ba'al Hatanya replied that he once heard a beautiful Torah thought from the Mezritcher Maggid and since then he was so inspired and overcome by those thoughts that his ability to taste food had disappeared.

(*Ma'aseh Hashem Dinov*, p. 101)

Challah in the Soup

There are those who put pieces of challah into their soup. The soup then contains *yoch*, soup; *beblich*, beans; and *koilitch*, challah, which forms the acronym of *yud*, *beis*, *kuf*, one of the names of Hashem. These letters are also an acronym of phrase in Tehillim (20:10), *ya'aneinu b'yom kareinu*—"He will answer us on the day we call," and also have the same numerical value as several names of Hashem.

(*Even Yisrael*, vol. 2; *Darkei Hayashar V'hatov*)

On Friday night, seven pieces of challah are put into the soup, and on Yom Tov, five pieces, corresponding to the number of people called up to the Torah. (*Elyah Rabbah*, 167:2)

Reb Hillel of Kalamaya once spent Shabbos with the Divrei Chaim of Sanz. On Friday night, he was surprised to see the Rebbe putting challah into the hot soup, since according to halachah one may not put a baked dish into a hot cooked dish that is still *yad soledes bo* (very hot).

The Sanzer Rav replied that the soup was no longer so hot. He placed Reb Hillel's hand into the soup to prove it to him, but Reb Hillel quickly jumped away because the soup was too hot for him to touch. (*Magen Avos*, p. 242)

There are those who place the challah in their mouth and not directly into the soup, since the soup is hot, and ideally one should not put a baked food into it, even if the soup is already in a *kli sheini* (second vessel).

(Based on *Shulchan Aruch, Orach Chaim* 318:5)

There was once a guest of the Butchatcher Rebbe who placed challah into his boiling soup. The Rebbe publicly chastised him for violating the halachah. Although there is a *minhag* to eat soup, beans, and challah together, he held that one should not place the challah directly into the soup.

(*Zemiros Shabbos Kadshecha*, p. 72)

Reb Menachem Mendel Hager of Vizhnitz would put pieces of challah into his soup while eating it. The number of pieces he put in it, and his intentions in doing this, are not known.

(*Tzava'as Abba, Keren Zayin, Hakehunah*, sec. 6)

How to Eat Soup

A pious person does not bend toward the soup but rather lifts the spoon towards his mouth, as it is not fitting for a person to lower himself to his food. (See *Igra D'pirka*, sec. 16)

One should eat in a dignified manner and be careful to cut the *lokshen* into small pieces so that it should not fall off the spoon. (*Magen Avos*, p. 241)

Several *talmidim* once ate at the Friday night *seudah* of Reb Benzion of Bobov. One of the *talmidim* tilted the soup plate away from him so that he could finish his soup.

The Rebbe turned to the *talmid* and told him, "Don't tilt the plate like that—lift the other side, which is further away from you, so that the food comes towards you.

"If you wonder what the difference is, I will tell you. Tilting the plate away from you is considered mannerly by those who wish to be modern and progressive; therefore, it is proper for someone who possesses fear of Heaven to do the opposite.

"In truth, there are many behaviors which a person should avoid, although there is no prohibition against them in the Torah. How does a person know if he should distance himself from something if it is not written in the Torah? If he sees an issue that *resha'im* are working hard to strengthen, he can clearly know that although it is not an outright prohibition, he should distance himself as far as possible from it.

"We see this concept in the words of Rashi in *Parshas Vayishlach*, where Rashi states, 'I lived with Lavan and kept the 613 mitzvos, *v'lo lamaditi mima'asav hara'im*, and I did not learn from Lavan's wicked ways.'

"*V'lo*— I knew that whatever was *not* included in the 613 mitzvos, *lamaditi*—I learned, *mima'asav hara'im*—from his bad deeds. By seeing what Lavan did, I knew what *not* to do." (*Pri Hakerem*, issue 16, p. 6)

Tzaddikim had special intentions regarding the amount of spoonfuls of soup that they ate. It has been said that if one does not eat more than 21 spoonfuls of soup, he will be able to learn after the *seudah* instead of falling asleep immediately.

(Elderly chassidim)

Reb Mordechai Chaim of Slonim would say that all sevens are holy: the seventh hour of the day—which is Minchah time, the seventh hour of the night—*chatzos*, the seventh day of the week—Shabbos, the seventh month of the year—Tishrei, the seventh year—*shemittah*. When the Rebbe would reach the seventh spoonful of soup he would stop eating.

(*Mizekeinim Esbonan*, vol. 1, p. 170)

The *Siddur Reb Shabsi* states that all of our eating on Shabbos, even if it is more than usual, is entirely spiritual, and one does not need to restrain himself in any way. However, in a different location in the siddur, he writes that one should break his desire for food and restrain himself from eating, even on Shabbos.

This contradiction can be reconciled as follows: One should decide in advance how much he will eat and then take pleasure in eating that amount. For example, one should decide how many spoonfuls of soup that he wishes to eat before he begins eating it.
(Divrei Torah Mahadura 2, sec. 2)

The Kolshitzer Rebbe once demonstrated how the Divrei Chaim of Sanz ate the soup. He held the spoon like a child, with his palms and not with his fingers. When he ate the soup, his hands shook from what appeared to be weakness, but it was in fact intentional, so that the soup should spill. He didn't place the spoon in his mouth, but poured it into his mouth, so much of it spilled. With all that, he only took three to four spoons of soup and would pause between each spoonful. This was to show that he ate with a lot of *yiras Shamayim*.
(Divrei Chanah, vol. 2, p. 356)

Reb Itzikel of Pshevorsk would only eat a half or quarter of a spoonful of soup at once—never an entire spoonful.
(Zichron Tzaddik, p. 193)

The Ruzhiner Rebbe said that a special *neshamah* comes to each person on Friday night, but if one is not careful, he can drown it in his soup. In other words, if one eats his soup gluttonously, he can lose his *neshamah yeseirah*.
(Ma'amar Mordechai, Slonim, vol. 1, p. 71)

Chapter 12
The Main Course

Meat on Shabbos

On Shabbos, the *nitzotzos* (holy sparks) which are in the food that is eaten are rectified and the food itself is uplifted. This is especially true with the meat. Since it is the most favorite food, it therefore contains more significant *nitzotzos* than other foods and can be brought closer to Hashem.

(Me'or V'shemesh, Haftoras Shabbos Rosh Chodesh)

It is written in the *Shulchan Aruch* that on Shabbos one should serve as much meat, wine, and delicacies as he is able. One who honors the Shabbos more, whether with his actions, his clothing, or with eating and drinking, is praised. One should increase the quantity of the meat he prepares, even if he does not need that amount and will only eat a small portion. *(Nimukei Orach Chaim 271:1)*

When Hashem gave the Jews the *slav* (meat) in the *midbar*, the *pasuk* in *Bamidbar* (11:19) states: *You shall eat it not one day, not two days, not five days, not ten days, and not twenty days. But even for a full month...*

Why does the *pasuk* not immediately state that they would have it for a month? Rabbi Yehudah Hachassid explains that all the numbers in the *pasuk* total 68, which corresponds to the 68 days of the year when we are required to eat meat: The 52 Shabbasos of the year, the six remaining days of Pesach and seven days of Sukkos, one day of Shavuos, and two days of Rosh Hashanah.

(Rabbeinu Ephraim, Beha'aloscha; Chayei Yitzchak)

The Gemara states that Reb Abba would purchase meat from 13 butchers for Shabbos *(Shabbos* 119a). Rashi explains that he wanted to have the best possible meat for Shabbos, so he bought a large quantity to see which was the best. The Gemara states that Shammai Hazakein ate meat in honor of Shabbos all his life. Whenever he would find a choice animal during the week, he would set it aside for Shabbos. If he later found a superior animal, he would eat the first one during the week and save the new one for Shabbos.

From this one can conclude that the main *oneg Shabbos* is from meat. *(Likutei Maharich*, vol. 2, p. 38b)

Meat can cause a person to be haughty. Chazal state that a person should minimize his intake of meat so that his heart is humble before Hashem. However, on Shabbos, Yom Tov and Rosh Chodesh, it is a mitzvah for a person to increase his intake of meat. Since on these special days the *Shechinah* rests between us (as explained in the *Zohar*), one does not need to be concerned that he will come to haughtiness. Similarly, the *kohanim* ate a large amount of meat from the *korbanos*, and the *Shechinah* protected them from haughtiness.

(Nefesh Yeseirah, Ma'areches Shin, sec. 43)

The Sifri states about the *pasuk* in *Beha'aloscha* (10:10), *On the days of your rejoicing,* that this refers to Shabbos. Many say that it follows then that one must eat meat on Shabbos just like he does on Yom Tov. The Gra and others opine that this does not refer to Shabbos, because on Shabbos there is no obligation to be joyful, but only to have *oneg*, pleasure. Rabbeinu Yonah states that though one does have to rejoice on Shabbos, there is still no obligation to eat meat on Shabbos.

Indeed, Shabbos is a day on which a person can feel a special joy, which is a happiness that Hashem bestows upon him regardless of his actions. Accordingly, there is no obligation to eat meat on Shabbos, because there is no obligation to rejoice. The joy that exists on Shabbos is a gift from Hashem.

(Dvar Tzvi Shabbos, sec. 62)

Another reason for eating meat on Shabbos is based on the Gemara in *Bava Kamma* (71b): *Rava asked Rav Nachman a question and Rav Nachman answered him. The next day, Rav Nachman came back to Rava with the opposite reply. Rav Nachman explained that the reason that he did not tell him this reply the day before was because he had not eaten meat from an ox.* The commentaries explain that eating meat from an ox brings a person serenity so he can better understand Torah. Since Shabbos is a day for the *neshamah*, we eat meat in order to have tranquility so we can learn Torah properly.

(*Rabbi Dovid Meisels*)

The Chazon Ish once related the following story about the Bach, Reb Yoel Sirkis, and his son-in-law, the Taz. The Bach had pledged to support his son-in-law, and as part of the agreement, he served him a portion of meat each day so that he should have the strength to toil in Torah and the service of Hashem.

As time passed, the Bach became impoverished and he did not have the means to serve his son-in-law meat as he had promised. He purchased the lung of an animal, which was less expensive, and served that in the place of meat. To everyone's astonishment, the next day the Taz took the Bach to a *din Torah* for breaking their agreement. The *beis din* ruled in favor of the Bach, that the lung is considered meat.

The Taz then explained why he acted in such a startling manner. On the day that he was served the lung of an animal, he felt weak and was unable to learn as he usually did. This caused an accusation in Heaven to be brought against the Bach. Therefore, the Taz was forced to bring his father-in-law to *beis din* so that if the *beis din* would rule that the lung is also considered meat, then the Bach would be exonerated from the accusations in Heaven.

The Chazon Ish concluded that from this story we can see how precious one moment of Torah learning in depth is considered in Heaven. (*Pe'er Hador*, vol. 2, p. 342)

There are those who eat two kinds of meat on Shabbos: either roasted and cooked chicken, or chicken and meat.

The Ba'al Hatosafos cites the *Midrash Shochar Tov*, that every aspect of Shabbos is double. Therefore, it is appropriate to eat two types of meat. (*Darkei Chaim V'shalom*, sec. 394, He'aros)

One should eat chicken before meat, lean meat before fatty meat, and cooked meat before roasted meat, since one should first eat that which is easier on the digestive system.

(*Kaf Hachaim* 157:38)

Basar (meat) is comprised of the words *ba sar*, the minister came, meaning it is an important food. It is said that Shabbos without meat is like a king without his ministers (see *Rambam, Hilchos Shabbos* 30:1). Shabbos provides food for the seven days of the week. (*Nifla'os Misorasecha, Orah V'simchah, Megillas Esther*, p. 55)

The Kol Bo states that everything in this world has a spiritual *sar*, an angel, appointed over it. During the first Friday night of creation, Hashem sat on His Throne and called to all the *sarim* to come before Him. Then Hashem rose from His Throne and placed the *sar* of Shabbos on it. When the *sarim* saw this they all stood up and recited song and praise to the *sar* of Shabbos.

Therefore, we eat *basar* on Shabbos because it consists of the words *ba sar*, alluding to the great honor of the *sar* of Shabbos. Perhaps that is why we sing *zemiros* after we eat the meat, to hint to the fact that the songs were only sung after the *sar* of Shabbos sat on the Heavenly Throne.

(*Rabbi Dovid Meisels*)

Not Eating a Lot of Meat

One should not eat an excessive amount of meat, even on Shabbos. (*Maggid Meisharim, Azharos V'sikunim V'siyagim*, sec. 6)

Reb Moshe, the son of the Ba'al Hatanya, did not eat meat on Shabbos. When asked if it is a mitzvah to eat meat on Shabbos, he replied that one is not obligated to do so, and in general, it is not so terrible if one minimizes mitzvos that involve eating and drinking. *(Igros Kodesh, Admor Hareitz,* vol. 7, p. 18)

Meat with Challah

The *minhag* of *tzaddikim* is to eat the meat with bread or challah, and not by itself. This can be derived from the words of the Rosh *(Brachos, Keitzad Mevarchin, Siman* 26) who gives meat as an example of something which is *machmas seudah*, connected to the *seudah*, because meat is eaten with bread. Reb Baruch of Gorlitz was accustomed to doing so.

(Baruch She'amar, p. 289)

When Reb Mordche of Nadvorna would celebrate a *bris,* he would serve the following meal: challah, fish, fish sauce, meat, and then fried meat. The Rebbe instructed that the challah should be distributed together with the fried meat. He would quip—playing on the words of the *pasuk, Hu nosein lechem l'chol basar*—"He gives bread to all flesh"—that one should give [eat] bread every time he eats meat. *(Raza D'avda,* p. 152)

All Parts of the Chicken

Chassidim say that one should honor the Shabbos by eating from every part of the chicken over Shabbos. On Friday night, one should eat the chicken bottoms, the liver, and *gedishechtz*— which is made from the wings and the necks of the chickens (which some eat on Erev Shabbos as *russil*). At the day *seudah,* one should eat *p'tcha* and *galaretta*, made from the legs and the heads of the chicken. After the kugel, one should eat the tops of the chicken called *kalte oif* (cold cuts), as a *segulah* that the week should be filled with *kol tuv*, everything good (similar in sound to *kalte oif*). (As heard from elderly chassidim)

Sucking the marrow from the bones alludes to pulling out *kedushah* from evil forces. *(Panim Yafos, Vayechi)*

Several *tzaddikim* would distribute the chicken bones *(bein* in Yiddish) as a *segulah* to be blessed with a son *(bein* in Hebrew).
(Shalsheles Spinka, p. 448; *Ro'eh Even Yisrael*, Pshevorsk, p. 165)

On Friday night, prior to reciting *Birkas Hamazon*, they served the Sanzer Rav a roasted male chicken. He would eat a small piece from under the wings and he did not distribute *shirayim* to anyone. The chicken was then put away for the day *seudah*, when the Rav ate from it after reciting *divrei Torah*.

On the Shabbos of a *shalom zachor*, the Rebbe distributed some of the chicken to the family of the newborn.

(Darkei Chaim, Sanz, Hanhagos, sec. 71)

Chrein with the Meat

Belzer chassidim had the *minhag* of eating *chrein* with the meat. Reb Shea of Belz explained that all eating on Shabbos corresponds to the *avodah* in the Beis Hamikdash, and the Shabbos *seudah* corresponds to the *korbanos*. The *kohanim* ate the *korbanos* with mustard or other condiments, and therefore meat on Shabbos is eaten with *chrein*.

(Shulchan Aruch, Yoreh De'ah, 61:2)

The *Sefer Likutei Yosher* writes that the Mahariv would ensure that there was *chrein* on the table on Shabbos and Yom Tov, comparing it to the *Korban Shelamim,* which the *kohanim* were required to eat with mustard. *(Otzar Yad Hachaim*, sec. 1, 045)

Meat should be flavored with sharp seasonings similar to the meat of *matnos kehunah*, which the *kohanim* ate with mustard. Perhaps this is the intention of the Gemara in *Brachos* that states that a *seudah* which does not include a sharp appetizer is not considered a *seudah*.

Chassidim mention another reason for eating *chrein* with meat. In case there is a doubt about its kashrus, the *chrein* takes away some of the taste of the meat, so one is not benefiting directly from the meat, but from the meat and *chrein* together. *(Magen Avos*, p. 242)

The Imrei Chaim of Vizhnitz was accustomed to serving *chrein* in remembrance of our Exodus from Mitzrayim, similar to the *maror* eaten on Seder night *(Shulchan Menachem, Re'eh)*

Meat with Compote

There are those who eat every bite of chicken together with compote. *(Zemiros Tiferes Tzvi, p. 114)*

The Satmar Rebbe, Reb Yoel, would eat compote with every spoon of meat. He did not recite a *brachah* on the compote, even if it contained whole fruit, since the compote was secondary to the meat, which was secondary to the bread.

(Zemiros Divrei Yoel, p. 96)

Reb Moshe Aryeh Freund did not eat the meat together with the compote. He first ate the meat and then the compote.

(Zemiros Ateres Yehoshua, p. 100)

Kugel on Friday Night

It is written that in several locations they were accustomed to eating a *pashtidah*, pastry filled with meat with a crust on the top and the bottom, on Friday night, in commemoration of the *mann* that was covered with dew on the top and bottom *(Maharil)*. However, the Rema states that in his country of residence they did not have this custom. (Today, we eat kugel, which also has a crust on the top and the bottom, for this reason.)

(Shulchan Aruch, Orach Chaim, 242, Rema)

The *Sefer Yosef Ometz* states that although the Rema writes that in his country the *minhag* of *pashtidah* was not practiced, he was speaking in reference to Poland. However, in Germany, where people prepare kugel for an important visitor, they should definitely do so in honor of Shabbos.

(Yosef Ometz; see *Zemiros Divrei Yoel, p. 96)*

Why is *pashtidah* eaten on Friday night in commemoration of the *mann*, if the *mann* did not fall on Shabbos? Tosafos writes that we replicate the *mann* to compensate for the fact that it did not fall on Shabbos. The *Toras Chaim (Eruvin 73b)* states that Shabbos is compared to *Olam Haba,* which is also called "Shabbos," and where Hashem serves *mann* to the *tzaddikim*. Therefore, we eat foods that remind us of the *mann* on Shabbos. *(Beis Menuchah, p. 57b)*

There are those who are accustomed to eating stuffed chicken neck filled with meat, since that is the kugel to which the Rema (242:1) is referring.

(Shiras HaShabbos, p. 219; See Nimukei Orach Chaim 272:2)

Rebbe Avraham Yehoshua Heschel of Kopishnitz related the reason why there is the *minhag* in Kopishnitz to eat kugel on Friday night: His mother once told him that one of the grandchildren fell, and she promised to add one additional food each Friday night in the merit that the child should be healed. The child recovered, but she did not know which food to add. She considered adding *tzimmes* but was not sure if she would be able to obtain its ingredients every Erev Shabbos. In the end, she decided to add kugel to the Friday night *seudah*.

(Zemiros Shirei Malchus Ruzhin, p. 141)

Drinking after Eating

The Rambam writes that one should only drink a small amount of water while eating, which should be mixed with wine. Once the food starts being digested, he should drink as much as necessary, but not too much. According to this Rambam, one should be careful not to drink until after eating meat. *(Rambam, Hilchos Dei'os 4:2)*

There are those who are accustomed to drinking after eating the meat. The reason for this is stated in the Gemara that one who drinks large quantities of water after eating will not suffer from digestive problems *(Brachos 40a)*. *(Shabbos 41a)*

Drinking Wine during the Seudah

After the Buhusher Rebbe would sing *Kah Echsof*, quality wine would be brought to the table and the Rebbe would recite the blessing of *Hatov V'hameitiv* over it (see *Shulchan Aruch* 175:1). *(Zemiros Beis Buhush, p. 14)*

The Munkatcher Rebbe would drink a small amount of wine between each course at the Shabbos *seudos*. He would also dip several slices of challah into his cup of wine and then eat them. *(Darkei Chaim V'shalom*, sec. 398)

Some Rebbes had the custom of placing wine on the table and announcing the names of those who contributed to its cost. In Sanz, they placed wine on the table, and in Shiniva they used beer.

There were those who placed seven bottles of beer on the table to correspond to the seven people who are called up to the Torah on Shabbos. *(Zemiros Divrei Yoel*, sec. 59)

The source for placing wine on the table of *tzaddikim* and contributing toward its cost is derived from the words of *Chazal*, that one who wants to pour *yayin nesech* on the *Mizbe'ach* should fill the throats of *talmidei chachamim* with wine *(Yuma* 71a). *(Zemiros Tiferes Tzvi*, p. 112)

The Yerushlayimer Rav, Reb Moshe Aryeh Freund, would fill cups with beer and distribute them to all present. To those who were married he would give cups that were entirely full, and to the *bachurim* he would give cups that were partially full. *(Zemiros Ateres Yehoshua*, p. 107)

Chazal explain how great and precious *oneg Shabbos* is and how great is its reward, and conversely, how great will be the punishment for decreasing it *(Shabbos* 118a).

A *nazir* abstains from wine for a period of 30 days *(Nazir* 5a), which includes several Shabbasos. *Chazal* comment on the *pasuk* in *Bamidbar* (6:3), *from new wine and aged wine he should abstain,* that a *nazir* is prohibited to drink wine for a mitzvah just like he is prohibited to drink any other wine, and he must definitely abstain from wine which is only for the purpose of *oneg Shabbos,* and not for Kiddush or Havdalah. Although the *neshamah yeseirah* longs for the pleasure of wine, and if one does not fulfill this desire he brings sin upon himself, a *nazir* still may not drink wine on Shabbos.

Therefore, the *pasuk* (ibid. 6:11) states in regard to the *nazir, He shall prepare...offerings to atone on his behalf for sinning on his soul.* The soul here refers to the *neshamah yeseirah,* the additional soul that one is granted on Shabbos. A *nazir* needs atonement for depriving his *neshamah yeseirah* of its *oneg Shabbos* through wine. (*Noam Megadim, Re'eh,* s.v. *Ki yarchiv*)

Other than drinking wine after the fish, the Rebbe of Setchin did not drink during the *seudah*, and he did not bring any beverages to the table. (*Mishmei D'Reb Tanchum,* sec. 18)

The Gemara in *Pesachim* (105a) states that honoring Shabbos during the day takes precedence over honoring Shabbos at night. Therefore, if there is not a lot of wine left after reciting Friday night Kiddush, it should be reserved for the day *seudah*. (*Likutei Maharich, Seudos Leil Shabbos Kodesh*)

Tzimmes

Tzimmes refers to a dish that simmered for a long time.

The word *tzimmes* is similar to the word *tzomes*, which means joined. This alludes to the fact that Hashem, Shabbos, and Bnei Yisrael are all connected. (*Sefer Matamim, Inyanei Shabbos*)

In Dzhikov they ate two types of *tzimmes*: *farfel*, which was known as the Ba'al Shem Tov's *tzimmes*, and a rice dish known as Ruzhiner *tzimmes*. (*Nitzotzei Hakodesh,* p. 111)

Chassidim eat *farfel* on Friday night and *lokshen* kugel on Shabbos day. The author of the *Chiddushei Maharya* heard from his father that these two dishes have their source from the Ba'al Shem Tov.

The Ba'al Shem Tov explained that *farfel* alludes to the hope that one's sins should be *farfalen*, fall away, since Erev Shabbos is a time of *teshuvah. Lokshen* kugel, which is comprised of the words *lo kashin*, signifies that one should not question the ways of Hashem because everything He does is good.

(*Chiddushei Maharya, Nedarim* 50b)

The Shiniver Rav would eat four types of *tzimmes* after the meat in the following order: *farfel*, carrots, cooked fruit, and liver. (*L'ateir Pesora*, p. 42; *Sichos Yekarim Antwerp* 5757, p. 14)

One should first eat the compote, since a *brachah* is recited upon it, before eating the carrot *tzimmes* and the *farfel*, which are a part of the *seudah* and do not require a *brachah*.

On Rosh Hashanah, when the *brachah* of *Ha'eitz* is recited on the apple dipped in honey, and one does not recite another *brachah* on the compote, the carrots are eaten first.

(*Magen Avos*, p. 251)

Carrots and *farfel* are brought to the table at the same time, on one tray but on two separate plates. The Bobover Rebbes placed the carrots on the right side of the tray and the *farfel* on the left side. Elderly chassidim explain that this is because the first letters of the words *mehren tzimmes* and *farfel tzimmes* allude to the Name of Hashem of *yud, keh, vav, keh* using the system of *At-Bash* (a system where the first letter of the *aleph-beis* corresponds to the last letter, the second letter corresponds to the second-to-last letter, etc.). *Mem* corresponds to *yud*, *tzaddi* to *heh*, *feh* to *vav*, and *tzaddi* to *heh* again, forming *yud, keh, vav, keh*. The Rebbes were careful to place the food in the correct order so that the Name of Hashem should be in the proper order from right to left. (*Magen Avos*, p. 254)

The Bobover Rebbe, Reb Shlomo, first ate from the carrot *tzimmes*, distributed *shirayim*, and then ate the *farfel*, for the abovementioned reason.

However, there are those who are accustomed to eating the *farfel* first, since it is similar in sound to the Yiddish word *farfalen* (to fall away) which alludes to one's sins falling away. Only then do they eat the carrot *tzimmes*, which in Yiddish is called *mehren,* which also means, "to increase." The carrot *tzimmes* alludes to increasing our merits, thus fulfilling *sur meira va'asei tov*—turn away from the bad and then do good. *(Dvar Tzvi, Veitzen)*

Belzer chassidim ate three types of *tzimmes*: *farfel*, carrots, and plums. *(Dibros Kodesh, p. 62)*

The students of Reb Yosef Shaul Natansohn were once discussing the fact that the Sanzer Rav eats 13 types of *tzimmes,* and they frowned upon this practice. Reb Yosef Shaul heard their discussion and added, "But the Rav also runs to the *mikvah* 13 times, and each time he needs to remove his bandages." (The Sanzer Rav suffered from ailments on his feet).
(Siach Zekeinim, p. 232)

The Sanzer Rav considered carrot *tzimmes* to be the most significant of all Shabbos foods. In Dzhikov they called it *goldene rendlech* ("golden coins," signifying their importance and because carrots are golden). *(Hakdamas Sefer Toras Aish)*

They would serve the Buhusher Rebbe "*kinder tzimmes*" (children's *tzimmes*) that consisted of rice and raisins. The *minhag* in Buhush was that this dish was called by the name of the youngest child and was a *segulah* for good children.
(Zemiros Buhush, Hanhagos Kodesh, p. 15)

Farfel

The Rebbe of Rodishitz was accustomed to eating *farfel* on Friday night after all other courses. Like most *tzaddikim,* he called it the Ba'al Shem Tov's *tzimmes.*
(Nifla'os HaSaba Kaddisha, vol. 1, 29a)

Farfel is known as the Ba'al Shem Tov's *tzimmes* because in his youth, the Ba'al Shem Tov was destitute and he lacked the money to buy fish for Shabbos; he sufficed with eating *farfel,* which was inexpensive. *(Magen Avos, p. 253)*

Reb Dovid Tzvi Shlomo of Lelov would eat *farfel* at the end of the *seudah*. He would call it the Ba'al Shem's *tzimmes,* since the Ba'al Shem Tov was accustomed to eating the *farfel* as the sixth dish of the *seudah*, which is a *segulah* known to those who understand the deeper secrets of the Torah.

(*Tiferes Beis Dovid*, p. 111)

The Ba'al Shem Tov instituted the *minhag* of eating *farfel*. The *pasuk* in *Yeshayah* (56:2) states, "One who keeps the Shabbos, *meichalelo*, from being desecrated." *Chazal* explain that one should read it *machol lo*; one who keeps the Shabbos is forgiven for all his sins. Therefore, we eat *farfel* which is similar to the word *farfalen*, fell away, because our sins should fall away.

Reb Pinchas of Koritz said that *farfel* is an allusion to being happy with what one has. *Farfel* is comprised in Yiddish of the words, *par* (a few) and *feel* (a lot), alluding to someone who has little but views it as a lot. (*Imrei Pinchas, Sha'ar Dalet*, sec. 509)

Farfel is similar to the word *farfillen*, that Hashem should fulfill our hearts' desires. Indeed, *Chazal* have said that one who delights in the Shabbos will be granted his heart's desires, as the *pasuk* in *Tehillim* (37:4) says, *You should delight in Hashem, and He will give you what your heart desires.*

(As heard from elderly chassidim)

Reb Shlomo of Bobov said that the word *farfel* is derived from the word "*farfal*," to fall, in commemoration of the *mann* which fell from the Heavens. (*Magen Avos*, p. 253)

It is cited in the name of the Ba'al Shem Tov that eating *farfel* is a *segulah* for livelihood. (*Zemiros Nata Aharon*, p. 116)

The Maharam Schick was always in a good frame of mind on Friday night. During the week, unless it was absolutely necessary, he would not speak at a meal (perhaps because the table at which one eats is like a *Mizbe'ach* and he did not want any mundane talk to be combined with that which is holy). On Shabbos, however, he would converse with his family.

Once, when the *farfel* was served, the Maharam Schick's married daughter said that she does not serve *farfel* at the *seudah*. She felt that by the time it came to the *farfel*, they were already satiated from the previous courses.

When the Maharam Schick heard this, he was very displeased. He told her that even the previous generations ate *farfel* every Friday night since it is one of the Shabbos foods eaten in honor of Shabbos. *Farfel* has a numerical value of 410, and it is in commemoration of the first Beis Hamikdash which stood for 410 years. (Feh, ayin, reish, vav, vav, ayin, lamed, plus the seven letters of the word and the word itself total 410.)

(*Od Yosef Chai*, p. 32)

Reb Elimelech of Rudnick once ate a *seudah* at the home of a wealthy person. The host had prepared a large *seudah* in honor of Reb Elimelech, at the end of which he served a bowl of *farfel*. Although Reb Elimelech usually ate a small amount and distributed the rest as *shirayim*, this time he ate the entire bowl. He then asked if there was more and ate two more bowls of *farfel*. It was very strange in the eyes of those present.

Later, it became known that the Jewish maid had mistakenly poured paraffin into the *farfel* instead of oil, and it was almost impossible to eat. If the matter would have been known she would have been terribly embarrassed and perhaps even dismissed from her job. In order to avoid any embarrassment or pain to be caused to the maid, Reb Elimelech ate all the *farfel* himself. (*Toldos of the Rebbe of Reisha*, chap. 1)

The Sanzer Rav ate the first spoon of *farfel* with challah so as not to have questions of whether he was required to recite a *brachah*. (*Likutei Maharich, Seder Birchas Hamotzi*, p. 161)

The Chozeh of Lublin said that the *farfel* should be so hot that it emits steam. Reb Yissachar Dov of Belz explains that the Shabbos dishes correspond to the *avodah* performed in the

Beis Hamikdash. *Farfel* is in commemoration of the *Lechem Hapanim*. The *Lechem Hapanim* were as warm when they were removed from the *Shulchan* as when they were placed there (*Chagigah* 26b).

Belzer chassidim eat *farfel* twice, once in the soup and once as a separate dish. By the time the *farfel* is eaten it is already cold, so therefore it is first eaten it in the soup. Because they do not eat it hot, Belzer chassidim specifically eat square *farfel*, to correspond to the *Lechem Hapanim* that had four sides. (*Kuntris Dibburei Kodesh*, p. 35)

Reb Yissachar Dov of Belz would say that a Jew is required to walk a *techum* (2,000 *amos*) to have *farfel* on Shabbos, and it is only considered *farfel* if it emits steam.

(*Seudasa D'Malka*, Belz, chap. 4)

The Chozeh used to say that when he inhaled the steam of the *farfel* he was absorbing inspiration.

(*B'kedushaso Shel Aharon*, p. 240)

Stuffed Cabbage

Several *tzaddikim* ate stuffed meat, chicken neck, or stuffed cabbage as a remembrance to the *mann* that was surrounded above and below with dew. (*Minhagei Komarno*, sec. 234)

In Ropshitz they ate stuffed cabbage on Friday night instead of *farfel*. The Rebbe of Nassad had this custom as well, and he said in the name of the Ropshitzer Rebbe that stuffed cabbage is a food of *talmidei chachamim*.

(*Gedulas Yehoshua*, vol. 1, p. 44, sec. 43; *Tehillos Chaim*)

When Reb Shalom Eliezer of Rotzfert once could not obtain carrots, he instructed that stuffed cabbage be made instead, since stuffed cabbage is a food of *tzaddikim*. (*Magen Avos*, p. 253)

Reb Yozif Nanisher would travel to Kalev to spend Shabbos with the Kalever Rebbe. The Kalever Rebbe would eat stuffed goose and stuffed cabbage at the Shabbos *seudah*. Reb Yozif was not accustomed to eating these dishes out of concern for *kashrus*. When he came to Kalev he would eat the stuffed goose, but he did not eat cabbage even in Kalev.

The Kalever Rebbe once asked him why he did not eat the stuffed cabbage. Reb Yozif replied that when he saw the Kalever Rebbe eating the goose, he knew that it was definitely kosher and could be eaten. However, with the cabbage, it is possible that on the Rebbe's spoon there were no insects while on his spoon there were insects. The Kalever Rebbe agreed with Reb Yozif's reasoning. (*Chemdah Genuzah*, vol. 2, p. 137)

During special Shabbasos, stuffed cabbage is served at the end of the meal. The Rebbe of Salka once said that stuffed cabbage has a special importance and is therefore eaten last.
(*Minhag Pri Eliezer*, p. 224)

Gedishachtz

Gedishachtz is a dish made from chicken wings and necks. The Satmar Rebbe, Reb Yoel, would eat some *gedishachtz* and then distribute *shirayim*. (*Zemiros Divrei Yoel*, p. 97)

Gelingelech

Gelingelech is a dish made of thinly sliced lungs (derived from the word *lingen* in Yiddish). When there were no lungs available, it was made from liver fried in fat and onions. The Satmar Rebbe would distribute the *gelingelech* to specific people.
(*Halichos Kodesh*, p. 79)

Liver

Rabba bar Rav Huna came to the home of Rabbah bar Rav Nachman on Shabbos. The Gemara states that they found a piece of liver that was questionable. From this we can see that that liver was served on Shabbos in the times of the Gemara.
(*Chullin* 111a)

Kaveid, liver, has a numerical value of 26, equivalent to the *Shem Havayah*: *yud, keh, vav, keh*. (*Zemiros Nitei Aharon*, p. 117)

The Sanzer Rebbe would distribute *shirayim* of the liver (*kaveid*) to his wealthy chassidim, explaining that one should give wealthy people *kavod* (honor). (*Halichos Kodesh*, p. 79, sec. 52)

Reb Shlomo of Bobov gave several ideas related to word *leber* (Yiddish for liver):

The numerical value of the word *leber (lamed, beis, reish)* is 232. This is the same total numerical value of the different forms of the *Shem Havayah*.

Leber is an acronym for *l'holid banim rabbim*, having many children. Reb Shlomo related that his father, the Kedushas Tzion, would distribute liver to the young men as a *segulah* for having children.

Reb Shlomo of Bobov would distribute liver to the *bachurim* who were of marriageable age. In his later years, he would give it to *chassadim* as a *segulah* for children.

Eating liver arouses the merit of our Imahos, since liver contains a large amount of iron, *barzel*, which is an acronym for Bilhah, Rachel, Zilpah, and Leah. While eating liver, one can have in mind that the merit of the Imahos should stand him in good stead. (*Magen Avos*, p. 257)

The Gemara states that one who eats three *seudos* on Shabbos will be spared from the birth pangs of Mashiach and the war of Gog and Magog. From the words of the *Agra D'pirka* (*Remez* 256) we can understand that when Mashiach comes, iron will no longer be used for weapons of war, but for peace. Therefore, we eat liver, which contains a large amount of iron, on Shabbos, to signify that the *Geulah* will come in the merit of Shabbos, and then iron will only be used for peaceful purposes. (*Rabbi Dovid Meisels*)

Many are accustomed to eating the liver at the end of the *seudah*. This is alluded to in a play on words of the phrase, *sof hakavod lavo* (at the end, the honor that a person deserves will come to him). Therefore, at the end of the *seudah*, *kaveid*, liver, is eaten.   (*Rabbi Dovid Meisels*)

Reb Itzikel of Pshevorsk once said that the Gemara in *Brachos* (3b) states that the Rabbis went to Dovid Hamelech complaining that the Jews need a livelihood. Dovid Hamelech advised them to take up arms (literally, to stretch out your arms). [They should conquer enemy territory which will give them land or acquire booty from the enemy.]

We see from this Gemara that livelihood arrives by stretching out one's hand. Similarly, liver is a *segulah* for livelihood and should be taken by stretching out one's hand (i.e. grabbing it).
        (*Siach Yitzchak*, p. 49)

A person once grabbed liver at the table of the Kedushas Zion of Bobov and burned himself in the process. The Rebbe explained that one who grabs *kavod* (honor) gets burned.
        (*Beis Tzaddikim Ya'amod*, p. 63)

Liver with Challah

Reb Mendel of Stropkov would distribute *shirayim* of the liver with a piece of challah. He would say in the name of his grandfather, the Shiniver Rav, that this alludes to an honorable *parnassah*, since bread hints to *parnassah* and *kaveid*, liver, hints to the word *b'kavod*.   (*Noam Siach*, p. 159)

The reason for eating challah with liver at the end of the *seudah* may be because the Gemara states that for every prohibition stated in the Torah, the Torah permits something similar. Since the Torah forbade eating blood, the Torah permits eating liver, which is saturated with blood.

Similarly, if a person does *teshuvah* out of love, his transgressions become merits. Shabbos is a time of love between us and Hashem, as the Bnei Yissaschar writes in the name of the Ateres Tzvi of Ziditchov, that Shabbos has the same numerical value as *ahavah b'chol lev, ahavah b'chol nefesh, ahavah b'chol me'od*—love with all of one's heart, love with all of one's soul, love with all of one's possessions. It is for this reason that Shabbos has the power to turn sins into merits. We eat liver on Shabbos to symbolize this idea.

The Bnei Yissaschar writes that one can only recite a *brachah* on food that is in its original form. However, once the form of a food is changed, and it is no longer recognizable as the original food, its value is decreased and its *brachah* is *Shehakol*. However, when wheat or grapes are changed into bread or wine, the value is increased, and they have their own special *brachah*. Therefore, wheat and grapes allude to *teshuvah* done out of love since the change they undergo increases their value.

Thus, challah and liver both symbolize *teshuvah* performed with love. Hence, it is fitting that they be eaten together at *seudas Shabbos,* which atone for our sins and is a time of love.

(*Rabbi Dovid Meisels*)

There are those who advise refraining from eating liver since it is among the foods that our Sages have advised can be harmful for those carrying children or nursing.

(*Mizmor L'asaf*, p. 88b)

It is told that the Sanzer Rav never ate potatoes or liver. While he did distribute liver to the guests on Friday night, he did not eat it, although he dipped his challah into it. The only exception was Erev Pesach when he ate potatoes cooked with liver.

(*Toldos Chaim Sanz*)

Karsh

There is a custom to eat cornmeal bread that is called *karsh* on Shabbos. Prior to baking *karsh* it is very liquidy, but as it cooks it congeals and hardens. This is eaten because Rashi states (*Bereishis* 1:6) that although the sky was created on the first day, it was not firm until Hashem commanded, *"yehi rakia"* on the second day. At that point, *nikrash*, it hardened. We should learn from this that just like the *rakia* became hard when Hashem commanded it, Hashem also commands us to "harden" our souls to fear Him. As it says in *Devarim* (10:12): *What does Hashem ask from you? Only to fear Hashem, your G-d.* (For the same reason, many eat jellied fish sauce on Shabbos).

(Minhagei Vizhnitz; Divrei Ephraim)

Garlic

It is one of the institutions of Ezra to eat garlic on Erev Shabbos; some say it should be eaten on Friday night. The garlic should preferably be roasted, but can perhaps also be cooked; it should not be eaten raw.

(Magen Avraham 280; *Elyah Rabbah* ibid.: 2)

Compote

The custom to serve compote and dessert at the end of the *seudah* is to enhance one's Torah study.

The midrash states on the *pasuk* in Rus: *And Boaz ate and drank, and gladdened his heart,* that Boaz gladdened his heart by eating sweets, so as to enhance the voice of Torah study (*Rus Rabbah* 5:15).

Similarly, the *Yerushalmi* states that for 40 years before Bnei Yisrael were exiled to Bavel, they planted dates in Bavel, so that when they arrived there they would have a craving for sweet foods which would promote their Torah study (*Ta'anis* 4:5).

The Gemara states that a person's innards expand to make room for a sweet food (*Eiruvin* 82b). Hashem created the world in this way so that a person should always be able to eat sweets and enhance his Torah study even when he is already satiated.

(V'darashta V'chakarta, Orach Chaim, sec. 36)

Some serve a second compote in honor of Shabbos, as the *Zohar* writes that on Shabbos one is required to have an additional dish. (In the name of the Sfas Emes)

The Belzer chassidim ate compote after the day meal, but the Rebbes only ate compote on Friday night. It is possible that the reason for this is because the Rebbes of Belz would only eat four cooked dishes at the *seudah*; at night, compote was one of the four dishes. During the day, however, they ate four cooked dishes without the compote. Therefore, compote was not considered part of the *seudah* and those who ate it recited a *brachah*. At the Friday night *seudah*, the *minhag* was to eat the compote with challah in order to exempt it from a *brachah*.

In Poland, they were not accustomed to eating compote during the week. Since it was not usually part of the meal, when it was eaten a *brachah* was recited.

(*She'eilos Uteshuvos Chelkas Yaakov, Orach Chaim* 50)

The *minhag* of the Belzer Rebbe was that when he ate apple compote he did not recite a *brachah*. During the week, he definitely did not recite a *brachah* and ate the compote with bread. On Shabbos, even without bread he did not recite a *brachah*. (*Pekudas Elazar, Teshuvah* 11)

Those who do not recite a *brachah* on the compote because they consider it part of the *seudah* have this *minhag* by every *seudas mitzvah*, not only Shabbos.

The *Mishnah Berurah* (178:10) states that one must make a *brachah* on compote served at the end of the meal. However, Rav Rottenberg, *rosh yeshivah* of Beis Meir in Bnei Brak, says that his father heard from the Chafetz Chaim himself that he no longer *paskened* this way, and in practice, one does not have to make a *brachah* on it because it is considered part of the *seudah*. (*Rabbeinu Hagadol Amro*, ch. 16)

Reb Itzikel of Pshevorsk related that during the first Shabbos after the passing of the Sanzer Rebbe, his children, rebbes in their own right, ate the Shabbos *seudah* together. When the compote was served, the Shiniver Rav requested that they bring him a piece of apple. Since that differed from what the Sanzer Rav used to do, his brother, the Kishinover Rebbe asked him if he was following the *minhag* of Belz, since the Shiniver Rav had traveled to Belz. The Shiniver Rav replied, "In truth we should recite a *brachah* on the compote, as our father did. However, the Belzer Rav was outstanding in his knowledge of *hilchos brachos*, and he did not recite a *brachah* on the compote. Since I am not an expert in these *halachos*, I resolve this question by reciting a *brachah* on a raw piece of fruit."

(*Shulchan Rabboseinu*, p. 182)

The Ba'al Bnei Sheleishim holds that one should eat the compote with challah in order to eliminate any doubts about reciting a *brachah*. (*Halichos Kodesh*, p. 48)

Aside from eating compote with the meat, the Satmar Rebbe, Reb Yoel, also ate some compote which contained whole pieces of fruit at the end of the meal. Since it was eaten for pleasure, it was not exempted from a *brachah* by the recitation of *Hamotzi*, and he would recite *Ha'eitz* on it.

(*Zemiros Divrei Yoel*, p. 97)

Reb Hershel of Spinka ate compote a second time at the end of the meal. Both times, he would put pieces of challah into it and did not recite a *brachah*.

The first compote always consisted of apples. During the summer, the second compote contained summer fruit in order to rectify those fruits by eating them at the Shabbos *seudah*.

(*Zemiros Tiferes Tzvi*, p. 116)

Apples

One should eat apples on Friday night, because the Friday night *seudah* is known as *seudasa chakal tapuchin kaddishin*, a feast of the field of sacred apples, among other reasons.

(*Nefesh Yeseirah B'Shabbos*)

The Maggid of Kozhnitz would say that if one eats apples at the Friday night *seudah*, which is referred to as *chakal tapuchin kaddishin*, he is guaranteed to have livelihood that week. (*Sifsei Tzaddikim, Kisvei Ratzad Glaser*, p. 76, sec. 3)

Tosafos, on the words *borei nefashos rabbos v'chesronan*, states the following: Regarding, "Hashem created many people and their lack," that "lack" refers to the necessities without which the world can't exist, such as bread and water. *Al kol mah shebarasa*—"on everything that You created," refers to everything else, such as foods we could live without, for instance apples, which were created just to give us *oneg*, pleasure. Therefore, we eat apples on Friday night for *oneg Shabbos*. (*Sefarim*)

The Amshinover Rebbe once visited the Imrei Emes of Gur. The Imrei Emes served him fruits but the Amshinover Rebbe declined to eat, saying that fruits and wine are harmful to his health. The Imrei Emes replied that apples are a cure for every illness. (*Imrei Emes, Likutim*, p. 120)

The Sanzer Rebbe once gave the Kaminka Rebbe an apple during his *tish*. He explained that *tapuach*, apple, is an acronym for *tigalun pisgamin v'seimerun chiddusha*—one should uncover hidden secrets of the Torah and recite *chiddushei Torah*. He requested that the Kaminka Rebbe eat the apple and then recite *divrei Torah*. (*Darchei Chaim Sippurim*, p. 131)

The *pasuk* in *Shir Hashirim* (2:3) compares Hashem to an apple, as it says: *As an apple tree among the trees of the forest, so is my beloved among the sons...* The *Zohar* states that just like an apple is a remedy, Hashem is the cure for every illness; just like an apple has a delicate fragrance, the *pasuk* in *Hoshe'a* (14:7) states in regard to Hashem, *Its fragrance like the Levanon*, and just like an apple has a sweet taste, *Shir Hashirim* (5:16) states (regarding Hashem), *His palate is sweet*. (See *Zohar*, vol. 3, p. 74a)

When an apple is cut in half, one can see 10 spots. *Chazal* say that *tzaddikim* give existence to the world, which was created with 10 *ma'amaros* (utterances), by fulfilling the Torah, which is encompassed in the *Aseres Hadibros*.

(Zera Kodesh, Parshas Toldos, on the *pasuk Re'eh Rei'ach B'ni)*

The *Shechinah* is referred to as *chakal tapuchin kaddishin*, and the Jews are referred to as a *tapuach*, an apple, and the *Shem Havayah—yud, keh, vav, keh* is found in an apple. If one cuts an apple across there are 10 red spots which corresponds to the *yud*. The five seed cavities correspond to the letter *heh*, and the stem is the letter *vav*. When the apple tree blossoms there are five small petals, which correspond to the final *heh*.

(Halichos Kodesh, p. 82)

The apple should be cut into five parts because five times the word *tapuach* has a numerical value of 2,470. With the inclusion of the word as one, and five times the word (corresponding to the five pieces of apple) it equals 2,476, which is the numerical value of *Shema Yisrael Hashem Elokeinu Hashem echad* and *Baruch Shem k'vod malchuso l'olam va'ed*.

(Halichos Kodesh, p. 82)

While the Modzhitzer Rebbe was once eating the Shabbos day *seudah*, after they finished singing *Asadeir L'seudasa*, the door burst open and a woman came in, clearly very agitated. She told the Rebbe that her son had a bad fall and had stopped talking. She begged the Rebbe to help her. The Rebbe took an apple from the table and instructed her to give it to the child to eat and he would be healed. Indeed, the child ate the apple and his speech returned.

The Modzhitzer Rebbe's students asked him what lay behind this *segulah*. The Rebbe replied with wisdom and a play on words. "We just sang *Asadeir L'seudasa*, in which we said, *kadam Ribon almin, b'milin sisimin, tigalun pisgamin, v'seimrun chiddusha*—Before The King of all worlds, [you should speak] with sealed words, unveil matters, and express new [Torah] insights. The first letters of the words *tigalun pisgamin, v'seimrun chiddusha* spell *tapuach* (apple). This is to show us that if the *milin*, words, are *sisimin*, sealed, then *tigalun pisgamin*, his power of speech will be revealed, *v'seimrun chiddusha*, with new speech, if he eats an apple."

(*Imrei Shaul*, Modzhitz)

Eating Challah at the End of the Meal

The Shelah would leave over a small amount of the *Hamotzi* and eat it at the end of the meal, either plain or with a beverage, so the taste of the *Hamotzi* would remain in his mouth.

(*Shelah Hakadosh, Sha'ar Ha'osiyos Kedushas Ha'achilah*)

Some are accustomed to eating the leftovers of the *Hamotzi* slice at the end of the *seudah* before washing *mayim acharonim* to express their love for the mitzvah. This is similar to the Gemara that Rabbi Yochanan would gather the crumbs of a *seudas mitzvah* to demonstrate that the leftovers of a mitzvah have special importance. This idea is also found in the Yalkut, which states that when leaving Mitzrayim, the Jews took along with them the remaining matzah and *maror*, out of their love for the mitzvah. (See *Yalkut*, Bo, *Remez* 208)

When reciting *Birkas Hamazon* with 10 people, some hold that the 10 people should eat a slice of bread together prior to washing *mayim acharonim* to ensure that there is a definite obligation of reciting *Birkas Hamazon* with a minyan.

(*Zichru Toras Moshe, Shemini*)

The Pri Megadim and the Tzlach state that one is required by Torah law (*d'Oraisa*) to recite *Birkas Hamazon* only if he became satiated from bread itself and not from other foods as well.

The Keren L'Dovid explains that if one eats a *kezayis* of bread at the end of the *seudah*, then the bread combines with all the previous foods eaten during the meal to make up an amount that is enough to satiate a person, and consequentially require *Birkas Hamazon d'Oraisa*. However, if one ate the bread at the beginning of the *seudah,* it is not definite that the food eaten later combines with the bread. Therefore, at a meal that does not consist mainly of bread, it is proper to eat a *kezayis* of bread at the end of the meal so that he should have a Torah obligation to recite *Birkas Hamazon.*

(*Pri Megadim, Orach Chaim* 184, *Eishel Avraham* 8)

Leaving Over Shabbos Food

In *Tzur Mishelo,* sung on Friday night, we say, *We were satiated and we left over from the [Shabbos] food, as Hashem commanded.* One may wonder what command this is referring to. When did Hashem command us to leave over Shabbos food?

Eating until one is satiated is part of the mitzvah of *oneg Shabbos.* If a person leaves over food, he proves that he is satiated and that he has fulfilled the mitzvah of *oneg Shabbos.* (*Imrei Pinchas Sha'ar HaShabbos,* sec. 68)

Reb Dovid Yungreis ate whichever dish was served to him on Shabbos, without leaving any over.

(*Shulchan Menachem, Beshalach*)

Eating in Order to Recite Birkas Hamazon

In the song *Kol Mekadeish,* sung on Friday night, we say, *We eat three meals in order to praise and thank Hashem.* Reb Tzvi Hersh of Riminov says that this refers to those who eat three *seudos* only in order to be able to recite *Birkas Hamazon.*

(*Be'eiros Hamayim, Rosh Chodesh Elul*)

The *neshamah yeseirah* derives a special pleasure from *Birkas Hamazon.* Therefore, the main intent of the *seudah* should be the *Birkas Hamazon.* (*Igra D'kallah, Vayeira,* s.v *Ekchah*)

Reciting Birkas Hamazon Over a Cup of Wine

It is proper to recite *Birkas Hamazon* over a cup of wine at the three *seudos,* even if one is not accustomed to doing so during the week. This also helps one recite 100 *brachos* throughout Shabbos, since an additional *brachah* of *Hagafen* is recited. *(Mekor Chaim* 274)

Another reason we recite *Birkas Hamazon* over wine on Shabbos and Yom Tov is because there is wine on the table.

The *Sefer Ruach Chaim* states that although the *Shulchan Aruch* holds that one does not need to recite *Birkas Hamazon* over wine, one should do so because one who drinks wine during the *seudah* and does not recite *Birkas Hamazon* over wine has transgressed. Hashem will tell him, "For your own desires you drink wine, but for My honor, to recite *Birkas Hamazon* over wine, you don't?"

Indeed, *Chazal* say that you should honor Hashem *meihoncha* (with your possessions) which can mean *geroncha* (with your throat). One honors Hashem with his throat by drinking wine when reciting *Birkas Hamazon*. *(Magen Avos,* p. 546)

In Sibenbergen, the *minhag* was that if three people were reciting *Birkas Hamazon* then the cup was held with the fingers; if 10 people were reciting *Birkas Hamazon*, then the cup was held in the palm of the hand. *(Aleph Ksav,* sec. 602)

One should not drink less than a *revi'is* in order to eliminate any doubt of whether he should recite *Al Hagefen*.
(See *Shulchan Aruch* 190:3, *Taz,* ibid.:3)

Everyone present should drink a bit from the *kos shel brachah* (the wine upon which *Birkas Hamazon* was recited).
(Shulchan Aruch 190:4)

Rabbi Yaakov of Melitz would say that one should specifically drink from the original cup upon which *Birkas Hamazon* was recited. He explained that since this wine is known as *kos shel brachah* (literally, the cup of *brachah*), and not *yayin shel brachah* (the wine of *brachah*), it must be that the cup itself also brings *brachah*. *(Nezer Kodesh, Seudas Leil Shabbos,* sec. 117)

Chapter 13
After the Meal—Friday Night Oneg

Shehakol Cake after Birkas Hamazon

After the Friday night *seudah*, Reb Itzikel of Pshevorsk would eat fruits, a cake upon which *Shehakol* was recited, and a cake upon which *Mezonos* was recited. He would say several times that the *neshamah yeseirah* is a tranquil heart for rest and joy that is open wide, so one can eat and drink more than usual (*Beitzah* 16a; s.v. *Neshamah yeseirah*). (*Siach Yitzchak*, p. 49)

In Pshevorsk, there was once a winter during which it did not snow. One of the chassidim of Reb Moshe Yitzchak of Pshevorsk requested that the Rebbe *daven* for snow (since the lumber merchants transfer lumber on the frozen rivers). The Rebbe replied that if he sees a cake upon which *Shehakol* is recited, which is made with a "snow" (beaten egg whites), then there will be snow. This is the source for the *minhag* to recite *Shehakol* on cake after *Birkas Hamazon*.

(As heard from Reb Yankele of Pshevorsk)

Eating Fruit for 100 Brachos on Shabbos

One should eat more fruits and delicacies than usual and smell good fragrances on Shabbos so that he has more opportunities to recite *brachos*. In this way, he will be able to recite 100 *brachos* throughout Shabbos, beginning Friday night. (*Shulchan Aruch* 290:1; *Mishneh Berurah* ibid.:1)

It is preferable to recite as many *brachos* as possible on Friday night, so one can complete 100 *brachos* over Shabbos.

(*Mishneh Berurah* ibid.:1)

One should eat fruits after the *seudah* in order to complete 100 *brachos* on Shabbos so that the total *brachos* recited throughout the week is 700. Indeed, the word Shabbos is an acronym for 700 *brachos* (*tav* and *shin* have a numerical value of seven hundred and *beis* stands for *brachos*.) (*Sefer Matamim Hachadash*)

Shabbos is an acronym for **Shabbos b'peiros tivareich**, one should recite *brachos* on fruits on Shabbos (in order to recite 100 *brachos* throughout Shabbos). (*Devarim Nifla'im*, chap. 6)

One should eat dates, pomegranates, walnuts, and apples, which are all mentioned in *Shir Hashirim* as a parable to the Jewish nation. In regard to dates, the *pasuk* states, *your stature is like a palm tree* (7:8); regarding pomegranates it says, *your temple is like a split pomegranate* (4:3). About walnuts the *pasuk* says, *I went down to the nut garden* (a reference to Bnei Yisrael) (6:11); regarding apples it says, *As an apple tree among the trees of the forest, so is my beloved among the sons* (2:3).
(*Kaf Hachaim* 250:15)

Beans

After *Birkas Hamazon*, fruits, kugel, and beans were served, and the Spinka Rebbe would lead a *tish*. When he distributed the beans (*bandelech* in Yiddish) he would say, "**Banim atem laHashem Elokeichem**—'You are the children of Hashem, your G-d.'" (*Devarim* 14:1). (*Minhagei Spinka*)

The Kretchnifer Rebbe would invest much effort into eating beans. At times, he would say *banim atem laHashem Elokeichem* while eating them.

He would repeat the following thought in the name of the Sadigura Rebbe, on the *pasuk* in *Vayikra* (23:4), *Tikriu osam b'moadam*—"You shall designate them in their appointed time," referring to designating the Yamim Tovim. *Chazal* say that one shouldn't read it *osam*, but rather *atem*, you. This demonstrates that designating the Yamim Tovim is dependent on us, on when *beis din* chooses to proclaim the new month. Even if *beis din* mistakenly designated the new month on the wrong day, and even if they did so intentionally, it is still *atem*—the new month is dependent on *beis din*.

The Sadigura Rebbe would say that in the *pasuk* of *Banim atem laHashem Elokeichem*, where the word *atem* is stated outright, as opposed to in *Vayikra* where it is written as *osam*, we can definitely apply the previous concept. Even if we sinned, we are still *banim atem*, the children of Hashem.

(*Raza D'Shabbos*, p. 33)

Whiskey on Friday Night

After the Friday night *seudah*, the Munkatcher Rav would lead a *tish* where fruit and whiskey were served. They would dance and sing, including the song *Raninu Tzaddikim*; they termed this *Raninu Tzaddikim Broinfen* (whiskey).

(*Darkei Chaim V'shalom* sec. 408)

When one is about to enjoy a pleasure that does not have a designated *brachah*, one should recite *Shehakol* on another food or drink and have in mind that pleasure. Therefore, many *tzaddikim* would recite *Shehakol* over a cup of whiskey before retiring so that the *Shehakol* should include the pleasure of sleep. (*Maggid Ta'alumah Brachos*, on the words of the Rif, p. 28)

Friday Night Cholent

The *Zohar* (*Bereishis* 48b) states that the mitzvah of *to'ameha* refers to all the Shabbos food, and it should be done on Friday night and not Erev Shabbos. Accordingly, there are those who taste the cholent and kugel on Friday night as well.

One should only eat a small amount, less than a *kezayis*, because the honor of the day *seudah* takes precedence over the night *seudah*. (See *Nimukei Orach Chaim* 250)

Regarding those who eat cholent Friday night, Reb Shlomo of Bobov would say that the Shabbos foods have a set order according to the *Sheimos* (Names) of Hashem, and one should not mix up the order. (*Magen Avos*, p. 427)

Chapter 14
Shabbos Morning and Kiddush

Drinking Coffee Early in the Morning

The Ksav Sofer would awaken three hours after *chatzos* on Shabbos morning. He would wash his hands and recite *Birchos Hashachar* with tremendous excitement, crying tears of intense joy.

His family would awaken upon hearing him recite the *brachos* and they would also cry. The neighbors nearby would also wake up from his cries. Privileged were the people who witnessed it. He then called to two *bachurim* and one of his sons and they drank coffee. Then they would learn *Masechtos Shabbos* and *Eiruvin* with tremendous joy.

The Ksav Sofer would say of waking up, drinking coffee, and then learning with single-minded concentration, that sinners have no concept of this pleasure, and all their pleasure cannot compare to it. (*Ksav Sofer Al HaTorah, Hakdamah Ohel Leah*, p. 17)

Preparing the Challos before Mussaf

When Reb Aharon of Belz would go *daven Mussaf* he would instruct that the challos be placed on the table.
(*B'kedushaso Shel Aharon*, p. 443)

Pas Shacharis on Shabbos

A woman should eat *pas Shacharis*, even on Shabbos and Yom Tov, before she goes to *shul* (since her physical makeup is weaker than a man's). She should *daven brachos* and recite *Krias Shema* before eating.
(*Tzava'as Abba, Keren Dalet, Amud Bris Hashalom*, p. 29b, sec. 10)

Kiddusha Rabba

We find in the *Agra D'pirka* (sec. 190) that the second day of Yom Tov, which is *d'Rabbanan*, is greater than the first day. The reason for this is according to Kabbalah. Similarly, Kiddush recited by day, which is *d'Rabbanan*, has an advantage over Kiddush recited by night, and is therefore called *Kiddusha Rabba*, the greater Kiddush. *(Divrei Torah Mahadura Kama, sec. 43)*

Most *poskim* are of the opinion that the obligation to recite Kiddush takes effect after Shacharis. The Levush is of the opinion that the obligation to recite Kiddush takes effect after *krias haTorah*, and those who eat before *krias haTorah* are not obligated to make Kiddush. *(Magen Avos, p. 392)*

The Gra was particular only to recite Kiddush prior to a *seudah* on bread. Even during the day, he did not rely on the opinions that one can eat pastries or drink another cup of wine in lieu of a *seudah*.

(Biur Halachah 273:5, s.v. Kasvu hageonim; Binyan Olam, chap. 8)

Kiddush over Whiskey

The Taz states that one may recite Kiddush on whiskey since it is *chamar medinah*, a national drink (i.e. a popularly accepted drink) of the country. *(Kisvei Rabbi Yashe, Eirech HaTaz V'doro)*

The Yid Hakadosh of Peshischa was accustomed to reciting Kiddush on strong whiskey in order to demonstrate that the halachah follows the ruling of the Taz. *(Tiferes Hayehudi, sec. 18)*

Reb Yitzchak Isaac of Ziditchov gives another reason Kiddush is recited on whiskey. In Kiddush, we declare that Hashem created the world in six days and rested on the seventh. From what did Hashem rest? Only from speech, since He created the world through speech. Therefore, it is fitting to recite Kiddush on whiskey, which is *Shehakol*, the *brachah* in which we affirm that everything was created by the word of Hashem. *(Darchei Chaim, p. 134; Hadras Kodesh, p. 51)*

The Ropshitzer Rav would instruct his students to recite the day Kiddush on a small cup of whiskey, even though there was wine on the table, to demonstrate to them that one may recite Kiddush on whiskey.

(She'eilos Uteshuvos Maharsham, vol. 1, sec. 175)

Before his passing, the Sanzer Rav was extremely weak. His son, the Rebbe of Gorlitz, did not want his father to recite Kiddush on whiskey, as he was afraid it would adversely affect him. However, the Sanzer Rav did not agree to forgo Kiddush on whiskey, and replied, "What we learned from the Ropshitzer Rav, we perform even with *mesiras nefesh*."

(*Zemiros Ateres Yehoshua,* p. 262)

The following *rabbanim* are of the opinion that it is either preferable to recite the morning Kiddush on whiskey, or that one may recite it on whiskey without hesitation:

Reb Menachem Mendel of Riminov, the Chozeh of Lublin, the Ropshitzer Rav, the Yid Hakadosh of Peshischa, the Sanzer Rav, the Sar Shalom of Belz, the Kaminka Rebbe, the Kotzker Rebbe, the Shiniver Rav, the Chasam Sofer, the Rebbe of Stretin, the Minchas Yitzchak (Heller), the Spinka Rebbes, the Ba'al Imrei Yosef, and the Rebbe of Interdam, among others.

Among those who disagreed and were of the opinion that one should not recite Kiddush over whiskey are the Rebbe of Komarno, Reb Shimon of Yaroslav, the Lubavitcher Rebbes, the *talmidim* of the Gra, Reb Moshe Aharon Reichman, the Rav of Navotantz, and the Ba'al Lechem Hapanim.

The Komarno Rebbe once spent Shabbos with the Kol Aryeh. When it was time for morning Kiddush, the Kol Aryeh asked the Komarno Rebbe if he recited Kiddush on wine or whiskey. The Komarno Rebbe replied that one who drinks whiskey is ignorant of halachah. The Kol Aryeh responded that the Sanzer Rav recited Kiddush on whiskey.

The Komarno Rebbe then proceeded to recite Kiddush over what appeared to be wine. However, when he drank it he realized that it was whiskey. The Kol Aryeh then commented that it seemed like Heaven wanted to prove to the Komarno Rebbe that Kiddush over whiskey is not really wrong.

(*Toldos Kol Aryeh*)

The Ruzhiner Rebbe once asked Reb Elimelech of Rudnick which of the three *seudos* was most important. Reb Elimelech replied that it was the day *seudah*, since at that *seudah* they recited Kiddush on whiskey and were therefore in high spirits.

The Ruzhiner Rebbe took great pleasure in this answer and replied, "I did not know that Ropshitzer chassidim were that clever," alluding to the fact that these ideas are above our understanding. (*Siach Zekeinim*, p. 13; *Yud Gimmel Oros*, vol. 2)

Amount of Whiskey and Time Allotted for Drinking It

The Taz writes that a *brachah acharonah* is recited on the usual amount that people drink, even if it is less than a *revi'is*. Since most people drink only a small amount of whiskey, this amount is significant enough to warrant a *brachah acharonah*. Accordingly, it is also significant enough for Kiddush to be recited over it. Many people rely on this ruling and recite the Kiddush of Shabbos day over a small cup of whiskey.

(*Taz* 210:1)

Reb Aharon of Bendekovitz once came to the Sanzer Rav to see how he recited Kiddush—if he drank a *revi'is* of whiskey, or if he relied on the fact that the combined drinking of all the participants would equal a *revi'is*. However, the Sanzer Rav was accustomed to using a silver Kiddush cup, and Reb Aharon could not see how much he drank. As Reb Aharon was thinking these thoughts, the Sanzer Rav turned to him and said, "There are those who wonder why I do not follow the custom of the Ropshitzer Rav who recited the morning Kiddush using a glass cup. I use a silver cup so that I can do as I wish without the interference of other people's opinions."

(Magen Avos, p. 396)

The allotted time for drinking the required amount of a drink is considerably shorter than the allotted time for eating a *kezayis* of food. Therefore, if one finds it difficult to drink *rov revi'is* of whiskey in the allotted time, he may dip his cake into a *revi'is* of whiskey, until the whiskey is absorbed, and then eat the cake. Since the whiskey becomes part of the cake, the timeframe in which he can consume the whiskey is now the same as the timeframe in which one can eat the cake, which is *kedei achilas pras* (approximately four minutes).

(She'eilos Uteshuvos Haradad, Orach Chaim 8, s.v. Mei'atah)

The Ropshitzer Rav states that one may recite Kiddush on Shabbos day over whiskey, preferably by filling a large glass but only drinking a small amount. One may also fill a small glass and drink most of it.

Perhaps the reason it is preferable to fill a large glass is so that those present should also be able to drink from the Kiddush and the combined amount of all the participants is *melo lugmav* (a cheekful—the minimum amount required for Kiddush).

(She'eilos Uteshuvos Ginzei Yosef, vol. 2, sec. 62)

The Sanzer Rav and the Kaminka Rebbe would recite Kiddush on Shabbos and Yom Tov day on a small cup of whiskey. There are those who say that it contained a *revi'is*, and those who say that it contained, at most, a medium-sized *beitzah*, which is less than a *revi'is*.

(Nitzotzei Hakodesh, p. 127; Yud Gimmel Oros, p. 381)

Kiddush over Wine

The Shiniver Rav was accustomed to reciting Kiddush on wine, according to the Belzer *minhag*.

(Halichos U'minhagim, p. 17)

It was heard from Reb Aryeh Leib, the Rav of Cracow, that one should not recite Kiddush on whiskey since it is not considered a beverage. The midrash states that just like the Jews are above all other nations, oil rises to the top of every beverage. However, when one places oil into whiskey it sinks to the bottom. Thus, whiskey does not have the status of a beverage and Kiddush cannot be recited on it.

(Machatzis Hashekel 272:6)

The Magen Avraham writes that one should not recite Kiddush on whiskey, except in locations where most of the population drinks whiskey on a daily basis.

(Magen Avraham 272:6)

Participants Drinking from Kiddush

During the day, the participants are not obligated to drink from the Kiddush wine in order to have fulfilled the obligation of Kiddush, because the main mitzvah is the recitation of the *brachah* on the wine and not the actual drinking.

(Magen Avos, p. 399)

Conversely, the Brisker Rav, Reb Yitzchak Zev, was of the opinion that by day it is not sufficient just to hear the *brachah* of *Hagafen*; each listener must drink a sip of wine.

However, when the Chelkas Yaakov was with Reb Yissachar Dov of Belz, there were thousands of people present, among them *rabbanim*, chassidim, and pious people who were meticulous in their mitzvah observance, and all of them heard Kiddush from the Rebbe and did not drink wine afterwards; instead, they ate immediately.

It is written in the *Tosafos* *(Pesachim* 106a, s.v. *Havei gachin; Rosh* ibid.:16) that for Kiddush during the day, only one person is obligated to drink the wine. The reason for this is as explained by the Rashbam, that it is recited in order to praise Hashem, and praise is offered to Hashem over a cup of wine *(Rashbam* ibid., s.v. *Amar Rav Yehudah*). Therefore, the *brachah* over the wine is considered praise and is the main mitzvah, rather than the drinking. Accordingly, all who hear the *brachah* have fulfilled the obligation of Kiddush.

(She'eilos Uteshuvos, Chelkas Yaakov vol. 3, sec. 180, 193)

Not Wishing L'chaim

The Ba'al Minchas Elazar of Munkatch learned from his father, grandfather, and the Divrei Chaim, that one should not wish *l'chaim* at the Shabbos morning Kiddush.

The Nimukei Orach Chaim writes in the name of the Ba'al Darkei Teshuvah that this is because it shows a lack of respect to the Kiddush. Since at night one drinks wine and does not say *l'chaim*, if on Shabbos day he does say *l'chaim*, it appears as if the Shabbos day Kiddush is more important, which is not the case—reciting Kiddush at night is *d'Oraisa*, and during the day it is *d'Rabbanan*. *(She'eilos Uteshuvos Tiferes Adam, vol. 3)*

Covering the Cake

It seems that when reciting Kiddush on Shabbos morning one is required to cover the pastries, since the *brachah* of *Mezonos* usually comes before *Hagafen*. *(Shvilei Dovid 271:3)*

There are those who do not cover the pastries on the table during Kiddush. Since one may not recite Kiddush solely on pastries, we are not embarrassing the pastries by not reciting Kiddush over them. *(Eishel Avraham 182)*

The Kalashitzer Rebbe would not have the pastries on the table while reciting the morning Kiddush. They were only brought to the table afterward. *(Nitzotzei Hakodesh, p. 128)*

Pastries after Kiddush

Many *tzaddikim* were accustomed to eating pastries after the morning Kiddush, before the *seudah*, and only afterwards washing for the *seudah*, in order to recite more *brachos* on Shabbos. However, in order not to enter into a situation of doubt as to whether to recite a *brachah acharonah*, they ate less than a *kezayis* (the Sanzer Rav was accustomed to doing so).

(See *She'eilos Uteshuvos Maharsham* vol. 3, sec. 17)

The Yismach Moshe would eat cake before the morning *seudah*. He would recite *Al Hamichyah*, go outside for a bit, and then eat the Shabbos *seudah*.

(*Birchas Habayis, Sha'ar* 16; *Sha'arei Binah*, sec. 43)

The Ba'al Kedushas Yom Tov would eat a *kezayis* of a cookie which was made up of a large percentage of flour, so as not to have a doubt about whether or not to recite a *brachah acharonah*. In addition to the regular pastries, each person present also received a cookie that contained mostly flour, for this reason. (*She'eilos Uteshuvos Divrei Yoel*, 13:9)

One who recites Kiddush for others should eat a *kezayis* of cake or other grains, such as a flour-based kugel, in a short period of time (*kedei achilas pras*), so that he fulfills *Kiddush b'makom seudah* (reciting Kiddush at the time when one has a meal). At the very least, he should drink another *revi'is* of wine, aside from the Kiddush wine. For those who heard his Kiddush, one *revi'is* is sufficient. (*Otzar Halachos* 289:16)

The Ohr Zarua writes that it is a mitzvah to eat the *seudas Shabbos* with an appetite, and the challah constitutes the main part of the *seudah*. Therefore, one should not eat pastries prior to the *seudah*, since he will not be able to eat the *seudah* with an appetite. The Magen Avraham agrees with the Ohr Zarua and states that at the time that one may already eat the *seudah*, he should not fill up on other food.

The Darkei Moshe disagrees and is of the opinion that one may eat cake before the *seudah*. In practice, we accept the lenient opinion and do eat cake before the *seudah* (see *Shulchan Aruch Harav* 249:10, *Kuntris Acharon* 4, for more explanation).

People who are meticulous, wash immediately after Kiddush. Even one who does eat cake before the *seudah* should not eat too much, so that he can satiate himself with the bread at the *seudah*. *(Biur Halachah* 249, s.v. *Muttar)*

It is permissible to eat cake before the *seudah* because cake is *pas haba bakisnin*; if one eats a large quantity of it, he is required to wash. Therefore, it can be considered like bread, and constitutes part of the *seudah*.

Even if one eats cooked cereal, some say that since it requires a *brachah acharonah* which mentions Shabbos, it can also be considered *seudas Shabbos*. *(Tehillah L'Dovid,* 249: 3)

One is not supposed to eat a substantial amount of cake (a *kebeitzah*) before the *seudah* to ensure that the meal will be eaten with appetite. Yet, many people do eat cake after making Kiddush Shabbos morning.

We can find justification for this custom because the Shulchan Aruch Harav states that the requirement to eat the *seudah* with an appetite is not strictly necessary *(Shulchan Aruch Harav* 249:6). It is only a stringency, and one may be lenient. Furthermore, the Orchos Chaim is of the opinion that this restriction only applies on Friday night, because the person is satiated from eating on Friday. However, on Shabbos morning, after a night's sleep, a snack before the meal will not spoil his appetite. On the contrary, the snack might serve as an appetizer, to increase appetite *(Orchos Chaim* ibid.).

(Ohr Yisrael, Year 13, Issue 2)

The Rebbe of Nassad said that eating pastries after the morning Kiddush is a *segulah* for livelihood and *shidduchim*.

(As heard from elderly chassidim)

Whole Cookie

It is better to recite the *brachah* on a whole cookie, even if it is small, than on a slice of cake. *(Shulchan Aruch* 168:1)

Lechem Mishneh on Pastries

If one recites Kiddush on Shabbos morning on cake prior to the *seudah,* he should recite the *brachah* of *Mezonos* on two whole pastries.
(Kitzur Shulchan Aruch 77:17)

One is not obligated to recite *Mezonos* on two whole pastries. Even if one wishes to do so, it is sufficient to use two slices of cake. If one wants to recite *Mezonos* on two whole pastries, he should do so only at home.
(She'eilos Uteshuvos Minchas Yitzchak, vol. 3, sec. 13)

In practice, most people do not recite *Mezonos* on two pastries, since this is not the main *seudah*. *(Be'er Yaakov* 273:10)

Cake

Lekach (cake) is eaten after Kiddush since it alludes to the Torah, based on a play on words from the *pasuk* in *Mishlei* (4:2): *Ki lekach tov nasati lachem*—"for I have given you a good *lekach*" (i.e. the Torah).

Honey is also compared to the Torah, as it says in *Shir Hashirim* (4:11), *...honey and milk are under your tongue* (*Devarim Rabbah* 7:3). Therefore, many specifically eat honey cake after Kiddush on Shabbos. *(Zemiros Tiferes Tzvi,* p. 244)

Many have a custom to eat cake at Kiddush called, *Shidduchim Lekach* as a *segulah* for *shidduchim* for their children, to merit serving *lekach* at a *l'chaim* (engagement) soon. The connection between *lekach* (cake) and a *shidduch* is based on the *pasuk, Ki lekach tov nasati lachem* (*Mishlei* 4:2). Later in *Mishlei* (18:22), it says about a wife, *matza ishah matza tov*—"one who finds a wife finds good." Since the word *tov* (good) is used about *lekach* and about a wife, we eat *lekach* to symbolize one finding a wife. *(Zemiros Shirei Hamalchus,* P. 247)

Eating cake after Kiddush is a *segulah* for *parnassah*.
(Gedulas Yehoshua)

Seudas Rabbi Chidka

Chazal ask: How many *seudos* is a person required to eat on Shabbos? The Rabbis held that a person should eat three *seudos*, but Rabbi Chidka held that one should eat four *seudos*. Rabbi Yochanan said that both views were taken from the same *pasuk*, in which the Torah states the word, *"hayom"* three times in regard to eating the *mann* on Shabbos *(Shemos* 16:25). Rashi states that these three times refer to the three *seudos* of Shabbos. Rabbi Chidka holds that the word, *hayom* written three times only referred to the Shabbos day, excluding the night *seudah*, thus totaling four *seudos* to be eaten throughout Shabbos. The Rabbis held that three times *"hayom"* referred to the entire Shabbos, totaling three *seudos*. *(Shabbos* 117b)

It is said that eating after Kiddush on Shabbos morning fulfills the opinion of Rabbi Chidka who held that one should eat four *seudos* on Shabbos *(Shabbos* 117b).

There are others who are of the opinion that the reason is in order to say 100 *brachos* on Shabbos. *(Magen Avos,* p. 399)

There was a great person who received a visitor during his Shabbos *seudah*. He instructed his guest that if he already recited *Birkas Hamazon,* he should recite Kiddush and wash again in order to fulfill the *seudah* of Rabbi Chidka.

The Gaon of Brezahn held that it is forbidden for one to do so since the halachah is according to the *Rabbanan* and not Reb Chidka. However, having in mind to fulfill *seudas Rabbi Chidka* is permitted, as long as it is not stated explicitly.

(Michla D'asvisa, sec. 81)

On Shabbos morning, the author of the *Zichron Yehoshua* recited Kiddush while still wearing his *tallis* and he then ate fish and fruit preserves. He would say that this is in order to fulfill the *Seudas Rebbe Chidka*, who held that one should eat four *seudos* throughout Shabbos *(Shabbos* 118a).

(Zichron Yehoshua, Erech Seudah, sec. 7)

After eating cake, Reb Aharon of Belz would eat a small amount of compote on Shabbos morning. The chassidim believed that this was in order to fulfill *Seudas Rabbi Chidka*.

(*B'kedushaso Shel Aharon*, p. 442)

Compote before the Meal

The accepted *minhag* is to eat appetizers and fruit preserves before the *seudah*. (*Shulchan Aruch Harav, Kuntris Acharon*, 249:4)

The Bobover Rebbe would recite *Ha'eitz* on compote made of the *esrog* that was used on Sukkos. This was in order to be able to recite 100 *brachos* throughout the day. Since the *esrog* was used for a mitzvah, he used it to fulfill more mitzvos.

(*Magen Avos*, p. 401)

The *minhag* by Sanzer chassidim was that from Tu B'Shevat until Pesach they would eat *esrog* after reciting the morning Kiddush. (*Minhagei Sanz*)

There are those who are accustomed to eating other foods after the cake in order to recite more *brachos*. (*Minhagei Sanz*)

Yerushalmi Kugel

Although generally, there is a minimum amount required to be eaten in order to be regarded as a meal, because of the significance of Shabbos food, on Shabbos even a minimal amount can be considered a complete meal. If so, eating even a small amount of cake may obligate one to recite *Birkas Hamazon*. Perhaps this is the reason for the *minhag* of serving *lokshen* kugel after Kiddush which, even if one eats a large amount, does not require *Birkas Hamazon*. (*She'eilos Uteshuvos Maharach*)

The Chida disagrees with the abovementioned view and is of the opinion that one can eat cake on Shabbos and he is not required to recite *Birkas Hamazon*. This is the accepted practice. (*Birchei Yosef*, ibid.)

In Yerushalayim they were accustomed to eating noodle kugel so as not to enter into doubts of consuming too much cake, and possibly being obligated to recite *Birkas Hamazon*. However, the Chazon Ish states that although *minhag Yerushalayim* is sacred, if one eats a substantial amount of *lokshen* kugel, he faces the same dilemma regarding *Birkas Hamazon* as with cake. (*Ma'aseh Ish*, vol. 3, p. 121)

Shalom Bayis Kugel

The Kozhnitzer Maggid and his descendants had a *minhag* to eat a kugel that they termed *Shalom Bayis* kugel after the morning Kiddush. They then ate kugel again during the *seudah*.

To explain this *minhag*, they related the following story: A *din Torah* between a husband and wife once came before the Maggid of Kozhnitz. The husband requested that the Maggid grant them a *get*. He explained that his wife was extremely pious and honored him tremendously; however, he had one complaint.

He raised animals and fowl and had a stream with fish near his home. Thus, he was able to eat a meal of meat and fish on most days of the week. Since he ate such complete meals during the week, there was almost nothing different on his Shabbos menu, except for kugel. Therefore, he wanted it to be served immediately after he came home from shul so that he could eat it with an appetite in honor of Shabbos, and not towards the end of the *seudah*, when he was already satiated. However, his wife did not want to fulfill his request and serve the kugel earlier, and he therefore wanted to divorce her.

The wife then entered and presented her side. She stated that for the most part she had nothing against her husband. He was meticulous in his mitzvah observance and honored her greatly. However, he wanted to eat kugel immediately after arriving home from shul and she had never heard of such a custom. Since a *minhag* is sacrosanct, she wanted to divorce him.

The Maggid called them together and told them that the *beis din's* ruling is that the wife should cook two kugels each week. One should be eaten as soon as her husband returned home from shul, and the second one should be eaten during the *seudah,* as is the *minhag*. The couple went home extremely happy.

At the time of this *din Torah* there was a commotion in Heaven that this couple had agreed to the divorce solely for the sake of Heaven, since they were truly happy with each other. From that day on, the Maggid instructed that two kugels should be prepared each Shabbos. (*Vaya'an Yosef,* p. 24)

Eating Fish Prior to the Seudah

The Dinover Rebbe would eat fish before the *seudah,* after reciting Kiddush on Shabbos morning. Although fish is an essential part of Shabbos, we do not recite a *brachah* on it when it is eaten during the *seudah*. Therefore, the Rebbe ate it before the *seudah* so that he could recite the *brachah* of *Shehakol* on it. (*Divrei Torah,* vol. 3, sec. 9)

Reb Moshe of Dezh was once together with the Shiniver Rav on Shabbos. On Shabbos morning, the Shiniver Rav recited Kiddush on wine. He explained that although his father recited Kiddush on whiskey, he did not do so because he ate the fish prior to the *seudah* in order to be able to recite a *brachah* on it. If he would recite Kiddush over whiskey, he would no longer be able to recite a *Shehakol* on the fish.

(*Ma'amar Yechezkel,* Shiniva, p. 7)

The Minchas Elazar of Munkatch stressed the *minhag* of eating fish specifically during the *seudah*. He felt that since *tzaddikim* are *megulgal* in fish, in order to demonstrate that they do not need such a tremendous *tikkun*, it is not necessary to recite a *brachah* on the fish itself; the *Hamotzi* recited on the entire *seudah* is sufficient. (*Divrei Torah, Mahadura* 3, sec. 9)

On Shabbos day, Belzer chassidim do not serve the fish sauce, because the main reason for eating fish sauce is to dip the challah into it. Since they eat the fish after Kiddush, and not during the *seudah*, it is not possible to dip challah into the sauce. (*Halichos Hatzaddikim*, p. 329)

Meat Prior to the Seudah

The Ba'al Chakal Yitzchak was accustomed to eating fried chicken after Kiddush. (*Zemiros Tiferes Tzvi*, p. 245)

Brachah Acharonah after Kiddush

If one eats pastries after Kiddush on Shabbos morning, and he plans to wash on bread a short while later, he should definitely not recite a *brachah acharonah* since Kiddush is supposed to be *b'makom seudah*—together with the meal. The food eaten after Kiddush could be regarded as part of the *seudah* and does not require a separate *brachah acharonah*. (*Aruch Hashulchan* 176:8; *Birchas Habayis, Sha'ar* 16)

If a person eats a *kezayis* of pastries after the morning Kiddush and eats the *seudah* immediately afterward, he does not need to recite a *brachah acharonah*. He should have in mind when reciting *Birkas Hamazon* that it should include the pastries that he ate earlier.

It is written in the name of the *Sefer She'eilos Teshuvos Pe'ulos Tzedek* that if after Kiddush one eats fruits that he would recite a blessing over during the meal, the *Birkas Hamazon* exempts it from a *brachah acharonah*. Similarly, if one eats *Mezonos* prior to the *seudah*, he does not need to recite a *brachah acharonah* because Kiddush is considered the beginning of the *seudah*.

(*She'eilos Uteshuvos Maharsham*, vol. 2, sec. 17)

Chapter 15
The Shabbos Day Seudah

Being Ma'avir Sedrah Before the Seudah

The midrash states that before his passing, Reb Yehudah Hanasi instructed his children on three matters, among them that one should not eat the morning *seudah* on Shabbos until he has finished being *ma'avir sedrah* (learning the *parshah* by reading the *pesukim* twice and *targum* once) (*Mechilta, Bo*).

(*Tosafos, Brachos* 8b, s.v. *Yashlim parshiyosav*)

Eating Right after Davening

Over Shabbos, we say three *tefillos* which correspond to the three terms mentioned in the first *brachah* of *Shemoneh Esrei*: *Hagadol* (the Great One), *Hagibor* (the Strong One), and *Hanora* (the Awesome One). On Friday night, we say *Atah Kidashta,* which is proof of the creation of the world, corresponding to *Hagadol*. On Shabbos day, we say *Yismach Moshe,* which is a sign that Hashem runs the world constantly, which corresponds to the term *Hagibor*. During *Minchah*, we say *Atah Echad,* which demonstrates that in the future all the nations will recognize Hashem. This corresponds to the term *Hanora*.

The three *seudos* of Shabbos also correspond to these three terms. The first *seudah* corresponds to *Hagadol*, the second to *Hagibor*, and the third to *Hanora*. Therefore, one should eat the day *seudah* soon after *davening* to show the connection between *Yismach Moshe, Hagibor,* and the day *seudah*.

(*Kavei El Hashem*, chap. 15)

The Honor of the Day Seudah

The honor of the day *seudah* takes precedence over that of the night *seudah*, so one should eat better foods at the day *seudah*. This *seudah* is a very significant, elevated time. One should act as if he is eating before a king, and eat with holiness and modesty.
(Chemdas Hayamim)

Rashi explains that if one only has enough wine or enough of a certain delicacy for one *seudah*, he should reserve it for the day. The day *seudah* is greater than the night *seudah* because the holiness of Shabbos increases as Shabbos goes on.
(She'eilos Uteshuvos Chasam Sofer, Orach Chaim 17)

Another reason why the day *seudah* takes precedence is because we derive the concept of eating three *seudos* on Shabbos from the *pasuk* in *Shemos* (16:25), *ichluhu hayom*, which uses the word *hayom* three times, corresponding to the three *seudos*. Since the *pasuk* uses the word *hayom* (day), this demonstrates that the main *seudah* of Shabbos is during the day.
(Chasdei Dovid on Tosefta Brachos 3:12)

Another reason that the day *suedah* takes precedence is that the miracle of the *mann* was only noticeable on Shabbos morning. During the week, each night they ate the *mann* from that day, and thus Friday night was no different from any other night of the week. It was only in the morning that Bnei Yisrael realized that the extra *mann* did not become spoiled overnight, while during the week it would have.
(Rash Sirilau, Yerushalmi Brachos, end of ch. 7)

The Gemara states that the main *seudos* are eaten during the day and not at night (see *Tosafos Avodah Zarah*, s.v. *Bas yuma*). At night, one is already satiated from the food that he ate during the day. Hence, a person has a greater appetite at the Shabbos day *seudah* and his *oneg Shabbos* is greater.

In addition, the holiness of Shabbos was most recognizable in the Beis Hamikdash during the day, since the *Korban Mussaf* was sacrificed then. *(Aruch Hashulchan 289:2)*

Since the honor of the day *seudah* is greater, one should reserve one specific food for the day. *(Umkah Shel Halachah, p. 92)*

It is preferable that the clothing that one wears Shabbos day should be nicer than those worn at night to give greater honor to the Shabbos day. The *minhag* is to wear light-colored clothes at night, and dark clothes, which are more elegant, by day. *(Yafeh L'lev vol. 5, Kuntris Acharon, Orach Chaim 262)*

According to the Yismach Moshe, the second *seudas Shabbos* is the most elevated point of Shabbos.
(Shulchan Menachem, Beshalach)

The Yam Shel Shlomo writes that it is wrong not to differentiate between the night and day *seudos*. Some even make the night *seudah* more elaborate than the day *seudah* and eat special fish at night as the main course of the *seudah*. The Yam Shel Shlomo restrained himself and did not eat fish on Friday night since it is an important dish. In this way, even if the night *seudah* had many delicacies, the day *seudah* would still be superior, since it contained fish.
(Yam Shel Shlomo, Gittin 4:51)

Reciting Kiddush a Second Time

One who recites Kiddush prior to *Mussaf* does not need to recite Kiddush again afterward. However, there is room to be stringent and repeat Kiddush, because some are of the opinion that there is no obligation to recite Kiddush before *Mussaf*, so if one recited Kiddush at that time, he needs to recite it again. Another reason is because one is not permitted to eat a proper meal prior to *davening Mussaf*, and therefore, the Kiddush only exempts that which is eaten at the proper time, which is before *Mussaf*.

If one recited Kiddush after *Mussaf*, but only ate cake and the like, it is a commendable practice to recite Kiddush again prior to washing for the *seudah*. With this, one fulfills the opinion of the Gra that the morning Kiddush needs to be followed by a proper meal with bread. Reb Yosef Chaim Sonnenfeld agrees with this opinion. *(Middah Nechonah,* chap. 8, sec. 11)

Drinking before Washing

Although one does not need to recite a *brachah* on whiskey that one drinks in the middle of a *seudah*, the Magen Avraham states that if one drinks whiskey immediately at the beginning or the end of the *seudah*, a *brachah* needs to be recited. Therefore, it is proper for one to drink a small amount prior to washing for bread, with which one exempts any beverage he will drink throughout the *seudah*. If one drinks wine during the *seudah*, the *brachah* on the wine also exempts any other beverage and he does not need to recite another *brachah* on any beverage throughout the meal. *(Chelkas Yaakov* 163)

Covering the Challos

There are several *minhagim* regarding covering the challos during the day. Reb Menachem Mendel of Riminov, the Ropshitzer Rav, and the Sanzer Rav did not cover them, and the Chozeh of Lublin and the Shiniver Rav did. The Ba'al Shem Shlomo of Munkatch would cover the challos partially as a compromise. *(Lev Same'ach Hachadash, Ohr Chadash,* sec. 8)

Reb Mendel of Riminov once spent Shabbos with his Rebbe, the Chozeh of Lublin. On Shabbos morning, when Reb Mendel saw that the challos for the *seudah* were uncovered, he told those present to bring a challah cover and cover them. Although the *talmidim* of the Chozeh knew that their Rebbe was not accustomed to covering the challos, out of respect for Reb Mendel of Riminov, they abided by his request.

When the Chozeh arrived, he removed the cover from the challos. The next day, Rebbe Mendel of Riminov came to the Chozeh and apologized for unknowingly opposing the Rebbe's customs. *(Sichos Chaim,* p. 21b)

Challah for Shabbos Day Seudah

At the day *seudah* we use braided challos, since one should have dishes that are more special for the day *seudah*. One should cut into the large challah on the right side.

(Magen Avos, p. 407)

There are those who cut into two loaves of challah at the day *seudah* to demonstrate that the honor of the day *seudah* is greater than that of the night *seudah*.   *(Elyah Rabbah* 274:4)

On Friday night, one should cut a *kezayis* of challah for himself and a *kebeitzah* for his wife. However, on Shabbos day and *shalosh seudos* it is sufficient to give one's wife a *kezayis*. However, some are of the opinion that at all *seudos* one should give his wife a *kebeitzah*.

(Kaf Hachaim, Sofer, 167:20; *Kaf Hachaim, Palagi,* 36:48)

Rabbi Aharon Yeshayah Fisch of Hadas was wont to say that one who eats a large amount of challah before the cholent is a glutton and a drunkard. *(Noam Siach,* p. 220)

Menu and Order of Shabbos Day Seudah

Reb Shalom of Kaminka said that the names of Hashem are alluded to in our Shabbos food. He explained that for this reason his Rebbe, Reb Shalom of Belz, ate only four dishes at his Shabbos *seudah*, corresponding to the four letters in the *Shem Havayah*. He did not eat fish or compote during the day *seudah*, only eggs with onions, cholent, kugel, and meat.

(Yud Gimmel Oros, vol. 2, *Ma'areches Reb Shalom of Belz,* p. 235)

The *minhag* of Komarno is to eat the following menu on Shabbos day: gefilte fish and plain fish, eggs with chopped

onions, liver with chopped onions, warm *galaretta* (a dish made from calves' feet), cholent, potato kugel and another two kugels (one of them sweet), stuffed *kishke*, chicken, meat, *tzimmes*, and compote.
(Minhagei Komarno, p. 54)

The Shabbos foods are eggs with onions, *p'tcha*, cholent, and *farfel*, like that which is eaten at night.
(Minhagei Beis Alik, p. 363)

There are those who eat the *seudah* in the order of the words from *davening: Galei k'vod malchuscha*—"Reveal the glory of Your kingdom." They first eat *gala*, then *kaveid* (liver), then eggs, which allude to the *middah* of *malchus* *(Tikkunei Zohar, Hakdamah*, p. 2). (As heard)

It was said in the name of the Ba'al Hatanya that it was handed down from Moshe Rabbeinu that one should first eat cholent, then kugel, and then meat.
(Teshurah Misimchas Nisu'in, p. 45)

It is written in the name of *tzaddikim* that the order of the Shabbos food eaten at the *seudah* is handed down from Moshe Rabbeinu, and one must eat them in this order. Shabbos is our spouse, as the midrash *(Bereishis Rabbah* 11:8) states that Shabbos came before Hashem and complained that all the days of the week have a partner except Shabbos. Hashem replied that Bnei Yisrael is its spouse.

The Gemara states that finding one's *zivug* is as difficult *(kasheh)* as *Krias Yam Suf*. Therefore, we eat kasha cholent. Then, we eat *lokshen* kugel that is in the shape of a circle to allude to a wedding ring. The word, *lokshen* is comprised of two words, *lo kashin*, not difficult, since in the merit of Shabbos, the difficulty of finding a *zivug* will be eased. After that we eat meat *(basar)* to allude to the *pasuk* of *v'hayah l'basar echad* *(Bereishis* 2:24) which refers to marriage. (In the name of *tzaddikim*)

The Yismach Moshe ate the cholent, then the eggs, and then the fish at the end of the *seudah* prior to *Birkas Hamazon* (as is the *minhag* in Karlin). His *talmid*, Reb Tzvi Hersh of Liska followed this *minhag*.

In the *tefillah* of *Tikanta Shabbos*, recited in the Shabbos *Mussaf*, the first letter of each word goes according to the *aleph-beis* backwards, from *tav* to *aleph*. It thus ends with the letters *vav, heh, dalet, gimmel, beis*, and *aleph* which spells the words *v'hadag ba* (and the fish comes) at the end of the *tefillah*. This is an allusion that the fish should be served at the end of the *seudah* (Beis Yosef, Orach Chaim 286).
(Darchei Hayashar V'hatov, p. 22b; Zemiros Vayidaber Moshe)

The Yismach Moshe explained that he enjoyed eating fish more than any other food. Since he finished *davening* late in the day and was very hungry at that point, if he would eat fish immediately, it would be difficult for him to have the proper intentions of eating it in honor of Shabbos. Therefore, he left it for the end, when he was already satiated and could have in mind the correct thoughts. (Dvar Tzvi Kedushas HaShabbos 127)

Reb Yerachmiel Moshe of Kozhnitz was accustomed to eating the fish at the end of the *seudah*. He would lightheartedly say that the fish is like *afikoman*, and it is not proper to eat anything else after eating it.
(Sifran Shel Tzaddikim, Ma'areches 17, p. 38b)

The *minhag* in Ukraine was that first fried onions and radishes were eaten, then chopped liver with fried onions, and then *p'tcha* which contained vinegar.

The Shpole Zeide gave a reason for this *minhag*. The radishes, which are bitter, remind a person to *"beht ehrlich,"* (*daven* devoutly). The liver (in Yiddish, *leberlach*) remind a person to *"lehb ehrlich"* (live honestly), and the *p'tcha*, which was sour (in Yiddish, *zeierlech*), reminds a person to *zei ehrlich* (be pious).
(Ish Hapele, Shpole, p. 308)

The Vizhnitzer Rebbetzin was also accustomed to eating these three dishes for the same reasons.

(Meir Hachaim, vol. 2, 2:15)

Fish During the Day Seudah

The Maharshal ate fish only during the day since he derived pleasure from it. This demonstrates that if one has a special food, he should save it for the day *seudah*.

(Sha'arei Teshuvah 271:3:1)

Our Rebbes ate two types of fish during the day, just like at the night *seudah*. *(Magen Avos,* p. 407; *Zemiros Tiferes Tzvi,* p. 248)

Not Eating Fish at the Day Seudah

In the *Likutei Maharich* it is written that, according to the *Zohar*, the honor of the night *seudah* is greater than the day, and therefore one should eat fish only at night.

(Kovetz Iyun Haparshah, Issue 73, *Asichah B'chukecha,* sec. 62)

The Shiniver Rav held that it is not necessary to eat fish during the day *seudah*. However, he would dip his challah into the fish sauce, explaining that it was difficult for him to eat a *kezayis* otherwise. He related that his father also did not eat fish at the day *seudah* until several Rebbes from Poland visited him and, in their honor, his father served fish, as was their *minhag*. From then on, he always ate fish by day.

(Zemiros Shabbos Shalom Umevorach, p. 71)

The Yerushlayimer Rav, Reb Moshe Aryeh Freund, ate the head of the fish on Friday night and *shalosh seudos,* but not at the Shabbos day meal. *(Zemiros Ateres Yehoshua,* p. 268)

There are those who do not eat fish during the day. This idea comes from those countries where they were accustomed to eating hot fish, and could not tolerate eating it cold. Since it is not possible to eat hot fish on Shabbos day, they did not eat it at all.

In countries where fish is eaten cold, it is a mitzvah to eat fish on Shabbos day. Nevertheless, it is possible that there is a deeper meaning to this custom [of not eating fish during the day]. *(Shulchan Hatahor 242:8)*

There are those who do not eat fish on Shabbos day for Kabbalistic reasons, but one who eats fish and has in mind to honor the Shabbos will be blessed.
(Shulchan Hatahor 242, Hagahos Zeir Zahav sec. 5,8, Komarno)

At the Shiniver Rav's *seudah,* only the Rav ate fish, and not the other participants. *(L'ateir Pesora, p. 79)*

"Falshe" Fish

After World War I, there was a time when meat was available but fish was not. Therefore, they cooked *"falshe"* fish, imitation fish, which consisted of ground meat, cooked so that its taste and appearance were similar to that of gefilte fish.

Reb Yosef Tzvi Piller was once a guest for Shabbos and was served *"falshe"* fish. Reb Yosef Tzvi remarked that in his city it was not possible to obtain fish. His hosts laughed and told him that it was really meat. *(Ranu L'Yaakov Simchah, p. 144)*

Garlic

Several *tzaddikim* ate garlic during the Shabbos day *seudah*. (See *She'eilos Uteshuvos, Divrei Yatziv, Yoreh De'ah*, 105:3)

Onions

The Ba'al Shem Tov states two reasons for eating onions on Shabbos. First, onions are detrimental to a person's health. By eating onions on Shabbos, we demonstrate that Shabbos heals. Secondly, the seven layers of an onion allude to the seven days of the week.

(She'eiris Yisrael of Hagaon Yisrael Gorzicinzki)

Batzel (onion) alludes to the *tzila dimheimenusa*, Hashem's protection, as the *pasuk* states in *Tehillim* (91:1): ***b'tzeil Shakai yislonan***—"he will dwell in the shadow of the Almighty." Since Shabbos is symbolic of *tzila dimheimenusa*, we eat onions.
(Imrei Pinchas, vol. 1, Sha'ar HaShabbos, sec. 39)

We eat onions on Shabbos because they are bitter, and in Yiddish the word *bitterlach* is similar to the words *beht ehrlich*, ask *(daven)* devoutly.
(Yalkut Me'orei Ohr, Erech Shabbos)

The Neshchizer Rebbe relates in the name of the Karliner Rebbe that eating onions at *seudas Shabbos* can prevent certain heart conditions.
(Zikaron Tov, Inyanei Ma'achal, sec. 2)

Aside from eating eggs with onions, the author of the *Zichron Yehoshua* cut a piece from a whole onion and ate it. He would say that by eating onions all the *klipos* (negative spiritual forces) would be nullified. (*Zichron Yehoshua*, *Eirech Seudah*, sec. 11)

Reb Yechezkel of Kuzmir states a reason for eating onions on Shabbos, based on a Gemara in *Beitzah* (15b) that Hashem tell us that a person should borrow money in order to honor the Shabbos, and Hashem will repay him. The word, *betzalim*, onions, is similar to the Yiddish word *batzalin*, which means to repay. We eat onions in order to remind ourselves that Hashem will repay that which we borrowed to honor Shabbos.
(Ma'amar Yechezkel, Kuzmir, p. 140; Imrei Tzvi, p. 38)

Reb Avraham of Stretin says that *tzibeles* (Yiddish for onions, spelled *tzaddi, yud, beis, lamed, sin*) is an acronym for *yancheini bma'aglei tzedek l'ma'an shemo*—"He leads me in paths of righteousness for His Name's sake" (*Tehillim* 23:4).
(Reb Avraham of Stretin)

Reb Dovid Tzvi Shlomo of Lelov would say that Shabbos is an acronym for ***Shabbos batzel tochal***—on Shabbos one should eat onions. He would say in the name of *tzaddikim* that without onions, Shabbos would lose its flavor.

(*Tiferes Beis Dovid, Likutei Divrei Dovid*, p. 44)

In the times of *Chazal*, onions were an important food eaten only by the upper class (see *Rambam, Bartenura* on Mishnah, *Terumos* 2:5, s.v. *Ma'achal poiltikin*). In honor of Shabbos, the poor would eat onions as well.

Onions have special importance. We see from the Gemara in *Shabbos* (119a) that one should delight in the Shabbos with spinach, large fish, and garlic, which were important foods. Rav Chisda ate spinach in honor of Shabbos since it is a vegetable that is beneficial to the heart, the eyes, and the digestive system. So too, onions are good for the heart and are also a significant food eaten in honor of Shabbos.

Another reason for eating onions on Shabbos is to oppose the *Kera'im*. Onions are generally cut with a knife, and the *Kera'im* said that one is not allowed to use a knife on Shabbos, so the *minhag* is to eat onions to prove them wrong.

The word *oneg* has the same numerical value (counting the word itself as one) as *batzel* (onion). The word *batzel* is an acronym for *b'Shabbos tzarich l'achlo*—one must eat it on Shabbos.

(*Alim L'trufah*, issue 627)

An allusion to eating onion at the *seudah* is that we find in the chapter of *Tehillim* (23) of *Mizmor L'Dovid* that the first letters of the phrase *b'ma'aglei tzedek l'ma'an* spells *batzel*. The *pasuk* continues with the word *Shemo*, which can refer to Shabbos, since Shabbos is one of the names of Hashem.

(*Mattan Shabbos, Ma'areches* 2, sec. 24)

Belzer chassidim were accustomed to eating onions twice—with liver and with eggs. They did not mix them together but ate them side by side. This was also the *minhag* in Komarno.

(See *Magen Avos*, p. 422)

Raw Onions

We are not accustomed to eating raw onions since they are not conducive to good health. *(Ta'anis* 30a, see *Tosafos)*

The *poskim* state that it is possible that times have changed and raw onions are no longer harmful.

It is written in the name of the Ba'al Shem Tov that one should not eat raw onions. However, this is not accepted in practice and most chassidic communities do eat them.
(Ba'al Shem Tov Al HaTorah, Yisro)

Onions, garlic, mustard, and radishes are harmful and should only be eaten in very small amounts during the winter season. During the summer one should not eat them at all.
(Rambam, Hilchos Dei'os 4:9)

One who travels from one location to another should eat onions so that the change in the atmosphere does not adversely affect him. *(Refuos Usegulos Meihalevushei Serad)*

Reb Nosson of Breslov would not eat raw onions, even mixed with fat or eggs. He was of the opinion that raw onions, even on Shabbos, are harmful both physically and spiritually.
(Sichos HaRan 265, *Ba'al Shem Tov Al HaTorah, Yisro,* sec. 46)

It is written in the *Sefer Ba'al Shem Tov* that, as a *segulah* for preventing illness, one should not eat raw onions, even on Shabbos and even if mixed with fat or eggs.

The Rambam mentions onions among foods that are detrimental to one's health, and the Gemara mentions several times that onions are harmful (see *Aruch, Os Nachash,* that this only refers to certain onions). The Gemara in *Eiruvin* states that a person should not eat onions because of snakes in them, which Rashi explains as poison. The Ritva states that some say that this refers to a worm that is created in the onion, which is as harmful as the poison of a snake.

The Gemara in *Pesachim* states that there is a harmful substance in lettuce, and it should therefore be dipped into *charoses*. The Gemara continues by stating that Rav Asa says that the remedy to the toxins found in some vegetables is warm food. Similarly, eating warm food removes the detrimental effects of onions. Since our *minhag* is to eat cholent after the eggs with onions, the onions are not harmful. There are those who cook the eggs in the cholent, so that they should be warm. There were *tzaddikim* who ate every spoon of eggs with onions with some cholent or *p'tcha*. (Rabbi Dovid Meisels)

Reb Shalom of Kaminka did not eat raw onions, even on Shabbos. He explained the onions are not considered a food since they do not have any content, only layers of peel. Instead of onions, he ate borscht.

Reb Shalom of Belz once asked him why he did not eat onions, since the word *batzel* has a *mispar kattan* of 14, which is twice seven. The Kaminka Rebbe replied that he eats borscht (*beis, reish, shin*) which has a *mispar kattan* of seven. To make up for the other seven, he would eat any other food (*ma'achal* [food] has a numerical value of 91, which is 13 times 7), but not onions, since he did not consider them a food.

(*Oheiv Shalom*, vol. 2, p. 46; *Nitzotzei Hakodesh*, p. 130)

Cutting Onions

Onions allude to *klipos* (literally peels, but can also mean negative spiritual forces). Reb Shlomo of Bobov said that the Sanzer Rav cut the onions himself, to destroy the negative forces.

(*Magen Avos*, p. 412)

The *minhag* is to use the bottom part of the onion. It should be placed face down and cut into small pieces.

(*Magen Avos*, p. 419)

The Kedushas Tzion once said that the reason for cutting the eggs and onion into small pieces is because the words, *dak, dak* (thin, thin, meaning very small), have the same numerical value as the word Yitzchak, and the Shabbos day *seudah* corresponds to Yitzchak. *(Magen Avos, p. 420)*

One should first cut off the leaves of the onion to allow the toxins to escape. *(Divrei Tzaddikim)*

There are seven Shabbos dishes corresponding to the seven attributes. Onion is the second food, and corresponds to the attribute of justice. We cut the onions to cut away retribution and negative decrees. *(Pnei Shabbos, p. 203)*

The Shiniver Rav would peel the onions himself. On one occasion, when his son wanted to help him, he asked with wonder, "You also know how to peel onions?" [His intention was to ask his son if he also understood the holy reasons behind peeling the onions.] *(Divrei Yechezkel Hachadash, p. 350)*

Eggs and Onions

The *minhag* is to eat hard-boiled eggs at the Shabbos day *seudah* since Moshe Rabbeinu died on Shabbos and hard-boiled eggs are customarily eaten during the mourning period. *(Knesses Hagedolah 288:8)*

Reb Pinchas of Koritz would say that if we knew the deep meaning behind eating eggs with onions on Shabbos, we would be prepared to pay a *rendel* (a large sum of money) if necessary, for each egg. *(Siach Zekeinim, vol. 4, p. 96)*

Beitzim (eggs) is an acronym for the *pasuk* in *Yirmiyahu* (14:8): *Mikvah Yisrael moshia b'eis tzarah*—"The Hope of Yisrael, their Savior at times of trouble." *(Kedushas Naftali, vol. 2, p. 240)*

Reb Avraham Azulai states that in *galus*, it is not generally appropriate to rejoice with drinking wine and eating meat. However, because we eat an egg, and thereby remember

the *Churban*, we are permitted to partake of meat and wine afterward.
(*Chasam Sofer, Revia'ah L'Pesach*)

An egg comes from a chicken and can bring forth another chicken. So too, Shabbos receives the effects of the preparations that were done in its honor, and it also brings bounty and blessing to the following week (*Zohar*, vol. 2, chap. 8a).
(*Damesek Eliezer*, p. 128)

Regarding the abovementioned reason for eating eggs, the Kedushas Tzion of Bobov explains that we need to eat something on Shabbos that is also eaten during the week, so that the blessing should have on what to rest. Since eggs are commonly eaten during the week, we eat them on Shabbos as well.
(*Zichronos Mimei Kedem*, p. 39)

Accordingly, it is possible that this is why some eat eggs and onions together with challah, because both allude to the fact that Shabbos has an effect on all the days of the week.
(*Rabbi Dovid Meisels*)

The Ropshitzer Rav would say that we eat *ei'er* (eggs) because *eider* (before) the world existed, Shabbos already existed.

The Kedushas Tzion explains that without Shabbos the world would not be able to exist. In truth, Shabbos already existed before the first of the six days of creation. On the *pasuk: And Hashem finished His work on the seventh day* (*Bereishis* 2:2), the Ramak explains the reason that the *pasuk* doesn't state that Hashem finished His work on the sixth day. This is because, in truth, Friday was the seventh day, because Hashem already created Shabbos before Sunday, the first day of creation.
(*Magen Avos*, p. 417)

It is written in the *Sefer Sifsei Kohen* that a *bas haya'anah* (ostrich) lays her eggs and places them on a high spot. She then watches them from a distance, without taking her concentration off them for even a moment. If any animal blocks her view, the *bas haya'anah* kills it. It is this gazing that enables the birds to come into existence and to emerge from the egg. Therefore, the eggs of a *bas haya'anah* are hung up in the *beis haknesses*, to remind us that in order for our prayers to produce results there can't be any obstacles between us and Hashem.

It is written in the *Sefer Kav Hayashar* that our sense of sight is so strong that when a person sees something holy, he brings holiness unto himself; when he looks at unholy sights, he brings impurity unto himself. A person should connect everything he sees to a Torah thought. The Kav Hayashar brings the *bas haya'anah* as proof of the strength of the power of sight, because the *bas haya'anah* can create a hole in her eggs just by gazing at them.

We eat eggs on Shabbos to remind us of these concepts.

(Rabbi Dovid Meisels)

Another reason for eating eggs with onions on Shabbos is that the Gemara states that if a person refrains from sinning, it is as if he has performed a mitzvah. However, this is only applicable when a person was put to the test, and controlled himself. Most of the *melachos* of Shabbos, such as digging and weaving, are not likely to be transgressed. However, when preparing eggs one could possibly transgress many *melachos*, including *borer* when peeling the eggs, *tochen* when mashing them, *lash* when mixing the oil, and *me'abeid* when salting them. When one prepares the eggs according to halachah, he receives a reward as if he has performed the positive commandment of keeping Shabbos, and a food which was prepared according to halachah contains a tremendous amount of holiness.

Another reason is because the honor of the day *seudah* takes precedence over the honor of the night *seudah*. However, one can assume that most dishes were simply left over from the night before, as it is not clear that they were prepared especially for the day *seudah*. However, eggs and onions cannot be prepared in advance, so it is clear that they were prepared in honor of the day *seudah*. (*Alim L'terufah*, issue 636)

In the time of the Ropshitzer Rav, a certain Rebbe became known, and it was unclear whether he was truly holy or only appeared so. When they asked the Ropshitzer Rav, he replied that they should verify two things: whether he cuts his nails in honor of Shabbos, and whether he eats eggs with onions on Shabbos. Indeed, it came to light that he did not do those two things. (*Noam Siach*, p. 25)

Preparing the Eggs

There are some who lift the eggs (once cooked) to the light to inspect them for blood spots. (*Dvar Tzvi L'Shabbos*)

The *minhag* of the Rebbe of Kossen was to cut the egg into four parts. He explained that four times the word *beitzah* (egg) has the same numerical value as *Chasoch* (lit. to cut), which is the name of the angel appointed over livelihood.
(*Bnei Sheleishim, Ohr Malei, Cheilek Hashmaos*, p. 106)

There are those who cut the egg into four parts on their palms since the end letters of the *pasuk, Posei'ach es yadecha*—"Open up Your hand," spell the name *Chasoch*, to allude to this *pasuk* which symbolizes livelihood.
(*Minhag Ziditchov; Noam Siach*, p. 220)

The Sanzer Rav was accustomed to cutting the egg into two equal parts. One part he would cut into small pieces, of which he ate one piece and distributed the rest to his children and grandchildren. The second part he cut into very small pieces and mixed with onions.
(*Pi Tzaddik*, p. 255, *Darchei Chaim Minhagei Sanz*)

It was heard from the Satmar Rebbe that the Chozeh of Lublin and the Sanzer Rav would cut the eggs and onions with great concentration and elevated thoughts. Although eggs with onions were not eaten in earlier times (and are not mentioned in the *Zohar*), the *tzaddikim*, with their intentions, turned them into holy foods. *(Zemiros Ir Hatamarim,* p. 190)

A person is required to delight in the Shabbos with every type of pleasure that exists. Shabbos food has the taste of *mann,* and encompassed the taste of every food and drink in the world. By eating it, a person could fulfill the directive of enjoying every pleasure in the world. However, the *mann* did not have the taste of onion and garlic (so as not to harm those carrying children), so we eat eggs with onions on Shabbos to complete our *oneg* Shabbos.

Since our Shabbos foods automatically have the taste and holiness of the *mann,* they do not require special preparation. However, the onions, which were not included in the taste of the *mann,* need special intentions while being prepared, and therefore the Divrei Chaim prepared the eggs and onions himself.

A person can elevate all the Shabbos foods along with the eggs and onions. This is because by preparing the eggs with onions a person demonstrates that he would like to imbue all the Shabbos dishes with his holy intentions, and he doesn't only eat them because they are already inherently holy.

We find that Moshe Rabbeinu commanded the generation of the *Midbar* to cook and bake in honor of Shabbos *(Shemos* 16:23). Why did he need to tell them this, if they already knew that one is not allowed to cook and bake on Shabbos, and must complete their preparations before Shabbos? Moshe Rabbeinu's intention was to teach them that by preparing for Shabbos and having in mind that the foods are in honor of Shabbos, the holiness of Shabbos will enter the Shabbos foods. *(Dvar Tzvi Shabbos,* sec. 128)

Eggs and onions symbolize *din* (retribution). We cut the eggs to remove the *din*.
(*Magen Avos*)

The Kedushas Tzion gave another reason for cutting the onions himself. All the Shabbos dishes have a numerical value or *mispar kattan* of seven. However, onions, *batzel,* have a numerical value of 14. In order to get to seven, one needs to cut the onion in half, since half of 14 is seven. Since the main connection of the onion to Shabbos is through it being cut, the Kedushas Tzion wanted to do it himself.
(*Zichronos Mimei Kedem*, p. 36)

Adding Fat to Eggs

The Sanzer Rav was accustomed to mixing *schmaltz* (chicken fat) into the eggs. If there was no *schmaltz* in the house, he would send someone to borrow from a neighbor.
(*Magen Avos*, p. 411)

Reb Shlomo of Bobov said that the *minhag* of mixing a large amount of chicken fat into the eggs with onions has a reason rooted in Kabbalah, hidden in the *pasuk* in *Bereishis* (32:6), *Vayehi li shor vachamor*—"And I have gained oxen and donkeys," and in the words of the *Zohar* on *Parshas Beshalach*, "regarding the *slav*... ."
(*Magen Avos*, p. 421)

Chicken fat is used because it congeals and, according to several opinions, the *melachah* of *lash*, creating a mixture, does not apply with it.
(*Magen Avos*, p. 421)

The Kedushas Tzion would put a large amount of fat into the eggs with onions because the Rambam writes that *oneg Shabbos* refers to preparing a dish with a large amount of fat.

The *Zohar* states that one should increase his food and drink on Shabbos from that of during the week. This can also mean that the food itself should contain more fat than during the week.
(*Dvar Tzvi Kedushas Tzvi*, sec. 18)

Pepper and Salt

There are those who put salt into the eggs three times and pepper once. Hashem commanded that the trees and the fruit they bear should taste alike, but most did not obey. The Gemara states that the pepper tree tastes like its fruits (*Sukkah* 35a). The Tosafos Hashaleim states that because the pepper obeyed the command of Hashem, it merited being used in Shabbos food.

(See *Magen Avos*, p. 422)

Liver

There are those who are accustomed to mixing liver into the onions. (*Tehillah L'Dovid* 321:25)

An allusion to eating liver and eggs with onions can be found in the mishnah in *Shabbos* (19b) which mentions meat, onions, and eggs consecutively. (*Machma'ei Shabbos*, p. 187)

There are those who only eat liver at the night *seudah* and not at the day *seudah*. (*Magen Avos*, p. 423)

Eating Eggs with the Cholent

There are those who cook the eggs in the cholent and eat some of the eggs with it. The Shabbos foods correspond to the seven attributes. Eggs are the fourth dish and correspond to the fourth *middah, netzach*; cholent is the fifth food and corresponds with *hod*. These two *middos* are connected, so the two foods should be eaten together. (*Pnei Shabbos*)

There is a *minhag* to eat eggs, onions, and beans on Shabbos, because these are all foods of mourning and three *tzaddikim* died on Shabbos: Moshe Rabbeinu, Dovid Hamelech, and Yosef Hatzaddik. (See *Sefer Divrei Tzaddikim* 2:4)

Many years ago, a Jew from Baghdad converted to Islam. According to the law, his conversion was not valid until the *chacham* of the Jews would attempt to persuade him to remain a Jew and he would refuse. The *Chacham* tried to convince him, but nothing he said made a difference. Then, a childhood friend of this man came to see him. This friend knew that he had a tremendous liking for eggs that were cooked in the *chamin*, and would eat many of them each Shabbos. The friend told him, "If you convert, how will you eat those eggs again, since that special taste is only for Jews who keep Shabbos?" This made an impression on the Jew and he returned to his faith. *(Ben Yehoyadah, Shabbos 119b, s.v. V'nimtza min hatavshil)*

Galaretta and P'tcha

There is a *minhag* to make a warm dish consisting of calves' feet for the Shabbos *seudah*.
(Knesses Hagedolah, sec. 318, Hagahos HaTur)

The *minhag* is to eat *galaretta*, a dish which is made from calf or chicken feet, with one's hands. *(Magen Avos, p. 409)*

They served the Spinka Rebbe *p'tcha*, which was made from feet, necks, gizzards, and other parts of the chicken, cooked with garlic. *(Zemiros Tiferes Tzvi, p. 250)*

Reb Moshe of Kobrin once exclaimed in the middle of eating *p'tcha*, "A king from his kingdom and a wealthy person from his affluence do not experience as much pleasure as I do from eating a piece of *p'tcha* in honor of Shabbos."

After that he ate another small amount and said, "If all the pleasure seekers of the world would taste *p'tcha*, they would forgo all their other desires to eat *p'tcha*." *(Imros Moshe, p. 38)*

Reb Avraham Yitzchak Kohn, the Ba'al Divrei Emunah, would say that *p'tcha* has a special significance and is a fundamental part of his Shabbos day *seudah*.
(Zechor L'Avraham 25:9)

The Shabbos foods correspond to the ten *sefiros* and *p'tcha* corresponds to *netzach hod*. *(Mishmeres Shalom 26:7)*

We eat beef feet on Shabbos because feet symbolize *emunah,* and we want to strengthen our *emunah.* (*Imros Tehoros*, p. 38)

Shabbos is symbolic of *emes* (truth), as the *Yerushalmi* states that on Shabbos, even an unlearned person is trusted. The Gemara states that falsehood does not have feet, meaning it does not last. We eat beef feet on Shabbos because Shabbos is connected to the *middah* of *emes,* which has "feet," meaning permanence. (*Imrei Pinchas, Sha'ar HaShabbos*, p. 488)

On Shabbos, one is able to elevate the physical and mundane. Therefore, we eat the feet which is the lowest part of the animal. (It is also for this reason that we eat onion, which is the most inferior vegetable, and kasha, the most inferior grain. Similarly, a *shtreimel* is made from the tails of an animal and is elevated to be worn on the head.) (*Sifran Shel Tzaddikim, Ma'areches Reb Pinchas Koritzer*, p. 139)

Our *tzaddikim* have ascribed deep meaning and intentions to the custom of eating *p'tcha.*
(*Divrei Torah Mahadura Kama*, sec. 101)

The midrash (*Bereishis Rabbah* 8:5) states that falsehood said that the world should be created and truth said it should not be created [since it is a world of falsehood]. On Shabbos, falsehood is banished from the world and truth has a pleasant existence in this world. We eat beef feet on Shabbos to demonstrate that Shabbos has a connection to truth. Feet symbolize truth, because (as mentioned above) falsehood has no feet.

Regel (foot) has the same numerical value (including the word itself as one) as the words Shabbos and *emes* together.
(*Vayidaber Moshe L'Shabbos*)

The seven Shabbos foods correspond to the seven *middos*. Onion, the second food, corresponds to the second *middah* of *gevurah,* and therefore we salt the onions. *Galaretta,* which is made from the feet of fowl, corresponds to the *middah* of *tiferes*, the *middah* of Yaakov Avinu. The *pasuk* states about

Yaakov, *Vayisa Yaakov raglav* (Bereishis 29:1). Since the *pasuk* mentions the word *raglav*, feet, we eat *galaretta* which is made from the feet.

(*Pnei Menachem Inyanei Shabbos*)

Another reason for eating beef feet is to remind us not to speak of mundane topics on Shabbos, as *Chazal* state that one's speech on Shabbos should not be like one's speech during the week (*Shabbos* 113b). We find that the removal of the legs of the serpent came about because of his sinning with speech, by persuading Chavah with his words. Thus, feet allude to speech.

Eating beef feet also reminds us of the Gemara that one's walking on Shabbos should be different than his walking during the week (ibid.).

(*Vayidaber Moshe L'Shabbos*)

Reb Pinchas Eliyahu Rottenberg of Piltz once asked the Sfas Emes why beef feet are eaten on Shabbos. The Sfas Emes asked Reb Pinchas his opinion. He replied that it is based on the *pasuk* in *Yeshayah* (58:14): *If you restrain your foot because of the Shabbos*, which teaches us that one should not walk on Shabbos like he walks during the week. The Sfas Emes said that we eat beef feet to allude to the concept that Shabbos elevates even the lowest elements.

(*B'shishim Chachmah*, p. 149, sec. 5)

Rabbi Baruch Mordechai of Koidinov would cut the beef feet himself in honor of Shabbos. It is possible that with this action he was alluding to fact that we are at the heels of Mashiach.

(*Mishmeres Shalom*, vol. 1, 24:7)

Reb Eliezer Zev of Kretchnif said several times that through *p'tcha, ein potzeh peh umetzaftzeif al Yisrael*, our prosecutors will not open their mouths and slander us. (*Raza D'avda*, p. 42)

P'tcha is made from something which at first is not so pleasant, but once it is cleaned and cooked, it is fit for the table of kings. This shows us that whatever situation a Jew is in, even if he sinks into impurity, with the power of Shabbos he can elevate himself to the highest levels.

(*Dibros Kodesh*, Strikov, *Toldos*)

Galaretta is made from a foot of a calf or kid, and is eaten warm with the challah during the Shabbos day *seudah*. To make *galaretta,* the foot of the calf is seared in fire, the hair is removed, and it is placed in a pot with the cartilage and loosely attached meat. It is spiced with onions and garlic and placed in the oven until it is well cooked. It should be removed from the oven when it is boiling. It then congeals and appears similar to the waves of the sea. This brings to mind several ideas:

The Gemara states that the Beis Hamikdash that was reconstructed by Hordus was made of blue, white, and green marble, built so that one row of stones protruded and the next row was set in. Hordus wanted to fill the holes with gold but the Rabbis advised him to leave it since it looked like the waves of the sea.

The commentaries explain that *Chazal* wanted it to appear like the waves of the sea to allude to the Jews who were *olei regel* and came to the Beis Hamikdash for Yom Tov and had a desire to be elevated, like the waves, which have a desire to reach upwards. With this, Hashem demonstrated how beloved it was to Him that the Jews were *olei regel*.

Another idea is that just like the waves are constantly reaching upwards, a person who strives to elevate himself and strengthens his *emunah* will be able to ride the waves of his life with tranquility. Therefore, we eat *gala*, which means waves and has the appearance of waves. (*Rabbi Dovid Meisels*)

The Shiniver Rav did not eat *galaretta* or *p'tcha*. He said it is a food eaten by noblemen and did not feel it was appropriate for the Shabbos *seudah*. If it had been prepared, he ate it after the eggs. *(Divrei Yechezkel Hachadash)*

Many *tzaddikim* have the *minhag* to eat beef feet at the Shabbos day *seudah*, and many also put in chicken or beef heads. It is mentioned in the Gemara that Rav Safra prepared the head of an animal for Shabbos, but there does not seem to be a source for eating the feet. However, everything our *tzaddikim* do has a reason.

As explained previously, the Gemara states that falsehood does not have feet (permanence) but truth does, so we eat beef feet because Shabbos is symbolic of the *middah* of truth.

A head also symbolizes truth, as the *pasuk* in *Tehillim* (119:160) states: *Rosh devarcha emes*—"The beginning of Your word is true." Indeed, we find that the letters which come after the letters of the word *rosh* (reish, aleph, shin), are *shin*, *beis* and *saf*, spelling Shabbos. Therefore, we eat beef head on Shabbos to symbolize *emes*. *(Yalkut Avraham, Orach Chaim 289:63)*

P'tcha as a Segulah

It is said in the name of the Sar Shalom of Belz that one who suffers from illness in his lungs should eat *p'tcha* and he will be completely cured. *(Segulos Yisrael, Ma'areches Shin, sec. 59)*

It is known to those well-versed in medicine that eating animal feet is a cure for illnesses of the lungs.
(Likutei Moharan, sec. 277)

Once, on Shabbos Chanukah, when Reb Shlomo of Bobov distributed *shirayim* of the *galaretta*, he gave some to a person who had an infection on his leg. Reb Shlomo told him that since Chanukah is like a Yom Tov, which can be referred to as *regel*, and he is eating Shabbos food made from feet, it is a *segulah* that his foot should be healed. *(Magen Avos, p. 409)*

P'tcha (spelled *peh, tzaddi, ayin, yud*) is an acronym for *amcha Yisrael tzrichin parnassah*, Klal Yisrael needs livelihood, so eating it is a *segulah* for *parnassah*. We eat *p'tcha* on Shabbos because Shabbos is the source of blessing for one's livelihood for the entire week. *(Hayashar V'hatov, p. 43, sec. 5)*

Shabbos is a time of *emunah*, since we give testimony to the fact that Hashem created the world in six days and rested on the seventh. In the merit of our *emunah* we will be granted livelihood. We therefore eat *p'tcha*, which is made of beef feet and symbolizes *emunah*, on Shabbos.

This is based on the *Sefer Rav Tuv, Parshas Behar*, which cites the midrash that Dovid Hamelech asked in what merit he can ask to be blessed with livelihood. The midrash brings the *pasuk* in *Tehillim* (119:59): *Chishavti derachai v'ashivah raglai el eidosecha*—"I thought over my ways and returned my feet to Your testimonies." *Chishavti derachai*—Dovid Hamelech thought over his ways to see if he fulfilled the Torah properly, and realized that he was lacking. *V'ashivah raglai el eidosecha*—since he kept Shabbos, which is an *eidus* (a witness) to the creation of the world, in the merit of that *emunah* he can request livelihood.

This midrash demonstrates that the word *regel*, which can mean foot, refers to Shabbos and *emunah*. We see that the word *regel* can refer to *emunah* and we see that in the merit of *emunah*, we receive livelihood. *(Rabbi Dovid Meisels)*

Chapter 16
The Main Course—Cholent

Chamin—Hot Food on Shabbos

The *minhag* across the world is to eat *chamin*, a warm dish, in honor of Shabbos. The Ba'al Hamaor states that our Sages have instituted that one should delight in the Shabbos with *chamin*. One who eats *chamin* is a believer in the words of our Sages and will merit seeing Mashiach.

(Ba'al Hamaor Shabbos, perek 3, p. 16 of the Dafei Harif)

On a simple level, the Ba'al Hamaor states that we eat *chamin* in order to delight in the Shabbos. Nevertheless, if there weren't secrets and high spiritual intentions behind eating *chamin,* the Ba'al Hamaor would not express himself in such strong language.

(Likutei Maharich, Seder Seudas Shacharis D'Shabbos, vol. 2, p. 71a)

It is a mitzvah to prepare and eat *chamin* on Shabbos, since by doing so one honors and takes pleasure in the Shabbos. One who does not believe the words of our Sages and forbids eating *chamin* on Shabbos is suspected of being a heretic.

(Rema 257)

The nature of a person is to think that he is in control of his life and the results depend on his efforts. We cook cholent for many hours without our interference. This demonstrates that Hashem is the one Who is in control, and this brings a person to *emunah*.

With this we can understand the words of the Rema: One who does not eat *chamin* (i.e. does not understand this idea), is suspect of being a heretic.

(Hayashar V'hatov)

In our generation, due to our sins, we find that there are those who refrain from the mitzvah of eating *chamin* on Shabbos, and by trampling on the words of our Sages they later come to transgress. A person should not turn away from the *minhag* of preparing *chamin* for Shabbos, and he should fulfill the mitzvah of *oneg Shabbos* as his parents and generations before him did. *(Mishnah Berurah 257:49)*

The *Kera'im* believed that one may not have a fire burning on Shabbos, even if it was lit before Shabbos. They did not light Shabbos candles or eat warm foods on Shabbos, even if it was kept warm off the fire, lest someone think he lit a fire on Shabbos. Therefore, our Sages instituted that it is a mitzvah to delight in the Shabbos specifically with warm food. On Friday night, we eat hot soup, and we serve cholent, which is a special food, at the day *seudah,* since the honor of the day *seudah* takes precedence over the night *seudah.*

One who does not desire cholent should train himself to eat and enjoy it, so that he can delight in the Shabbos in the manner that our Sages have taught us. (See *Sefer Ha'itim*, sec. 16)

We eat hot food on Shabbos to commemorate the *Lechem Hapanim,* which were kept warm until they were laid on the *Shulchan* on Shabbos.

The *poskim* say that whoever refrains from eating hot food on Shabbos is guilty of heresy. At the end of *Parshas Emor,* the Torah relates the story of the *megadeif* (blasphemer). The midrash states that the *megadeif* ridiculed the fact that the *Lechem Hapanim* were warm (warm bread was not considered appetizing). Thus, someone who doesn't commemorate the *Lechem Hapanim* by serving some hot food on Shabbos follows the view of the *megadeif.* *(Zemiros Zachor V'shamor)*

Even though during the week extremely hot food can harm a person's health, on Shabbos, hotter food is better. On Shabbos, a special light spreads over the world, and the heat of this light enters the Shabbos food. Therefore, there is a special significance in eating hot foods.

(*Zemiros Avodas Halevi*, p. 76, in the name of his great-grandfather)

Eating cholent is an important *minhag*. Since during the week a person eats warm foods, he should definitely eat warm food on Shabbos as *oneg Shabbos*. (*Sefer Ha'itim*, p. 880)

In Morocco, they ate *chamin* which they called *sechinah*. They would say that a Jew without *sechinah* is like a king without a kingdom. (*Yahadus Hamagrav, Mesoros Uminhagim*)

Cholent

The *minhag* is to prepare a dish which cooks for a long time in honor of Shabbos. This *minhag* is mentioned by the Rema (257). Perhaps a source for this *minhag* is the *Pesikta Rabbasi*, which asks to what extent a person needs to prepare in honor of Shabbos. Rav answers with meat, and Shmuel answers "*tochdimah.*" In another place, the Gemara states that many foods taste good if they are cooked *toch, toch*, meaning for a long time, and *di* means something repeated; hence "*tochdimah*" alludes to cholent which cooks for a long time. (*Hilchasa Rabbasa L'Shabbasa*, vol. 2, sec. 16)

The day *seudah* is the main *seudah*. Perhaps this is why cholent is eaten during the day. (*Yosef Ometz*)

The Spinker Rebbe's cholent consisted of beans, barley, and the parts of the chicken that are not usually eaten during the week, such as necks, feet, wings and gizzards.

(*Zemiros Tiferes Tzvi*, p. 251)

Reb Yaakov Yosef of Ostrow, the grandchild of Reb Yeivi, once said that as soon as it becomes light on Shabbos morning, the cholent is crying out in the oven, "Eat me!"

(*Sifran Shel Tzaddikim, Ma'areches* 336, p. 67, sec. 4)

When the cholent was placed before the Birchas Moshe he would sniff it and mention the Gemara which states that the emperor asked Reb Yehoshua ben Chananyah why the Shabbos food has such a good fragrance. Reb Yehoshua ben Chananyah replied that we have a spice whose name is Shabbos that we put into the food *(Shabbos* 119a).

He once said that Shabbos foods are a *segulah* for *yiras Shamayim* since the Gemara states that Shabbos foods have a good aroma and the word *rei'ach*, smell, alludes to *yiras Shamayim*, as it is written in *Yeshayahu* (11:3): *Vaharicho b'yiras Hashem*; we see that the concept of *yiras Shamayim* is mentioned near the word *rei'ach*. (*Birchas Moshe*)

Tzaddikim say that the fragrance from cholent that permeates the house on Shabbos is reminiscent of the fragrance of the *Ketores* that was burned in the Beis Hamikdash. (As heard)

Reb Yosef Yitzchak of Lubavitch instructed that one should not leave over any cholent on his plate; he should finish it entirely. (*HaShabbos B'kabbalah Uv'chassidus*, p. 771)

The Word "Cholent"

The name cholent is derived from the words *tzeli lan,* roasted overnight, since it is on the fire from Erev Shabbos.
(*Darkei Moshe* 253:7)

The word cholent is derived from the word *shalak*, which means something which is cooked for a long time and is an acronym for *l'kavod Shabbos Kodesh*. Cholent is an acronym for *Ta'am Shabbos hu nosen ta'am l'shvach*—"the taste of Shabbos is a good taste." (*Even Yisrael, Hashmatos* of vol. 1, sec. 4)

In Hungary, they called cholent, *shalet* (*Sha'ar Hakedushah* 15:77). When a person eats Shabbos food, the fat created in his body will not turn into worms at the end of his life. It is called *shalet*, because by eating it a person is *sholet* (in control) over the worms. (*Hilchasa Rabbasa L'Shabbasa*, vol.1, *Toldos*, p. 35)

The Angels Guard the Cholent

It is said that that there is a specific angel appointed over the cholent and kugel. *(Sichos Talmidei Chachamim, p. 285)*

Reb Meir of Premishlan said that every bean in the cholent has an angel presiding over it.

It is told in the name of the Ruzhiner Rebbe that we do not blow shofar on Rosh Hashanah which falls on Shabbos because the angel that is appointed over the shofar is also appointed over the cholent, and one angel does not perform two missions at once.

Perhaps we can say that this is alluded to in the *Yehi Ratzon* that is recited prior to *tekias shofar,* in which the angel by the name of *tav*, *shin*, *beis*, *shin* is mentioned. The names of the angels refer to their mission and the word Shabbos is found in these letters, since this angel is appointed over the Shabbos food. The remaining *shin* refers to the shofar.

(Raza D'Shabbos, p. 90)

Cholent as a Segulah

The Shem Shlomo of Munkatch states that cholent is a *segulah* for *emunah* and *emunas chachamim*. This is based on the words of the Rema that one who does not eat cholent, and in fact forbids it, is suspect of being a heretic. *Chazal* state that a good *middah* is many times stronger than a bad *middah*, so if one *does* eat cholent, not only is he not a heretic, but it brings him to *emunah*.

Cholent is also a *segulah* for livelihood, as the Rema writes that eating cholent is *kavod* and *oneg Shabbos*. One who fulfills *oneg Shabbos* merits abundant livelihood. This can be seen in the Gemara that asks in what merit the wealthy people in locations outside of Eretz Yisrael merit wealth. The Gemara answers that it is in the merit of honoring Shabbos.

(Chamishah Ma'amaros, Ma'amar Toras Shabbos, Bechukosai, p. 51)

The Satmar Rebbe, Reb Yoel Teitelbaum, once said that a person is required to educate his children in the mitzvah of eating cholent. Every person should educate even his little children to taste the cholent, since it brings *emunah*.

(Zemiros Divrei Yoel)

The Spinka Rebbe would ensure that his family ate cholent. He said that eating cholent brings a person to *emunah,* and a person should do his utmost to have as much *emunah* as possible. *(Zemiros Tiferes Tzvi, p. 252)*

When Reb Elimelech of Rudnick would eat cholent, he would tell those who did not yet merit having children to take a bone (*bein,* which can mean both bone and son), and those people would merit having a son the following year.

(Sefer Zichron Asher, sec. 13)

Reb Shalom of Belz said that food that is kept warm throughout Shabbos is a *segulah* for healing. *(Dover Shalom)*

Reb Shaya of Kerestir once served an ill person cholent. The man was afraid to eat it lest it to exacerbate his condition, but Reb Shaya kept on serving him more. Reb Shaya explained to him that this dish is called *sha'alet,* comprised of the words *sha'ah* and *let. Sha'ah* refers to the time that this is eaten, and the remaining letters, *lamed* and *tes,* are the first two letters of the word *l'tovah,* for the better. When one eats cholent, his situation can be improved. Reb Shaya had this in mind, and indeed the man was cured from his illness.

(Batei Avos Kerestir, p. 298)

Cholent Is Not Harmful

Throughout the week, any *mann* that was left over until the morning spoiled, but on Shabbos, the holiness of Shabbos prevented it from spoiling. It also enhanced the taste of the *mann,* so that it was tastier than during the week.

As a remembrance to the *mann*, we eat cholent, which cooks for many hours. Naturally, cholent should spoil and be detrimental to one who eats it. However, we have been eating this dish for two thousand years, and it does not harm us. Rather, it gives us strength for the entire week. The word, "cholent" alludes to this concept, since it is an acronym for *ta'am Shabbos hu nosen ta'am l'shvach*—"Shabbos gives a good taste." *(Matamim,* p. 193, sec. 79)

A person should not base his *emunah* on knowledge and proofs but on that which he heard from his parents. If a person understands the world according to his own understanding, then the cholent can harm him, since cholent is detrimental according to nature. But if a person serves Hashem with *emunah*, the cholent will purify him like the *mann* and heal him. *(Ohr L'Meir, Ha'azinu)*

It is said in the name of the Lisker Rav that by eating the Friday night *seudah,* a person can merit blessings that are in line with nature, and by eating the day *seudah* he can merit blessings that are above nature. Therefore, we eat cholent, which is cooked in a manner that is above nature (since it should spoil and be detrimental to a person's health) at the day *seudah*.

(Yatzav Avraham, Parshas Naso, p. 27)

The Gemara states that Reb Yehudah and Reb Shimon sat together, and a fig that was difficult to digest was brought to them. Reb Yehudah ate it, and Reb Shimon did not eat it. Reb Yehudah asked Reb Shimon why he did not eat the fig. Reb Shimon replied that such figs don't get fully digested. Reb Yehudah told him to eat it, because the fig would satiate him for the next day as well.

We can understand from Reb Yehudah's words that a food that is not well digested is not a disadvantage. Rather, it is an advantage since it satiates a person the next day. Therefore, it is not a good excuse to say that one cannot eat cholent because it is difficult to digest. On the contrary, it will satiate him longer.

Even if one wishes to behave like Reb Shimon who did not eat the fig, one should not refrain from eating cholent because this only applies to weekday food. Reb Shimon would have definitely eaten Shabbos food, with which one fulfills the mitzvah of *oneg Shabbos*, even if it was difficult to digest.

Although the Magen Avraham writes that one who is harmed by warm food may eat cold food, if it takes a person a day or two to digest his food, that does not fall into the category of being harmful, as we see from the words of Reb Yehudah. However, this depends on the person. If eating cholent causes a person to feel pain, it is not *oneg Shabbos*, and he is not required to eat it.

A man once came to the Ach Pri Tevuah of Liska and complained to him that cholent was causing him digestive problems. The Rebbe replied that, in truth, the Shabbos food was not causing him difficulties. Rather, the food that he was consuming on Sunday and Monday was the cause. The Rebbe explained that Shabbos food contains a blessing and continues to sustain a person for a day or two after Shabbos. Therefore, on those days one does not need to eat much. However, if one does eat on Sunday and Monday, that food will cause him digestive difficulties. (*Chiddushei Maharya Landau, Nedarim* 48)

Liquid from the Cholent

The Gemara states that a meal without soup is not a meal (*Brachos* 44a). It is for this reason that many *tzaddikim* have the *minhag* to eat soup at every *seudas mitzvah*, including the Shabbos day *seudah*. There are those who eat the liquid from the cholent on its own to fulfill this. (*Zemiros Tiferes Tzvi*, p. 251)

Reb Itzikel of Pshevorsk would say that *tzaddikim* eat the cholent with the liquid and the regular people eat dry cholent without liquid.

The Satmar Rebbe would be served two plates: one of soup and one of cholent, and he would eat one spoonful of both together and then he ate the cholent.

(Zemiros Divrei Yoel, vol. 1, p. 161)

Cholent with Beans

Most Jews are accustomed to eating cholent containing beans. This does not contradict the *minhag* mentioned by the Magen Avraham that one should not eat beans on the days that *Tachanun* is not recited (since those are days of *simchah*, and beans are a food of mourning), since Moshe Rabbeinu passed away on Shabbos (see *Shiyarei Knesses Hagedolah*).

(Tosafos Shabbos 290:1; see *Pri Megadim,* ibid., *Eishel Avraham* 1)

The *Midrash Rabbah* states on the words in *Bereishis* (25:34), "*nezid adashim,*" that lentils represent both mourning and joy. When Yaakov prepared the lentils, he was mourning Avraham Avinu's death, but he was also happy that he received the rights of the firstborn. Rashi explains that lentils can be associated with joy since they are eaten at festive meals. Perhaps this is the reason that beans are eaten on Shabbos and Yom Tov.

(Agra D'kallah, Toldos)

The Chessed L'Avraham writes that on days of *simchah* (on which *Tachanun* is not recited) one should first eat an egg to remember the *Churban* before eating meat. We eat eggs and beans at the Shabbos *seudah* for this reason.

(Toras Moshe, Shir Ma'on, Vayikra, p. 8)

One should eat beans on Shabbos to give them importance, since beans are inexpensive and people look down upon them. The Magen Avraham writes in the name of the *Yerushalmi* that a person will need to give a reckoning for having seen food but not having eaten it. There was a *Tanna* who ate every type of food throughout the year for this reason. Therefore, in order that beans should not be disparaged, we eat them on Shabbos.

Additionally, there is a custom to eat cholent made from beans, in order to honor Shabbos specifically with inexpensive food. The source for this is the *Midrash Tanchuma* (Bamidbar 27), in which Rabbi Levi quotes the *pasuk*, *Don't steal from the poor man because he is poor* (Mishlei 22:22). If everyone eats cholent made from inexpensive food, the poor people can eat the same food that rich people are eating on Shabbos and feel satisfied with their Shabbos *seudah*. Otherwise, the poor people will feel badly about the food they serve, and it will be as if their Shabbos is "stolen" form them.

(*Hilchasa Rabbasa L'Shabbasa*, vol. 2, sec. 16)

There is a component found in the ground that can cause sadness, as it says in *Bereishis* (3:17): *Arurah ha'adamah ba'avurecha, b'itzavon tochelenah*—"Cursed is the ground because of you, in sorrow you shall eat from it." This enters beans as they are growing, which is possibly why beans are a food of mourning and why, in some places, beans aren't eaten on Shabbos and Yom Tov.

Nevertheless, most do eat beans on Shabbos, because Shabbos is a blessing from Hashem and the *pasuk* in *Mishlei* (10:22) states, *Birchas Hashem hi ta'ashir v'lo yosif etzev imah*—"The blessing of Hashem enriches and one need not add sadness to it." This can be interpreted to mean that since Shabbos is a blessing from Hashem, there will be no sadness.

(*Tehillah L'Dovid Butchatch*, Tehillim 4:14)

It is said in the name of Reb Pinchas Koritzer that the maximum height of a beanstalk is shorter than other plants. We eat beans on Shabbos to demonstrate that Shabbos elevates even the lowest elements.

(*Tiferes Avos, Minhagei Maharyav*, sec. 226)

Reb Yissachar Dov of Belz once spent Shabbos in the city of Rotzfert where the local *minhag* was to eat cholent containing beans. The Belzer Rav himself ate a cholent with kasha. When one of the children at the *seudah* saw this, he exclaimed in wonder, "The Belzer Rav does not eat cholent?" From that day on the Rav started eating two types of cholent, one consisting of beans and one consisting of kasha. *(Gilyon M'be'er Rabboseinu)*

There is a Yemenite bean dish called *lasis* eaten on Shabbos. It requires a very long cooking time and would cook from Erev Shabbos until Shabbos morning, which enhanced its taste. They would say that Shabbos without *lasis* is like a king without his servants. (Shabbos is referred to as a king, since it provides sustenance for the seven days of the week, like a king distributes food to all his servants.) *(Orah V'simchah, Megillas Esther, p. 52)*

Cholent with Kasha

It is told that eating kasha on Shabbos is a *minhag* that was handed down for many generations from Sinai, and many *tzaddikim* praised this *minhag*. *(Zichron Shmuel, Zalmanov, p. 59)*

Reb Yitzchak Moshe of Pshevorsk was accustomed to saying, "Shabbos day, when we eat cholent, the Name of Hashem of *yud, beis, kuf*, is formed, as an acronym for *yoch* (sauce), *babalach* (beans), and kasha." If he did not have kasha, he dipped a slice of challah (in Yiddish called *koilitch*, which also starts with a *kuf*) into a spoonful of soup (specifically a spoonful, which is a *kli shlishi* and does not pose a problem of *bishul*).

(Divrei Chanah, vol. 2, p. 106)

Reb Yehudah Tzvi of Rozla was once at the home of Reb Hersh of Riminov for Shabbos. Reb Yehudah Tzvi instructed the attendant to prepare a dish consisting of beans, kasha, and sauce for him, thus fulfilling the intention of the Name of Hashem of *yud, beis, kuf* (see above). The attendant forgot to put beans in the dish. The Rebbe of Rozla told Reb Hersh that he could not form this Name of Hashem. Reb Hersh handed him a piece of the *bilkele* (challah roll) and told him, "Now you have the *beis*; your formation of the Name of Hashem is complete."

The Rebbe of Rozla then asked Reb Hersh, "And what would you do if I didn't have kasha?"

Reb Hersh replied, "I would give you a piece of the braided challah, which is called *koilitch*."

The Rozla Rebbe had great pleasure from these responses.

(*Tzvi Latzaddik, Zemiros Shabbos Kadshecha*, p. 75)

There are elevated ideas regarding eating kasha on Shabbos. Kasha *(kaf/kuf, aleph, shin, yud)* is an acronym for ***shema koleinu Hashem Elokeinu***—"Hear our voice, Hashem, our G-d, and for *Ki Sheim Hashem ekra*—"When the Name of Hashem I will call."

Therefore, it is fitting to make cholent with kasha, which alludes to us reaching out to Hashem, and cholent is the Name of Hashem of *yud, beis, kuf,* which is an acronym for *Ya'aneinu b'yom kareinu*—"Hashem should answer us in the day that we call to Him." (*Nachalas Tzvi*, p. 114)

The Tzemech Tzedek says that *seudas Shabbos* of *tzaddikim* and the kasha eaten at the *seudah* can accomplish more than discussions in Torah by *geonim*. (*Migdal Oz*, p. 259, sec. 31)

When Reb Aharon of Belz spent Shabbos in Pest, there was a Jew from the city of Rotzfert there. This Jew's father had brought kasha from Vienna to Reb Aharon's father, Reb Yissachar Dov of Belz, when he was in Rotzfert during the First World War. Now this Jew went in the ways of his father and brought kasha to Reb Aharon, even though it was difficult to do so.

This was the first Shabbos that Reb Aharon ate kasha in several weeks. Reb Aharon showed this man great honor and told him, "Father said that one should eat food that was eaten by *tzaddikim*, even with *mesiras nefesh*. You too displayed *mesiras nefesh* by smuggling in this kasha."

(*Reshimos Reb Yehoshua Heschel Deutsch*, Rav of Freiman)

Kasha as a Segulah

In many locations, the *minhag* was to eat kasha cholent, rather than cholent made from beans (as mentioned in the *Magen Avraham* that there are those who do not eat beans on Shabbos and Yom Tov). The Skulener Rebbe would say in the name of *tzaddikim* that eating kasha on Shabbos eliminates all *kushiyos* (difficulties) and negative spiritual forces.

(Kuntris HaShabbos, Noam Haneshamos, p. 99)

Reb Uri of Strelisk states that by eating kasha on Shabbos, all *kushiyos* are answered. The Bnei Yissaschar states that Shabbos has the same numerical value as *kashya rafya*—difficulties become softened and they are no longer difficult.

(Imrei Kodesh Hashaleim, Likutim, sec. 3)

Reb Mordechai of Lechovitch would say that eating kasha on Shabbos is a *segulah* to rid oneself of the *middah* of anger.

(Toras Avos, Inyanei Shabbos, sec. 8)

Reb Asher Hagadol of Stolin remarked that, in truth, there is no source for kasha being a *segulah* to rid oneself of anger. However, if the Lechivitcher Rebbe said so, even if this was not the case before, it now contains this power and is a wondrous *segulah*. *(Toras Avos, Shabbos 1:8, p. 210)*

The son of Reb Yeshayah Thumim, a chassid of the Lechivitcher Rebbe, once fell ill with fever. Reb Yeshayah said, "The Rebbe said that eating kasha is a *segulah* against anger, and anger is essentially negative energy." He fed his son a spoon of kasha cholent and he became well. *(Ibid., sec. 13)*

Chapter 17
Kugel—More Than a Side Dish

Preparation for Eating Kugel

It is said that Reb Shmelke of Selish would immerse himself in the *mikvah* prior to eating the kugel. *(Noam Siach, Salka 145)*

The Skulener Rebbe, Reb Eliezer Zusya, would say, "*L'kavod Shabbos Kodesh*; this a remembrance to the *mann*, which was also covered above and below it," prior to eating the kugel.

(Kuntris HaShabbos, Noam Haneshamos, p. 104)

Importance of Eating Kugel

Reb Mordechai of Nadvorna said that a Jew should have *mesiras nefesh* to eat kugel.

(Gedulas Mordechai, p. 40; Oros Mordechai)

Kugel is eaten at the end of the *seudah* when one is already satiated, because one should have *mesiras nefesh* for eating kugel on Shabbos. (Reb Leibish of Pshevorsk)

The Ba'al Hatanya once said that eating kugel on Shabbos is a Torah obligation and is a mitzvah like blowing shofar on Rosh Hashanah. *(HaShabbos B'kabbalah U'vachassidus, p. 751)*

The Lubavitcher Rebbe, Reb Shalom Dov Ber, once said that eating round kugel symbolizes the wedding ring. (The word kugel comes from the root of *k'igul*—like a circle, the shape of a wedding ring.) He said it should be eaten before the meat, similar to the ring that is given to the *kallah* before the meal.

(Halichos Uminhagim, Inyanei Shabbos Kodesh, p. 21)

Kugel is the main addition to the menu in honor of Shabbos. *(Mishmeres Shalom* 28:7)

The main significance of the kugel is that it is an addition that is prepared in honor of Shabbos, even more so than the meat, wine, and fish. Eating kugel is like a *hiddur mitzvah*, as one adorns the Shabbos meal with it. *(Zemiros Tiferes Tzvi,* p. 253)

When Reb Meir of Dzhikov, the Ba'al Imrei Noam, was six years old, his grandfather, the Ropshitzer Rav, asked him why we eat kugel on Shabbos. The child replied that the letters of the word kugel *(kaf, vav, gimmel, lamed)* are an acronym for *V'hu k'zera gad lavan (Shemos* 16:31—a description that refers to the *mann),* since kugel is in remembrance of the *mann.*
(Avnei Kodesh, p. 53; *Da'as Zekeinim,* chap. 12)

The acronym of *k'zera gad lavan (kaf, gimmel, lamed)* has the same numerical value as the word *"gan."* The end letters of the phrase spell *"Eden"* to indicate that Shabbos foods have a taste of Gan Eden. *(Sh'or Yashuv, Beshalach)*

Kugel is an acronym for *V'se'esof galuyoseinu l'chatzros kadshecha,* Hashem should gather all the people in *galus* to the Beis Hamikdash. (Heard in the name of *tzaddikim)*

Kugel is in remembrance of the *mann.* Just as the *mann* contained the taste of all different foods but always appeared the same, kugel contains many ingredients which are not recognizable. *(Derech Tzaddikim,* Reb Meir Shalom of Kalushin, 5:41)

The *minhag* is to serve the meat on a separate plate after the kugel is served so that it should be noticeable that the kugel is a special dish cooked in honor of Shabbos, and not just a side dish to the meat.

This idea is taken from the Ben Ish Chai that states that on Purim, one is required to place the two foods for his *mishloach manos* on separate dishes so that they are recognizable as separate foods. If he puts them on one plate it may appear to be one dish. Similarly, if one places the meat and kugel on one plate, the kugel will not be as noticeable.

(Zemiros Ateres Yehoshua, p. 273)

Round Kugel

The name kugel is taken from the word *k'igul*—like a circle. Kugel is usually made round, and in previous times it was made in round pans. *Chazal* state that the *mann* was round, *(Yuma* 75a) and kugel is in remembrance of the *mann*.

(Otzar Kol Minhagei Yeshurun, p. 287; Sefer Matamim)

Chazal state that in the future, Hashem will make a dance for the *tzaddikim* and sit between them in Gan Eden. Their pleasure will be without an end, just like a circle has no end point *(Ta'anis* 31a). Reb Moshe Aryeh Freund once said that we eat kugel, which is derived from the word "round," to allude to the circle of *tzaddikim*. *(Zemiros Ateres Yehoshua, p. 102)*

The abovementioned *Chazal* that Hashem will make a dance for the *tzaddikim* alludes to unity, because a dancing circle has no beginning or end. We eat kugel *(k'igul*—like a circle) which is round, to allude to unity among Jews.

(Zemiros Shabbos Kadshecha, p. 74)

According to the above, we eat *lokshen* kugel because *lokshen* signifies unity, since the noodles are intertwined with each other, as stated in the *Imrei Pinchas*. Shabbos is a time of *achdus*, since on Shabbos we connect to each other and to Hashem. *(Rabbi Dovid Meisels)*

We bake round kugel because a circle has no beginning or end and resembles a dance *(machol)*. *Chazal* say that if one keeps Shabbos properly, *mochlin lo al kol avonosav*—"He is forgiven for all his sins." The word *machol* (dance) and *mochel* (to forgive) share the same root letters. *(Rabbi Dovid Meisels)*

We make round kugel to demonstrate what the Ran states in the name of the *Yerushalmi,* that there are no squares in the natural world. The *sefarim* explain that Hashem created all the worlds in the form of a circle: the heavens and the earth are spherical; the orbits of the sun and the *mazalos* (constellations) are round. So too, a person's body is comprised of rounded parts: the head, the fingers, the hands, and the feet. This is to teach a person that Hashem is in the entire world. Just like all points of a circle are equidistant to its center, Hashem's supervision and involvement is equal to all His creations, as it says in *Tehillim* (145:18): *Hashem is close to all who call to Him.* (*Rabbi Dovid Meisels*)

Reb Itzikel of Pshevorsk said in the name of the Chozeh of Lublin that there is a special place in Gan Eden where reward is given to those who eat kugel on Shabbos. Even if one eats kugel to satisfy his own desires, he is still rewarded. He also said in the name of Reb Menachem Mendel of Riminov that eating kugel accumulates merit in Heaven for a person.
(*Ma'aseh Hashem, Dinov*, p. 440; *Zemiros L'ateir Pesora*, p. 82)

Lokshen Kugel

Many are accustomed to making the Friday night *lokshen* kugel with a large amount of garlic and pepper and calling it *"knobel* kugel," garlic kugel. The *lokshen* kugel served on Shabbos day is sweet, since the Torah, which is sweet, was given on Shabbos day. (As heard)

Reb Meir of Premishlan said that *"Lokshen* kugel is handed down from Sinai." The *minhag* in Galicia was to serve *lokshen* kugel. (*Panim Meirim*, p. 143)

Reb Mordechai of Nadvorna said the word "kugel" without any other descriptions refers to *lokshen* kugel.
(*Nezer Hakodesh*, p. 114)

The Shiniver Rav said that *lokshen* kugel is the main kugel; other types of kugel are simply nice dishes in honor of Shabbos.   (*Reb Leibish of Pshevorsk*)

The Gemara states that the livelihood of a person is as difficult as the splitting of the Sea. The Rebbe of Kretchnif said that if one eats *lokshen* kugel, his livelihood will come to him in a manner that is "*lo kashin*," not difficult.
(*Arba'ah Arazim*, p. 91, sec. 11)

Reb Yissachar Dov of Belz said that eating *lokshen* kugel is a *segulah* for *yiras Shamayim*.   (Reb Yisrael Brief)

The Gemara states that the livelihood of a person is as difficult (*kashin*) as the splitting of the Sea. *Lokshen* is comprised of the words "*lo kashin*," not difficult. We eat *lokshen* kugel to show that although earning a livelihood is difficult, money that one spends on Shabbos expenses is *lo kashin,* not difficult, because it will be returned to him. If he spends more, he will be given more; it is not included in the amount allotted to him on Rosh Hashanah.   (*Al Avoseinu V'al Yichusam*, p. 102)

Another reason for eating *lokshen* kugel is that *lokshen* are long strings which are similar to a measuring string (*kav hamiddah*) (*Sefer Ma'aseh Shoshan* states that a measuring string is a long string that forms a round ball when folded). The concept of *kav* means to gather a few things to become one, as it says *yikavu hamayim*, the waters should gather (*Bereishis* 1:9); all the separate bodies of water should become one large body.

According to this, we can say that we eat *lokshen* kugel to show that Shabbos is a time of unity; on Shabbos, all separate parts become one.

"Kugel" contains the same letters as the words *kav ugel,* a round line. Hashem first began creating the world with a straight line and then formed it into a sphere. We eat *lokshen* kugel, which is made of long "lines," baked in the shape of a circle. *(Rabbi Dovid Meisels)*

Mehl Kugel

The Sanzer Rav was accustomed to eating *mehl* kugel (lit. flour kugel) at the day *seudah*.

Reb Shlomo of Bobov once related that his mother worked as a cook in the royal palace in Austria. She once told him about a special dish that she prepared for the mother of the Kaiser. Once, when Reb Shlomo was ill, his Rebbetzin feared for his health and she asked him what she can take upon herself in his merit. The Rebbe advised her to bake another kugel in honor of Shabbos in addition to the two (*lokshen* kugel and potato kugel) she usually prepared. She took upon herself to make *mehl* kugel, similar to the kugel that his mother had described, and within several days the Rebbe recovered. This *mehl* kugel became known among chassidim as "*ma'adanei melach*," the delicacy of kings. *(Magen Avos, p. 430)*

Reb Tzvi Hersh of Spinka would eat *mehl* kugel that was made only of flour, oil, and salt. It is possible that this was supposed to be similar to the *Korban Minchah*, which contained only these three ingredients. *(Zemiros Tiferes Tzvi, p. 254)*

Challah Kugel

Challah kugel is prepared from the challah used for an *eruv chatzeiros* (an *eruv* that permits carrying from one's home to an enclosed yard); there are also those who use the leftover challah from the previous Shabbos. This is similar to the *Lechem Hapanim* that the *kohanim* ate on Shabbos from the previous week.
(Darkei Chaim V'shalom, Seder Erev Shabbos, p. 103)

Reb Aharon of Belz would only distribute *shirayim* of the challah kugel to those who washed for bread, because he held that it requires a *Hamotzi*. *(Kuntris Dibburei Kodesh)*

Potato Kugel

The Satmar Rebbe once said potato kugel is simply a food eaten in honor of Shabbos but should not be called "kugel." Only *lokshen* kugel should be given the title "kugel," since a dish must be made of flour to be called a kugel.

(See *Zecher Chassidim L'vrachah*, p. 612)

Reb Yisrael Chaim Hirsch from Kemetcha ate potato kugel on Shabbos. It seems to me that the reason may be because potatoes are referred to as *tapuchei adamah* and the word *tapuach* (apple) alludes to the love between Hashem and Bnei Yisrael, as the *pasuk* in *Shir Hashirim* (8:5) states: *Tachas hatapuach orarticha...* (*Birchas Yitzchak*, p. 17)

Helzel Kugel

The Komarno Rebbe served stuffed *kishke* at the Shabbos *seudah*. At night, they served *kishke* stuffed with chicken necks; during the day, the *kishke* was stuffed with ground *kishke*. (*Minhagei Komarno*, p. 234)

In Eretz Yisrael, some prepare *kishke* with flour and oil stuffing. (*M'be'er Rabboseinu*)

Number and Types of Kugels

The Komarno Rebbe would serve three kinds of kugel: potato kugel, sweet kugel, and a savory kugel, corresponding to children, life, and livelihood.

(*Minhagei Komarno*, sec. 234; *Darkei Chaim V'shalom*, sec. 454)

The Spinka Rebbe would serve four kinds of kugels each Shabbos: *mehl* kugel, potato kugel, *lokshen* kugel, and apple kugel. (*Zemiros Tiferes Tzvi*, p. 454)

In several chassidic courts, they serve as many kugels as the number of *simchos* being held there that week. (As heard)

Gezunter Kugel

In Slonim, chassidim would bring a kugel to the Rebbe's *tish* as thanks to Hashem for a salvation that they experienced. The Slonimer Rebbe, Reb Mordechai Chaim, would tell these chassidim that they should bring a *"gezunter* kugel" (lit. a healthy kugel). This referred to bringing a kugel to thank Hashem even without a specific reason. The Rebbe would say that if a week passed with no negative occurrences or tragedies, one should bring a kugel to thank Hashem; doing so prevents bad things from happening.　　　　　(*Olam Hachassidus*, Shevat 5763)

Kugel as a Segulah

It is told in the name of the Bobover Rebbes throughout the generations that kugel is a *segulah* for *parnassah*.

(*Magen Avos*, p. 432)

The Minchas Elazar once related that at the Shiniver Rav's *seudah,* a chassid climbed on to the table to grab *shirayim* of kugel. The Shiniver Rav was very disturbed by the incident and left the table. Those close to the Rav went to appease him. When the Rav returned to the table he said that it is accepted among chassidim that kugel is a *segulah* for livelihood. However, rather than grabbing kugel, one can also achieve those results with the *pasuk: Tevi'eimo vesita'eimo b'har nachalascha—* "You will bring them and plant them on the mountain of Your inheritance" (*Shemos* 15:17). The chassidim could not understand the Rebbe's words. Later, a chassid repeated the incident to the Darkei Teshuvah. The Darkei Teshuvah explained that in the *Siddur Arizal* this *pasuk* alludes to the eleven spices of *Ketores,* which is a *segulah* for livelihood.

(*Divrei Yechezkel Hachadash, Likutim*)

The Kalashitzer Rebbe would say in the name of his grandfather, the Shiniver Rav, that kugel eaten at the day *seudah* is a *segulah* for healing. He would add that whatever the Shiniver Rav said was passed down to him from previous generations. *(Divrei Chanah Hashaleim,* vol. 2, p. 173)

Reb Naftali Rothman was once traveling to the city of Debrecin. On the way, he collapsed. The doctors at the local hospital said that he had three days to live.

At that time, there was a fair taking place in the city of Darag. Reb Naftali's wife found someone traveling to the fair and asked him to inform the Imrei Shefer of Darag of Reb Naftali's situation. When the messenger came before the Rebbe, the Rebbe told him, "I have a piece of kugel that is left over from Shabbos, and I am sending it to Reb Naftali as a remedy." He instructed that it should be whispered into Reb Naftali's ear that Reb Shmuel of Darag, with the power of the Sanzer Rav, sent him the kugel and he should eat it and merit becoming well. Indeed, after the messenger told him these words, Reb Naftali awoke, ate the kugel, and was healed.

(Sippurei Shmuel, sec. 8)

Reb Moishele of Rozhvadov would distribute kugel to those who were being drafted into the army. He would say that the kugel is a *segulah* for being saved from the hands of gentiles. He would hold the plate in his hands and tears would stream from his eyes onto the kugel.

One Purim, there were several young chassidim present who were required to appear shortly before the draft committee. At the Purim *tish,* the song *Laminatze'ach Al Ayeles Hashachar* was sung. When they got to the words (Tehillim 22:19), *v'al levushi yapilu goral,* the Rebbe explained that the general decrees the *goral,* fate, of the *levush,* the clothes of those who come before him—if they will wear a *shtreimel* or an army hat, a *bekeshe* or a shield. We ask then (ibid.:22), *hatzilah micherev nafshi,* Hashem should save us from the battlefield filled with swords.

The Rebbe held the kugel and cried many tears. He distributed the kugel, saying that it was a *segulah* to be released from army service. Indeed, all those young men were freed from serving in the army.

It is told that Reb Shlomo of Bobov would also distribute kugel to those in danger of being drafted into the army. He would say that he does not have any of his own intentions by doing so, but is relying on what his uncle (Reb Moshe of Rozhvadov) did. (*Hachachmah Mei'ayin*, p. 127; *Magen Avos*, p. 431)

A man once came to ask the Tosher Rebbe for advice. He explained that although they were a family of *talmidei chachamim*, their youngest son had no interest in learning Torah. The Rebbe advised him that the mother should ensure that the child eats kugel each Shabbos.

(*Zemiros Shabbos Kadshecha*, p. 73)

When the Sanzer Rav once spent Shabbos in Baden, two non-observant men came to watch the Rav. When the Rav distributed *shirayim* of the kugel, he included those two men as well. One of them ate the kugel, while the other mocked him for doing so, and, "turning into a chassid." When the two men returned to their lodgings, the man who ate the kugel could not bring himself to eat anything. Several days passed, but his situation did not improve and the doctors could not advise him.

The man then realized that this strange illness had come since he ate the kugel of the Sanzer Rav. His wife traveled with him to Sanz, where they complained to the Rav about their situation. The Rav assured him that he did not suffer from illness. To prove his point, the Rav served the man a complete meal including soup, meat, and side dishes which the man ate ravenously, after not having eaten for several days. The Rav explained to the man that from the time that he ate the holy *shirayim*, his body could no longer tolerate non-kosher food. The Rav advised the couple to kasher their dishes and buy kosher meat. The man did so, and he eventually became a complete *ba'al teshuvah*. (*Divrei Menachem, Stropkov, Mikeitz*)

The Mittele Rebbe of Chabad, Reb Dov Ber Schneerson, once advised a chassid who came to him, beseeching him that he merit children, to bake a kugel in honor of Shabbos. In his great desire to follow the Rebbe's advice, the chassid baked two kugel*s*. The following year, his wife gave birth to twins. When the story was repeated to the Rebbe he replied, "What can I do if he baked two kugel*s*?" (*Olam Hachassidus*, Issue 116)

Flipping Over the Kugel

It is told in the name of the Chozeh of Lublin that the reason for flipping over the kugel before serving it is to turn over the *middah* of *din* (retribution) to *rachamim* (compassion).

(*Zemiros L'ateir Pesora*, p. 82)

Eating Kugel with One's Hands

The Gemara states that Rabba Bar Rav Huna saw Rav Huna eat porridge with his fingers. Rabba Bar Rav Huna asked Rav Huna why he is eating with his hands. Rav Huna replied that Rav said that porridge eaten with one's fingers tastes good. This Gemara provides a source for the *minhag* of *tzaddikim* and chassidim to eat kugel and *farfel* with their hands in order to enhance the taste of the Shabbos food.

Many *tzaddikim* were accustomed to eating their portions of Shabbos food with their hands and then distributing their *shirayim* (leftovers).

The Gemara (ibid.) states that one should not eat from a communal dish with one's hands because germs from the dirt under one's nails can spread to another person. However, we can justify the custom of *tzaddikim* because the Gemara is referring to a case where the food is not eaten during the course of a meal. But when the food is eaten during a meal, there is no concern of spreading germs because before every meal one is required to wash his hands, and before doing so he is required to clean his fingernails. Therefore, the *tzaddikim* who ate their food during the meal did so with clean hands and nails, and thus they could distribute *shirayim*.

One reason that *tzaddikim* distribute *shirayim* of kugel with their hands is because the kugel alludes to the *mann*, which symbolizes livelihood, and we wish to be handed livelihood easily. *(Chiddushei Maharya, Nedarim 49b)*

The Apter Rav once ate the *seudah* together with the Ruzhiner Rebbe. The Apter Rav ate all the Shabbos dishes with a spoon, except the kugel, which he ate with his hands. The Ruzhiner Rebbe did the opposite; he ate a bit from each dish with his hands except the kugel.

The Apter Rav explained that since all the foods receive their life force through an angel, he ate them with a spoon. The kugel, however, is a remembrance to the *mann* which received its power directly from Hashem, so he ate it directly with his hands.

The Ruzhiner Rebbe then explained why he did the opposite. He said that all the foods receive their life force from angels and he is not afraid of angels. But how can he have the audacity to touch a dish coming straight from Hashem with his bare hands? *(Irin Kaddishin, p. 648)*

This following story demonstrates that the Gra ate kugel with his hands: Reb Yechezkel Landau, the Rav of Vilna, related that on the Shabbos before his wedding, his father-in-law took him to the Gra to receive a blessing. The Gra was in the middle of eating kugel and wished to place his hands on the head of the *chassan* in order to bless him. The *chassan* stepped back so that the Gaon should not sully his new *shtreimel* with his hands which were greasy from the kugel. The Gaon placed one hand on his *shtreimel* and blessed him. Due to this blessing, Rav Yechezkel Landau lived a long life and learned until his last day with perfect eyesight, but he always regretted valuing his *shtreimel* more than the hands of the Gra.

(*Ma'asei Ilfas, Shalosh Seudos*)

The Bobover Rebbes were accustomed to eating kugel with their hands while it was still very hot. (*Magen Avos*, p. 431)

The first Reb Shlomo of Bobov once spent time in Frankfurt for health purposes. At the Shabbos *seudah*, many of the local *rabbanim* were present and the Rebbe distributed *shirayim* of the kugel with his hands into their hands.

This seemed offensive in the eyes of the German rabbis who were not accustomed to such conduct. Reb Shlomo, sensing their discomfort, told them, "You can take it from me; I am a *neki kapayim*," which refers to one's hands being clean from theft, but literally means "my hands are clean." (Ibid)

Kugel as Hachnasas Orchim

The Sar Shalom of Belz explains that the source for eating kugel on Shabbos is based on an incident that occurred during the times of Yehoshua bin Nun. After the Jews in Eretz Yisrael conquered and settled the land, they lived in peace and did not have any reason to travel from one place to another. Thus, there were no opportunities to fulfill *hachnasas orchim*.

A Jew once needed to travel to another location to arrange a *shidduch* for his child. When he arrived, all the residents of the city welcomed him and they each requested that he lodge at their home.

The Jew went to ask Yehoshua which offer he should accept. Yehoshua replied that he should stay at the home of the first person who invited him and everyone else should send him a kugel in honor of Shabbos. This was when the *minhag* of making kugel for Shabbos began.

The Shatzer Rebbe of London said that the Sar Shalom of Belz possessed old manuscripts from the days of the *nevi'im* where this story was recorded.

(*Zemiros Da'as Shalom*, p. 28; *Sichasam Shel Avdei Avos Belz*, p. 163)

Meat after Kugel

After eating the kugel, the *minhag* is to eat "*kalte oif*" (cold chicken tops) so that the week should be filled with "*kol tuv*" (which is similar in sound to *kalte oif*, and means, "all the best").

There is also a custom to eat round chicken meatballs, to allude to a *machol*, a circle dance which has no end, and also to the words *machol lo*, that Hashem forgives him.

(*Minhag Chassidim*)

They served the Satmar Rebbe warm meat with compote.

(*Zemiros Divrei Yoel*, vol. 1, p. 162)

Chapter 18
Dessert and Shabbos Afternoon Treats

Drinking Tea

There are those who drink a warm drink such as tea at the end of the *seudah*, according to the Gemara (*Shabbos* 36b) that one should prepare warm food and drink for Shabbos.

(As heard)

Reb Aharon of Belz would comment on tea, that it is a drink from Gan Eden, since it is neither too sour nor too sweet, and it warms a person.

(As heard)

Compote

There are those who do not eat compote at the Shabbos day *seudah*, and only eat it on Yom Tov so that it is considered like a third *seudah* on Yom Tov (*Magen Avraham, Orach Chaim* 529:2). (If it was eaten at every Shabbos *seudah* it would not be recognizable as a special addition in honor of Yom Tov.)

Reb Shalom Eliezer of Rotzfert once spent Shabbos in Etched where he was served compote at the day *seudah*. The Rebbe declined to eat the compote, saying that in Sanz the *minhag* is not to eat compote at the day *seudah*. Reb Shalom Eliezer's nephew was present and he asked his uncle why it bothered him to eat compote. The Rebbe replied, "I was still a young child when the Sanzer Rav passed away and I did not have a chance learn from him all the proper intentions one should

have in mind while eating. Therefore, I rely on my father's intentions, and a dish that he did not eat I do not eat either."
(*Noam Siach*, p. 155)

On Shabbos that falls on Yom Tov, compote is added to the day *seudah*. However, there are those who do not serve compote at the Shabbos day *seudah* at any time.
(*Irgun Tze'irei Vizhnitz*)

In the Beis Hamikdash, if the *Mizbe'ach* was not in use (all the daily *korbanos* were finished and there were no voluntary *korbanos* being sacrificed) during the week, there were special *korbanos* brought at that time, which were called *kayitz haMizbe'ach*, purchased from money that was previously set aside for this purpose. Rashi explains that *kayitz* means dried out figs that are eaten as dessert. The *korbanos* of *kayitz haMizbe'ach* were extra, "dessert," so to speak, for the *Mizbe'ach*.

On Shabbos, however, only the *korbanos* associated with Shabbos were sacrificed, and no additional *korbanos* were brought. Since on Shabbos the *Mizbe'ach* did not have its "dessert," we do not eat dessert at the day *seudah*.
(Heard in the name of Reb Yehoshua of Belz)

Oneg Shabbos for Children

Reb Aharon of Belz once said that one should give children *oneg Shabbos* to which they can relate, such as chocolate and sweets.
(*Halichos Hatzaddikim*, p. 342)

Eating Fruits before Minchah

One should eat fruits and sweets, and smell good fragrances on Shabbos afternoon in order to complete his recitation of 100 *brachos*.
(*Orach Chaim* 290:1)

Chapter 19
Shalosh Seudos—Equal to All Three Meals

Shalosh Seudos—the Importance of the Third Meal

One should be extremely meticulous to eat *shalosh seudos*. Even if one is satiated, he can fulfill this mitzvah by just eating a *kebeitzah*. If one is not able to eat at all, he is not required to suffer and eat. However, one who is wise should not satiate himself completely at the morning *seudah,* so that he is able to eat *shalosh seudos*.   (*Shulchan Aruch, Orach Chaim* 291)

Unlike the opinions that hold that one can fulfill *shalosh seudos* by eating other foods, the *Shulchan Aruch* is of the opinion that one is required to wash for bread. Heaven forbid that a person should make light of this, and it is a great sin to do so. One should be extremely careful with this, and there is no leeway unless one is ill. One who degrades *shalosh seudos* by not eating bread will face retribution in the future.
(*Aruch Hashulchan* 291:2)

Yemenite Jews are accustomed to calling the third *seudah* "*kiyum*." They use the phrase *l'kayeim es hakiyum*. Perhaps the reason for this is because often at *shalosh seudos* a person is not hungry and only eats in order to be *mekayeim* (fulfill) the mitzvah. Therefore, his reward is great, as *Chazal* have said, *Kol hamekayim* (one who fulfills) three *seudos* is spared from three evil happenings.
(*Shulchan Aruch Hamekutzar* sec. 59; *Einei Yitzchak,* sec. 59)

The greatness of eating three *seudos* is clear from the words of *Chazal*, as the Gemara states: *Rav Nachman said that he deserves reward for eating three* seudos *Shabbos*.

It seems that this reward refers mainly to the third *seudah*, *shalosh seudos*, since during the week a person also eats two meals a day.

Eating *shalosh seudos* is one of the great mitzvos. One who eats it will merit delighting in Gan Eden. One should be very careful about eating three *seudos*, especially *shalosh seudos*, which is the most elevated of all *seudos*. One does not need to be instructed to eat the first two *seudos*, because that is when he is hungry and will eat anyway. However, by *shalosh seudos*, when a person is satiated, he needs to be told to eat. One should know that the true reward for eating on Shabbos is for this *seudah*. *(Tzror Hamor, Bereishis)*

The meaning behind eating *shalosh seudos* is a deep secret. One should pay attention to the greatness of *shalosh seudos* and the reward that he will receive for eating it. One is required to eat bread at *shalosh seudos*, like at the first and second *seudos*. If one eats fruits as his third meal, this opportunity is lost. *(Sefer Hakaneh)*

The third Shabbos meal is called *shalosh seudos* (which literally means three meals), because during the first two meals, a person is hungry and derives pleasure from his food. However, by *shalosh seudos* it is clear that he is eating for the sake of Heaven, and by doing so, he demonstrates that he did so at first two *seudos* as well, even if he had not been hungry.

(Divrei Emes, Balak, s.v. Veyeired)

We have two main mitzvos on Shabbos: *oneg Shabbos* and honoring Shabbos. *Oneg* is fulfilled at the first two *seudos*; however, honoring the Shabbos is fulfilled mainly at the third *seudah*, which we eat solely in honor of Shabbos (since one is no longer hungry).

The third *seudah* corresponds to Yaakov Avinu, the "chosen one" of the *Avos*. It encompasses the first two *seudos* and is therefore called *shalosh seudos* (literally, three *seudos*). The main rectification occurs through this *seudah*.

(*Mishmeres Shalom*, sec. 29, he'arah 2)

Reb Moshe Cohen wrote that the reason for the obligation of *shalosh seudos* is that a person who eats gluttonously cannot eat another meal soon afterward. Therefore, when a person sees that it is a mitzvah to eat *shalosh seudos* he will not overeat at the other *seudos*, which will eventually cause him to eat for the sake of Heaven. His heart will remain free to study Torah, and he will have control over his desires.

(*Avudraham, Seder Minchah Shel Shabbos*)

One of the G-d-fearing, old-time residents of the Perushim of Meiron once came to the Satmar Rebbe when he was in Meiron, and tearfully related that he is constantly tormented by bad dreams, and he needed to fast even on Shabbos. (If one has a bad dream, he makes a *ta'anis chalom*—he fasts the next day to nullify any negative effects of the dream.) **He begged the Rebbe for salvation.**

The Rebbe asked him if he was careful about eating *shalosh seudos* on Shabbos. The man admitted that he did not have an appetite for eating *shalosh seudos* and did not do so. The Rebbe instructed him to eat *shalosh seudos* and then his bad dreams would cease. Indeed, that was the case.

Elders of Yerushalayim, who accompanied the Rebbe to Meiron, exerted much effort to comprehend the connection between bad dreams and *shalosh seudos*. Eventually, the elders of Teveriah found the following words of the *Zohar*: *Rabbi Shimon said upon himself that he never forgot to eat three* seudos *on Shabbos and therefore he never needed to fast on Shabbos.*

They also found the words of the *Maggid Meisharim* that the Maggid told the Beis Yosef that he did not need to fast a *ta'anis chalom* on Shabbos since he was careful to eat three seudos. (*Mibe'er Rabboseinu*)

Shalosh Seudos as a Segulah

Reb Pinchas of Koritz once said in the name of Reb Shmerel Varhivker that *shalosh seudos* is an auspicious time to *daven* for livelihood. (*Imrei Pinchas, Sha'ar HaShabbos*)

If a chassid came to the Rozhvadover Rebbe asking for a blessing for livelihood, he would give that person challah that was dipped into wine at *shalosh seudos* as a *segulah*.
(*Mishmei D'Reb Tanchum*, p. 250)

There was once an epidemic in a certain city and the people asked the Chasam Sofer for a *segulah* to stop it. The Chasam Sofer advised people to eat *shalosh seudos*.
(*Chasam Sofer, Haggadah Shel Pesach, Hosafos*)

Shalosh seudos corresponds to children. Therefore, during *shalosh seudas* we pray *V'yizku liros banim uvnei banim,* that we should merit seeing children and grandchildren who are engaged in Torah and mitzvos.
(*Sfas Emes, Parshas Ki Savo*, 5647, s.v. *Bamidrash*)

Eating Shalosh Seudos with Others

The Ba'al Shem Tov instituted eating *shalosh seudos* together with a minyan so that at the end of Shabbos, when the *neshamah yeseirah* leaves, it happens among Jews. This is similar to the halachah that when a person is dying and his *neshamah* is leaving his body, it is proper for this to occur among Jews, preferably with a minyan. (*Likutei Maharich*)

The Ba'al Shem Tov and his *talmidim* were extremely careful about eating *shalosh seudos*, and they were particular to eat together with others. (*Mishmeres Shalom* 29:2)

The *minhag* is to sit together at *shalosh seudos* and sing praises to Hashem. This is very praiseworthy, as it increases the honor of Heaven. Hashem should bless all who do so, and every person should take part in this. *(Siddur Yeshuas Yisrael)*

The Proper Time for Eating Shalosh Seudos

One should not eat *shalosh seudos* in the morning after the day *seudah* by dividing the day *seudah* into two meals, since then *shalosh seudos*, which is such an elevated time, is not clearly recognizable as its own *seudah*. *Shalosh seudos* should be eaten at the time when one can *daven* Minchah.

(Shulchan Shel Arba, Sha'ar Harishon)

Regarding the *mann*, the *pasuk* in *Shemos* (16:25) states, *And Moshe said, "Eat it today, for today is Shabbos for Hashem, today you will not find it in the field."* The word "today" is written three times, which teaches us to eat three *seudos* on Shabbos. Just as there is a separation between one "today" and the next, the three *seudos* also need to be separated from one another. This is another reason for not eating *shalosh seudos* in the morning. *(She'eilos Uteshuvos Min Hashamayim, sec. 14)*

It is written in the *Targum Yerushalmi* that a person is obligated to eat the three *seudos* of Shabbos at night, in the morning, and at Minchah time.

(Nefesh Yeseirah, Ma'areches Shin, sec. 11)

Shalosh seudos should be eaten at *bein hashmashos* (the time between dusk and nightfall). *Bein hashmashos* is day and night together. Thus, *shalosh seudos* is a combination of both Shabbos and weekday, and therefore it has the power to bring the holiness of Shabbos into the rest of the week.

Since *bein hashmashos* is a time without distinct boundaries, *shalosh seudos* corresponds to Yaakov Avinu, because he merited a portion without any boundaries. One who eats *shalosh seudos* also merits a reward without any boundaries.

(See *Maharid Mi'Belz, Sukkos*, p. 193)

Minimizing the Amount Eaten at Shalosh Seudos

It is sufficient to eat a *kezayis* of bread at *shalosh seudos*, but it should be eaten together with a cooked dish, such as fish.
(Maggid Meisharim, Tzav, p. 30)

One should be careful not to overeat at *shalosh seudos*, so that he will be able to eat *melaveh malkah*.
(Yesod V'shoresh Ha'avodah, sha'ar 8, chap. 12)

Some say that *To'ameha chaim zachu*—"those who taste it, merit life" (*Mussaf Shemoneh Esrei* of Shabbos), refers to *shalosh seudos* at which one only tastes (i.e. eats a small amount), since he is not hungry. One who eats *shalosh seudos* merits *Olam Haba*, the true life. *Chazal* say that one who eats three *seudos* on Shabbos will be spared from Gehinnom, which means that, consequentially, he will merit *Olam Haba*.
(Siddur Peirush Hatefillos, Rabbeinu Yehudah Bar Yakar)

Reb Mendel of Riminov quotes the *Zohar* that one who does not eat one of the three *seudos* on Shabbos will be punished greatly. Reb Mendel asks why at the first two *seudos*, which correspond to Avraham and Yitzchak, we eat meat, fish, and delicacies, whereas at *shalosh seudos*, which corresponds to Yaakov, the chosen of the *Avos*, it is enough to eat a *kezayis* of bread.

The Gemara in *Kesubos* states that one who provides for his wife through a third party should not give her less than two *kav* (a unit of measurement) of wheat, half a *kav* of beans, half a *lug* of oil, and a *kav* of dried figs. However, if the wife eats together with her husband, he is not required to provide her with all this, and she can eat whatever he eats. Since she is so happy to be together with her husband, she will be satisfied with whatever she is given.

Similarly, *shalosh seudos* is a time of *yichud*, being together with Hashem at the same table, so to speak. Thus, it is sufficient to eat a minimal amount of food.
(Imrei Tzaddikim, Cheilek Ta'am Hamelech, sec. 9)

The Chiddushei Harim once said in the name of the Rebbe of Peshischa, that *shalosh seudos* can be compared to the elevated days of *Selichos* during which one eats and drinks only a minimal amount. *(Siach Sarfei Kodesh, Erev Shabbos Kodesh)*

The three *seudos* Shabbos are derived from the *pasuk* in *Shemos* (16:25): *And Moshe said, "Eat it today, for today is Shabbos for Hashem, today you will not find it in the field."* The word "today" is written three times to teach us to eat three *seudos* Shabbos.

Why does one eat less at *shalosh seudos* than at the other *seudos* if all three *seudos* are derived from the same *pasuk*?

The first *seudah* is derived from the first time the word "today" is written, which is near the word *ichluhu,* eat it. The second "today" is written near the word Shabbos, which signifies honoring the Shabbos day by eating good food. The third "today," which corresponds to *shalosh seudos,* is written near the words "you will not find it," hinting that at *shalosh seudos* there isn't so much food to be found.

Shalosh seudos is a time of joy and *ra'ava d'ra'avin*, a very auspicious time, as we say in *Askinu Seudasa: Chadu hashta b'hai shata d'vei ra'ava d'ra'avin v'leis za'afin*—"we should rejoice in this time which is a very auspicious time, without any anger." Therefore, we minimize our food at this *seudah* so that it should be a time of spiritual joy without any distractions, and so that the holiness of Shabbos will continue.

(Magen Avos, pgs. 463, 464)

The Gemara *(Brachos* 20b) states that the angels asked Hashem why the Torah says that Hashem does not look away from sin. The angels claimed that Hashem does show favor to the Jews, as it says, *Yisa Hashem panav eilecha*—"Hashem will forgive you" *(Bamidbar* 6:26).

Hashem replied to them that He shows favor to the Jews because the Jews go above the letter of the law and do more than is required of them. The Torah states that Jews are required to recite *Birkas Hamazon* when they are satiated, but they recite *Birkas Hamazon* even when eating a *kezayis* or a *kebeitzah*.

The Bobover Rav explains that this applies when one is eating a *seudas mitzvah*, such as *shalosh seudos*. When eating *shalosh seudos* in the winter, soon after one finished eating the Shabbos day *seudah*, we are careful to eat a *kezayis* or *kebeitzah* in order not to enter into doubt of reciting a *brachah* in vain even though we are already satiated. In this merit of doing more than what is required of us, we deserve Hashem's favor (see also *She'eilos Uteshuvos Chasam Sofer, Orach Chaim* 49).

(*Dvar Tzvi Shabbos*, sec. 140)

Reb Henoch of Aleksander would say in jest that since *shalosh seudos* corresponds to Yaakov Avinu, and since Yaakov had twelve sons that he needed to support, he could not afford to feed them anything other than bread. Therefore, we fulfill eating *shalosh seudos* by just eating bread. (*Chemdas Tzvi*)

The *minhag* is not to dip the challah into the fish sauce at *shalosh seudos* like at the other *seudos*, in order to minimize one's eating at this *seudah*.

The custom is to drink less at this *seudah*, since the Rema writes (291:62) that one should not drink water on Shabbos between Minchah and Ma'ariv. (*Magen Avos*, p. 465)

Reciting Shehakol Prior to Shalosh Seudos

There are two opinions as to whether one needs to recite a *brachah* on drinks during a *seudah*. Some are careful to do this before *shalosh seudos*. Therefore, the *Shulchan Aruch* recommends that one recite a *Shehakol* on a drink prior to the *seudah* in order to avoid this difficulty. The Rema states that one does not need to be stringent in this matter.

(*Shulchan Aruch, Orach Chaim* 174)

The *Acharonim* write that if one drinks before the *seudah*, he should be careful to drink less than a *revi'is*. Otherwise, it becomes questionable whether or not he should recite a *brachah acharonah*, because it is possible that the *Birkas Hamazon* does not exempt this drink since it was not a part of the *seudah*.

(*Mishnah Berurah* 174)

Covering the Challos

Although the reason for covering the challos in remembrance of the *mann* is also applicable during *shalosh seudos*, most people do not cover the challos at *shalosh seudos*.

(*Aruch Hashulchan* 199:14; *Tosafos Chaim* on the *Chayei Adam* 6:116)

The Eishel Avraham writes that it is preferable to cover the challos by *shalosh seudos*.

The *sefarim* ask why it is not customary to the cover bread in memory of the *mann* during the week. The *Zohar* writes that the six days of the week are blessed through Shabbos, and for this reason we commemorate the *mann* only on Shabbos.

Hashem blessed the Shabbos with *mann*. A blessing only has effect on that which is hidden from the eye. Therefore, we cover the challos, which are in remembrance of the *mann*, with which Shabbos specifically is blessed.

According to this idea, it is appropriate to cover the challos at *shalosh seudos*, since saving the challos from embarrassment because of Kiddush is not the only reason.

(*Eishel Avraham*, end of sec. 271)

In the *Sefer Minhagim* of Rav Henich of Alesk (the son-in-law of the Sar Shalom of Belz) it is written that he covered all 12 challos at *shalosh seudos*.

(*Hagahos Zecher Chanoch* 108.)

We cover the challos as an allusion to the fact that wheat grows enveloped in a husk, which symbolizes modesty. Near the *Eitz Hada'as,* the word "naked" is written *(Eishel Avraham,* end of sec. 182). Eating challah rectifies the sin of the *Eitz Hada'as,* so we cover the challos at all the meals, including *shalosh seudos,* since this reason has no connection to the recitation of Kiddush. *(Rabbi Dovid Meisels)*

Braided Challos

The custom is that braided challos should be eaten at *shalosh seudos,* similar to the Shabbos day *seudah.* We cut the bottom third of the right challah, and then cut a *kezayis* from the smaller part. *(Magen Avos, p.459)*

Salt at Shalosh Seudos

There are those who have the custom not to dip the challah in salt at *shalosh seudos.* Since *shalosh seudos* is a time of *ra'ava d'ra'avin* (a very auspicious time), there is no need for salt, as the Rema explains that the salt protects from calamity (167:5). The Magen Avraham cites the Beis Yosef in the name of the Tosafos *(Brachos* 40a, in the name of the midrash) that while the Jews are sitting and waiting for each other to wash without performing any mitzvos, the Satan brings accusations against them, and the covenant of salt is what protects them. However, at the time of *ra'ava d'ra'avin* there is no need for its protection.

(Pri Yesha Aharon, p. 375)

Crumbs of Hamotzi

By *shalosh seudos,* when there is no spoon on the table, one should collect the crumbs with a knife and eat from them three times. *(Zemiros Divrei Yoel,* p. 185)

Wine at Shalosh Seudos

A person is obligated to eat three *seudos* on Shabbos: one in the evening at the time of Ma'ariv, one in the morning at the time of Shacharis, and one in the afternoon at the time of Minchah. All three *seudos* should include wine and two loaves of bread. *(Rambam, Hilchos Shabbos 30:9)*

It is a halachah in the *Shulchan Aruch* (*Orach Chaim* 291:4) that there is no need to make Kiddush at *shalosh seudos*. The Magen Avraham cites the *Tikkunei Shabbos* that one should drink some wine during *shalosh seudos* and recite *Hagafen* on it (ibid., sec. 109). It is also written in the *Be'er Heitev* in the *Sefer Hakavanos* (ibid., sec. 106): *There is no need to recite Kiddush, but one should make a* brachah *over wine and drink in the middle of the* seudah.

The Pri Eitz Chaim explains that the reason for this *minhag* is that drinking should come after eating *(Sha'ar HaShabbos*, ch. 18). *(Magen Avos, p. 465)*

There are righteous people who are accustomed to drinking wine at *shalosh seudos*. *(Minhagei Chasam Sofer 6:5)*

A person is required to eat three *seudos* and drink wine during all of them. *(Otzar Hachaim, vol. 2, p. 124)*

One is not obligated to make Kiddush over wine at *shalosh seudos* since he has already made Kiddush by the morning *seudah,* and Kiddush is made once by night and once by day. Nevertheless, one should take a cup of wine in his hand, for according to Kabbalah, one should make Kiddush over wine by *shalosh seudos* as well *(Sha'ar Hakavanos, Seudas Minchah)*.
(Siddur Shelah)

Since wine gladdens the heart, the Arizal drank wine at *shalosh seudos* to remove his sadness over the departure of Shabbos. The Rebbe of Luzvitza once expressed this concept by saying that Motza'ei Shabbos is like being thrown from a tall rooftop into a pit below. We say the *pasuk, Hinei Keil yeshuasi evtach v'lo efchad*—"My G-d is my salvation, I trust in Him and I shall not fear" *(Yeshayah* 12:2) in Havdalah on Motza'ei

Shabbos because a person may be afraid to leave the holiness of Shabbos behind, to enter the mundane week.

(Pri Tzaddik, Devarim, sec. 17)

The reason for eating bread and wine at *shalosh seudos* is because the Written Torah is referred to as "bread" and the Oral Torah is referred to as "wine." *Shalosh seudos* corresponds to Yaakov Avinu, who encompassed both Torahs.

(Zemiros Vayidaber Moshe, p. 499)

The Chiddushei Harim says that *shalosh seudos* is like a *Korban Chatas*, which did not atone for a person's sins unless he did *teshuvah*. If he did not regret his sins, the *levi'im* would sing until he was aroused to *teshuvah*. If he became depressed over his bad deed, the pouring of the wine would lead him to rejoice. This is also the reason that we drink wine at *shalosh seudos*.

(Siach Sarfei Kodesh, Erev Shabbos Kodesh)

Fish at Shalosh Seudos

The *minhag* is to eat gefilte fish (and not other fish) at *shalosh seudos*.

(Magen Avos, p. 464)

One should eat fish at *shalosh seudos* because the eyes of a fish are always open. Opened eyes are symbolic of unobstructed capacity, and at the time of *shalosh seudos* there is a spiritual light without any barriers. The *Zohar* (Adrah Rabbah, Nasso 129) discusses the auspicious time of Minchah on Shabbos, during which there is a Heavenly light that has no barriers. In Kabbalistic language, this is referred to as Heavenly eyes that have no eyelashes or eyebrows (i.e. barriers). The *Zohar* mentions this regarding the *pasuk* in *Tehillim* (121:3): *Hinei lo yanum v'lo yishan Shomer Yisrael*—"He will neither slumber nor sleep the Guardian of Israel," which can allude to fish that have no eyelashes or eyebrows and do not need protection for their eyes.

(Pri Eitz Chaim 318, ch. 21; Siddur R' Shabsi, Siddur Ba'al HaTanya 63)

Rebbe Meir Shalom, the *av beis din* of Parisov, said that one should eat fish during *shalosh seudos* because, according to Kabbalah, that is the most important time for fish to be eaten. He also added in jest that there is nothing else to eat at that time. *(Derech Tzaddikim*, p. 13)

Fish contain *gilgulim* of previous *tzaddikim*. Therefore, there is a mitzvah to eat fish on Shabbos, especially during *shalosh seudos*, to help the *neshamos* return to their resting places. *(Chareidim*, sec. 33)

It is a mitzvah to eat fish at Minchah time on Shabbos, as they symbolize the watchful eye that is revealed then.
(Duda'im Basadeh, Parshas Shelach)

An additional reason for eating fish during *shalosh seudos* is based on the *Rokeach* (sec. 354, from the *Shulchan Aruch*) that it is the custom to eat fish at a wedding *seudah* after *yichud*. Similarly, at *shalosh seudos*, when we enjoy a close relationship with Hashem, one should eat fish. *(Sha'ar Hakollel*, sec. 17, letter 25)

Rabbanim would recite the chapter of *Tehillim* 23, *Mizmor l' Dovid Hashem Ro'i*, three times at *shalosh seudos*. This may be based on the reason for eating fish on Shabbos. The Torah mentions *brachah* three times when describing three consecutive days during creation: On the fifth day, there was a *brachah* for fish, on the sixth day a *brachah* for Adam (mankind), and on the seventh day the *brachah* for Shabbos. Thus, a person who eats fish in honor of Shabbos is triply blessed with "the three-ply cord that is not easily broken." One should recite chapter 23 of *Tehillim,* which contains the number of letters with the numerical value of *brachah* three times for the triple blessing. There are also 57 words in the chapter, alluding to the numerical value of *dagim*—fish. In addition, it is symbolized by the acronym for the word "*(b'neos)* **deshe** *(yarbitzeini)*," **dagim, Shabbos, Adam,** alluding to the *brachos* for fish, Shabbos, and mankind.
(Bnei Yissaschar, Ma'amarei HaShabbasos 48, sec. 20)

Eggs and Onions

Eggs are a sign of mourning, and some have the custom to eat them specifically at *shalosh seudos* because Moshe Rabbeinu was *niftar* on Shabbos afternoon. *(Kaf Hachaim 36:54)*

Herring

Many people eat herring at *shalosh seudos*. The Chiddushei Harim is known to have done this.

There is an allusion to this found in the song *Azamer B'shvachin*, which was written by the Arizal and is sung on Friday night. In this song, we say the phrase *"v'nunin im rachashin."* Reb Yaakov of Posna defined *nunin* as large fish and *rachashin* as small fish eaten at *shalosh seudos*.

According to Kabbalah, one should have a small and large fish at each *seudah*. One can rectify more *neshamos* through small fish than large ones.

(Yosef Ometz, sec. 550; Chemdas Hayamim 8:34)

Herring nullifies one's negative desires.

(Sefer Chassidim, sec. 390)

The Belzer Rebbes would continue *shalosh seudos* after nightfall. Then, someone who already *davened* Ma'ariv would light candles on the table and they would continue singing. After that, they served fish once more at the end of the *seudah*, which they called *"lechtige fish,"* illuminated fish, because of the candles *(lecht)* that were on the table. Thus, we begin Shabbos with fish and end Shabbos with fish, just like the Pesach Seder ends with the *afikoman*. *(Halichos Hatzaddikim)*

Meat at Shalosh Seudos

Reb Yitzchak Eizik of Ziditchov said in the name of his Rebbe, the Ateres Tzvi, that one should eat meat at *shalosh seudos* as a *segulah* for *yiras Shamayim*.

(Hanhagos Maharya, sec. 75)

There are those who eat fish and meat at *shalosh seudos*. Perhaps this is according to the words of the Kli Yakar on the *pasuk* in *Bereishis* (1:20): **And Hashem said, "Let the waters swarm a swarming of living creatures, and let fowl fly over the earth, across the expanse of the heavens."** The Kli Yakar explains that there are three categories of Jews: *tzaddikim*, *resha'im*, and *beinonim*, those in between. The *resha'im*, who are pulled towards physical, earthly pleasures, are compared to animals. The *tzaddikim* are compared to water, which is more spiritual than earth, and to fish whose life force is water. The *beinonim* are compared to the birds who fly between heaven and earth which symbolizes their fluctuations between the spiritual and physical. Birds are also comprised of both earth and water.

Perhaps that is why we eat fish before we eat meat at the *seudos* on Shabbos, to demonstrate that we are not eating to fulfill our own earthly desires but to fulfill the command of Hashem.

It is written in the *Sefer Meichla D'Asvusa*, in the name of the *Zohar*, that one is required to eat meat at all three *seudos*. Perhaps for this reason, the Ziditchover Rebbe ate both fish and meat at *shalosh seudos*. (*Mattan Shabbos Ma'areches* 4, sec. 7)

Tzaddikim and chassidim did not eat meat at *shalosh seudos*, as is alluded to in the *Zohar*. The Magen Avraham writes that meat symbolizes *din* (retribution) (*Magen Avraham* 494:6). *Shalosh seudos* is a time of *ra'ava d'ra'avin*, an auspicious time, and therefore meat is not eaten.

It was said that the Ziditchover Rebbes were accustomed to eating meat because *shalosh seudos* is a time of *ra'ava d'ra'avin*, and they wanted to use it to sweeten the evil decrees. (*Yalkut Avraham, Orach Chaim* 291)

Dairy at Shalosh Seudos

From the Shabbos before Lag B'Omer until the month of Elul, the *minhag* in Sanz is to eat sour cream and to drink milk prior to eating the fish at *shalosh seudos*.

(*Sanzer Rav*, vol. 1, p. 224)

The Sanzer Rav would eat dairy at *shalosh seudos* during the long summer Shabbasos. (See *Zemiros Divrei Yoel*, p. 317)

Reb Shimon of Yaroslav was accustomed to having milk or sour cream at *shalosh seudos*. Perhaps the reason for this is according the Magen Avraham (494:6) that milk alludes to *rachamim* (compassion). He therefore ate milk products at *shalosh seudos*, a time of *ra'ava d'ra'avin* (a very auspicious time). (*Yalkut Avraham, Orach Chaim* 291; *Magen Avos*, p. 460)

On longer Shabbasos, when there is enough time between the day *seudah* and *shalosh seudos*, one should eat dairy at *shalosh seudos*, so that he eats dairy in honor of Shabbos, as well. On Shabbasos when there is not enough time, dairy is eaten at *melaveh malkah*.

During the summer days, the temptations of the street are greater, and the *yetzer hara* has a stronger effect. The antidote to this is to learn Torah, which is a weapon against the *yetzer hara*. Therefore, we eat dairy products since milk alludes to the Torah, as it says, *Honey and milk under your tongue* (*Shir Hashirim* 4:11). Dairy is eaten specifically at *shalosh seudos*, which is a time to ask for success in Torah learning, and *V'yizku liros banim uvnei vanim oskim baTorah uv'mitzvos*— "and we should merit seeing children and grandchildren occupying themselves with Torah and mitzvos" is commonly sung. *Tzaddikim daven* at *shalosh seudos* on behalf of their children and all who cleave to them, that they should succeed and grow in their Torah studies. (*Magen Avos*, p. 460)

The Gemara states that when Mar Ukva ate meat, he did not eat dairy for 24 hours. Perhaps this is the reason *tzaddikim* did not eat dairy on Shabbos and Yom Tov. Although they would not want to be more stringent than Mar Ukva, at holy times of the year we are more stringent in our service of Hashem. (The Orach Chaim writes about this concept in regard to eating *pas Yisrael* during Aseres Yemei Teshuvah.) (*Divrei Yesharim Shavuos*)

Pomegranates and Plums

It is good to eat pomegranate at *shalosh seudos,* and to have in mind that the word *rimon* (pomegranate) has the same numerical value as the words *ratzon* (will), *tzinor* (connection), and *mekor* (source). (See *Otzros Chaim Tikkun Seudah,* p. 111)

During the Second World War, the Klausenberger Rav took upon himself to add plums to his *shalosh seudos* menu. Perhaps the reason for this is because *tzaddikim* say that plums lead to *simchah.* The Rebbe wanted to demonstrate that even in such difficult times of war he wanted to arouse joy. (*Re'eh* 5772)

An Additional Kezayis at Shalosh Seudos

It is said that if *shalosh seudos* lasts until after nightfall and one eats another *kezayis* of bread at that time, this can be in the place of *melaveh malkah.* (*Aruch Hashulchan* ibid., sec. 3)

It is proper to continue *shalosh seudos* past nightfall, and to eat a small amount of bread— ideally more than a *kebeitzah,* and at least a *kezayis*—at that time. One should have in mind to fulfill with this the obligation of *melaveh malkah.* The *minhag* is to eat the fish while it is still day, in honor of *shalosh seudos,* and then once more after someone who has davened Ma'ariv lights candles. Nevertheless, one should eat *melaveh malkah* again after Havdalah. (*Mishmeres Shalom* 29:2)

Shalosh Seudos—a Segulah for Livelihood

Regarding the *mann* on Shabbos, the *pasuk* in *Shemos* (16:25) states: *Today you will not find it [the mann] in the field.* Rashi explains this to mean, "Today you will not find the *mann*, but tomorrow you will find it." We can explain this Rashi according to the words of the *Zohar*, that the *seudos* of Shabbos bring livelihood for the entire week. Today, you won't find *mann* in the field, but tomorrow you will find it, *because* of today. So too, we will have livelihood all week because of our *seudos Shabbos*.

This applies specifically to *shalosh seudas*. This *seudah* is inferred from the words *today you won't find [the mann] in the field*. The *minhag* is to continue *shalosh seudas* until after nightfall, which causes the blessing to continue into the week.

Reb Moshe Yosef Teitelbaum, the Rav of Uhel, compared eating *shalosh seudos* past nightfall to a wedding. At a wedding, one can tell who is truly close to the *chassan* and *kallah*. Some guests leave right after eating, the closer ones stay for dancing, and those who are even closer stay after dancing as well. So too, on Motza'ei Shabbos, some people immediately do *melachah*, whereas those who are closer to Hashem continue the *seudah* even after nightfall.

(Yatzev Avraham, Moadim, p. 5)

Drinking Wine after Birkas Hamazon

The *minhag* among Ziditchover chassidim was to drink the cup of wine after *Birkas Hamazon* at *shalosh seudos*. (That is not always the custom since drinking before Havdalah may be questionable.) The Ziditchover Rebbe said that one is required to display *mesiras nefesh* for this *minhag*, even when there is no *sheva brachos* (at which the *chassan* drinks the wine).

(Yalkut Maharya, p. 178)

For a while, the Divrei Shalom drank the cup of wine from *Birkas Hamazon* after *shalosh seudos*. Although his father did not do so, he did not know his father's reasons and it seemed to him that, according to the *Shulchan Aruch,* he should do so. After a while, he said that the reason why his father didn't drink the wine had been revealed to him.

Since his father recited Havdalah in the same place that he ate *shalosh seudos*, if he would recite a *brachah acharonah* after *shalosh seudos* and then make another *Hagafen* on wine in the same spot, it is possible that these *brachos* would be considered in vain. When the Divrei Shalom learned of this reason, he began to follow his father's custom. (*Divrei Shalom*)

The *minhag* of the Belzer chassidim is that at a *shalosh seudos* in which a *sheva brachos* takes place, whoever recites *Birkas Hamazon,* as well as the *chassan* and *kallah,* drink from the two cups of wine (one which was used to recite *Birkas Hamazon* and one which was used for the *sheva brachos.*)

Some leave over the wine from the *Birkas Hamazon* recited at *shalosh seudos* to use for Havdalah so that they do not have a question of drinking after *shalosh seudos*.

Another reason for saving the wine is because if a person uses something for a mitzvah, he should use it to perform more mitzvos. Once a person fulfilled the mitzvah of *Birkas Hamazon* with this wine, he should recite Havdalah with it as well. (*Zemiros Ateres Yehoshua*)

Chapter 20
Havdalah—Marking the Separation

No Eating before Havdalah

One may not eat or drink anything other than water from nightfall until he makes Havdalah. Ideally, women should also refrain from eating or drinking until they hear Havdalah.
(*Shulchan Aruch* 299; *Magen Avos*, p. 501)

It seems that by saying *Baruch Hamavdil* without Hashem's name, as is the custom of women immediately after nightfall so that they can begin their work, they are not prohibited from eating even if they did not yet hear Havdalah made over wine. Thus, after a Tishah B'Av which fell out on Shabbos or on Motza'ei Yom Kippur, in extenuating circumstances, there are some who allow women to eat before Havdalah.

(See *Magen Avos*, p. 501)

A Separation

Havdalah demonstrates the greatness and splendor of Shabbos. A person's soul becomes sanctified when Shabbos comes in, and the *neshamah yeseirah* is, so to speak, "wed" to the Shabbos. Hence, when Shabbos leaves, it receives a "temporary divorce" until the following Shabbos.

Indeed, we say in Havdalah, *Who differentiates between holiness and the mundane and between the seventh day and the days of the week...* The two phrases in Havdalah are actually one; the seventh day of the week has a special holiness that is unique to Shabbos and doesn't exist the other days of the week. (*Sha'arei Orah*, quoted in *Chok L'Yisrael Mussar L'yom HaShabbos*)

Not Reciting Havdalah Individually

Unlike Kiddush, when each person recites it for himself, by Havdalah one person should be *motzi* (exempt) everyone else. This is because Shabbos is in the realm of the Kabbalistic secret of *Achdus*, so every person can make his own Kiddush. In contrast, the week is in the realm of *Peirud* (division).

The solution is to cling to a *tzaddik*, who is always in the realm of *Achdus*. Therefore, one should enter the week clinging to a *tzaddik* by hearing Havdalah from him.

(Adir Bamarom, Mareich Naveh, p. 387)

Conversely, the Arugas Habosem would tell his students who were required to enlist in the army to make their own Havdalah on Motza'ei Shabbos, as a *segulah* to be saved from the gentiles.

(Aleph Ksav, letter 332)

The Havdalah Cup

There is a custom to spill some of the wine from the cup onto the ground. This custom is based on the Gemara (*Eiruvin* 65a) which states that a house where wine runs freely like water is a house with blessing. Thus, we do this as a good omen at the beginning of the new week.

(Shulchan Aruch, Orach Chaim, 296, fn. 1, in the Rema)

It seems that one should conduct himself according to that which is written in the *sefer Yesh Nochalin*, that when one fills the cup of wine for Havdalah, he should fill it all the way until the rim, and then continue to pour a bit more. This is the concept of "spilling on the ground"—the overflowing cup serves as the aforementioned "wine spilled like water," and no more wine need be spilled afterwards.

It seems that Chazal were not instructing us to actually spill wine. On the contrary, that is prohibited, as we find that care is taken that no wine should be wasted when brought to a *chassan*. "Wine spilled like water" must mean something else;

otherwise, why is it phrased retroactively, with the words, "wine is spilled" and not "every home in which people spill wine"? What Chazal meant is that a person should not become angry at home, even if wine was inadvertently spilled by one of the family members. The Gemara tells us that "a home in which wine is spilled" and it is not considered "like water" (i.e. he becomes upset about the loss of money), has no *siman brachah*. In *Maseches Sotah* it states that if there is anger in a home it is a sign of poverty, G-d forbid. Thus, Chazal's statement is not meant to serve as a directive to spill wine and waste it, even if the person's intent is to do it for the sake of a *siman brachah*, just as we do not waste wine in the case of a *chassan*, even though we have the same intention then. One should spill as little as possible from the cup of Havdalah, to avoid wasting the wine. (*Turei Zahav, Orach Chaim* 296, fn.1)

Raising the Cup

During Kiddush, the custom is that someone else lifts the cup for the person making Kiddush. During Havdalah, the person reciting Havdalah lifts it for himself. The reason for this is that on Shabbos, there is an elevation of *malchus Shamayim*. "*Malchus*" is also referred to in Kabbalah as "*kos*" (which can mean both kingdom and cup), and it requires something to help elevate it. During the week, the *malchus Shamayim* descends back to its place on its own.

(*Adir Bamarom, Mareich Naveh*, p. 386)

Havdalah over Wine

Havdalah is made specifically over wine because wine is derived from grapes. In the process of becoming wine, the grape separates from the shell. Even while still inside the grape, the wine is a distinct, more delicate part of it. In this way, it is comparable to Shabbos, which is completely separate and different from the days of the week. We are instructed to recite Havdalah over wine in order to demonstrate this distinction.

(*Maharal, Chiddushei Aggados, Shavuos*, p. 18b)

One who makes Havdalah over wine on Motza'ei Shabbasos will have children who are deserving of teaching Torah, as the Gemara in *Shavuos* (18b) states, *L'havdil, ul'horos* (literally, "to make Havdalah—and to teach").

There are several levels of knowledge. *Chachmah* refers to the strength of the mind and the ability to come up with novel ideas, according to a person's mental capabilities. *Da'as* is the ability to decide and rule between contradicting concepts, understanding which is truly correct. No matter what the issue is, a person will encounter doubts and different contradicting ideas. The stronger his mind is, the more points will be added to each contradicting side, but he still will not be able to know what the true conclusion is and provide a halachic ruling as to the proper way of acting. For that, one needs the ability to determine *(hachra'ah)*. After his mind has come up with all the different views and their supporting arguments, he can judge them and determine which is correct.

Havdalah is related to *da'as*, as explained in the *Yerushalmi* (*Brachos* 5:2), that Havdalah is in the *brachah* of *Chonen Hada'as*. The *Yerushalmi,* as well, states, *If there is no* da'as, *how can there be Havdalah?* When a person makes a proper Havdalah over wine, displaying that he has the attribute of *da'as*, this brings him to have children who are deserving of *hora'ah*, which also depends on *da'as*. His reward is measure for measure—since he recited Havdalah properly, which comes from the *da'as*, he will merit having children who have the *da'as* to determine halachic rulings.

(*Otzros Yosef, Drashah for Shabbos Shuvah*, p. 35a)

Besamim

We smell *besamim* on Motza'ei Shabbos because our bodies become weakened when the *neshamah yeseirah* leaves us, and [fragrant] smell strengthens the body.

Another reason is that on Shabbos, the fire of the Gehinnom ceases until Motza'ei Shabbos, when it begins to burn and reek again. We smell the *besamim* in order to mask the stench.

(*Tosafos, Beitzah* 34, s.v. *Ki havinan*; *Machzor Vitri* 345)

We make a *brachah* on the scent of the *besamim* before making a *brachah* on fire to draw the "scent" of Shabbos into the other days of the week. This, in turn, changes all the food that we will eat during the week to "soul food" as well.

(*Toras Shabbos*; *Likutei Moharan*, p. 8)

There was a story told of Reb Refael of Barshad, who once spent Shabbos in a small city near Kiev. After Shabbos, when he wanted to make Havdalah, the owner of the inn in which he was staying had no *besamim*. Messengers were sent to all the Jewish homes and stores in the city, but no one had *besamim* for the Rav. The Rav told them, "*Kedoshim*! Where are you?! This is a mitzvah that you can perform all year long for a price of three *perutos* [small coins], and you do not have it?! I will travel to every place in the world and tell everyone not to let their children marry yours!"

This is difficult to understand. Why would the people in that city deserve such a terrible punishment?

Along similar lines, a man's daughter had converted and married a non-Jew. The broken father traveled to Reb Dovid of Tolna to ask him to plead on his behalf.

When he came to the Rebbe and told him of the tragedy, the Rebbe asked the father whether he is careful to smell *besamim* when he makes Havdalah. The man admitted that he did not make Havdalah at all. Hearing this response, the Rebbe refused to speak to him, and only said to the others standing around him, "A person who always smells *besamim* during Havdalah is guaranteed never to have this tragedy occur with any of his descendants!"

There is a source for this in two places. The *Zohar* (part II, 208b and part III, 35b) states that on Erev Shabbos, the *neshamah* of the week leaves a person and the *neshamah yeseirah* takes its place. On Motza'ei Shabbos, the *neshamah yeseirah* leaves, and the *besamim* of Havdalah returns the weekday *neshamah* to the person. From this it seems clear that if a person does not smell the *besamim*, the *neshamah* of the week *will* not return to him, and the person will have no *neshamah* inside him and he will be left only with his *nefesh habeheimis*, animalistic soul. How can he draw down *neshamos* for his unborn children if he himself has none?

(*Likutim Yekarim* [Radivka], *Reb Refael of Barshad*, 8)

The Brachos of Havdalah

The *brachos* of Havdalah are in ascending order: *Hagafen* is first, because the sense of taste is less sensitive than the others senses, and only functions when coming in contact with something concrete. The sense of smell is finer; one can smell something even if it is some distance away. Sight is even more refined; one can see all the way to the stars in the sky. Finally, the *brachah* of Havdalah is the wisdom to differentiate between something which is holy and that which is not, which is why it was also inserted in the *brachah* of *Chonen Hada'as*. Our minds are even finer than the other senses; they can comprehend angels, beginning with the simpler levels and reaching deeper and deeper.

The senses are arranged in this order in the body as well. The tongue is all the way on the bottom. On top of that is the nose, and higher than that are the eyes. Finally, above them all is the mind.

(*Tashbetz, Sefer Ma'amar Chametz*)

Looking at One's Reflection in the Wine

The *minhag* is to drink most of the wine in the cup, even if it holds more than a *revi'is*. Then, one should look at the remaining wine by the light of the candle and see his forehead reflected in it. This is a *segulah* to be saved from harm.

The flame is extinguished in the wine, which is spilled on the table, and some more of the remaining wine in the cup is spilled over it to demonstrate that this candle was lit only for the sake of the mitzvah of Havdalah. (*Magen Avos*, p. 511)

One should make a separation between the cup and the light of the candle with his hand, look into the wine inside the cup to see his reflection, and then drink the wine. This is a *segulah* to be saved from all harm.
(*Remazei Shabbos*, 515, quoting the *sefer Shomer Shabbos* 8)

Many *tzaddikim* had the custom to look at their reflection inside the wine in the cup before drinking it at Kiddush and Havdalah.

It is said that a person once came to visit Reb Chaim of Zinkov to receive a *brachah*. Afterward, the man continued to stand there. Reb Chaim understood that it was not his righteousness that was prompting him to remain there, and asked him, "Why are you still standing here?"

The man responded that he wished to fulfill the mitzvah of gazing at the face of a *tzaddik*. Wisely, he immediately responded, "The *pasuk* in *Yeshayah* (60:21) teaches us that *Your nation, all are* tzaddikim. Therefore, you are a *tzaddik* too, so you should look at your own face!"

On Motza'ei Shabbos, after a person has said *Vayechulu*, testifying to Hashem's oneness, his sins are forgiven (*Shabbos* 119a) and he becomes a complete *tzaddik*. Since it is a mitzvah to gaze at the face of a *tzaddik*, he should look at his own face reflected in the wine. (Similarly, the Imrei Noam [*Vayechi*, s.v. *Hago'el*] states that it is customary for Jews to bless their children on Shabbos, because a person who keeps Shabbos with all of its details is forgiven for all of his sins—he is a *tzaddik*. Therefore, he can now acquire an abundance of *brachos* through this power of the mitzvah of Shabbos, which is the source of all *brachos*.) (*Kuntris Divrei Shmuel*, p. 58)

Drinking the Whole Cup of Havdalah

It is customary for the one who made the Havdalah to drink the entire cup of wine and not give any of it to his listeners. The simple reason for this is so that he can make a *brachah acharonah*.
(Zemiros Vayedaber Moshe, p. 559)

A *misnaged* who was a *talmid chacham* once came to Reb Refael of Barshad and told him that he is going through great distress. His only child, a girl perfect in every way, had lost her mind. The *tzaddik* responded, "I will share with you a *dvar Torah* that I just thought of this minute, and in the power of this *chiddush* (novel Torah thought), your daughter will be healed. *Chazal* say that on Shabbos and Yom Tov, we merit *hasagas hada'as*, attaining understanding. During the week, *da'as* brings us pain, as the *pasuk* in *Koheles* (1:18) states, *He who increases knowledge, increases pain*. That is why one must recite Havdalah on Motza'ei Shabbos and Yom Tov, in order to separate between the *kodesh* and *chol*, so that the *da'as* gained on Shabbos will not add pain during the days of the week. And so," said the *tzaddik*, "give some of the Havdalah wine to your daughter to drink, and she will be healed." The man followed the Rebbe's advice. From that moment, her condition began to improve, and shortly afterward she was completely healed.
(Kitzur Shulchan Aruch with Chassidic Stories, p. 196)

Generally, the person who made Havdalah drinks the entire cup of wine and does not give any to family members.
(Shibolei Haleket, Hilchos Kiddush)

Giving Havdalah Wine to Others

Some have a custom not to give the remaining Havdalah wine to others to drink, even to males, because this leads to strife. Reb Mordechai of Chernobyl would warn people not to give any of the Havdalah wine to anyone else, because this leads to hatred between people, G-d forbid.
(Likutei Torah, Likutim Avodas Hashem, p. 213)

The Rav of Shiniva warned, in the name of the Maharil, that one must be careful not to allow other family members to drink from the Havdalah wine, because this leads to fighting in the home. *(Divrei Yechezkel Hachadash, p. 76)*

A person who makes Havdalah over a cup of wine does not give any of it to family members. The reason for this is not known; perhaps there is a secret to the matter—yet a *minhag Yisrael* is considered Torah. *(Seder Hayom)*

Some people were not stringent in this and gave some of the Havdalah wine to other men or boys at home. The Chazon Ish would give the remaining wine in the cup to the children around him. *(Ma'aseh Ish, part I)*

Women Drinking Havdalah Wine

Another reason for the custom not to give Havdalah wine to family members is because women should not drink from this wine. It seems that in order not to shame them, it was determined that men should not drink from it either. Either way, when unsure it is best to do nothing. *(Kaf Hachaim 31:35)*

The reason given for why women do not drink from the leftover Havdalah wine is because they have no beard. Perhaps this is why there is a rumor that a woman who drinks from the wine of the Havdalah will grow a beard.

(Sefer Matamim, omissions)

Customarily, women would not drink from the remaining Havdalah wine. The Shelah explains that according to one opinion in the Gemara, the *Eitz Hada'as* was a grapevine *(Sanhedrin 70a)*. The midrash teaches that Chavah squeezed out grapes and served the wine to Adam to drink, and because of that she became a *niddah* and was separated from her husband. Therefore, the wine of Havdalah, which symbolizes a separation between Shabbos and weekday, is not fitting for a woman to drink. *(Shibolei Haleket; Shelah, Shabbos, Torah Ohr)*

Another reason is based on the opinion that women should not make Havdalah for themselves, only hear it from men. Therefore, the custom was not to give them from the Havdalah wine, so that they will not come to make Havdalah on their own. *(Likutei Chaver ben Chaim)*

If a woman has no one who can make Havdalah for her, there are those that rule that she should not make Havdalah at all. Rav Moshe Aryeh would say that this is what his holy father would regularly rule, and added wittily, "If they did not hear Havdalah this week, they will hear it next week…"
(Zemiros Ateres Yehoshua 355)

Some people are careful not to pour the leftover Havdalah wine back into the bottle, so that on the following Shabbos a woman should not drink from it. *(Minhagei Karlin)*

It is possible that the reason women do not drink from the remaining Havdalah wine is based on that which the Tur (end of 299) quotes from the *Yerushalmi*, that women generally do not perform work on Motza'ei Shabbos; their *minhag* is to extend Shabbos until the men finish reciting Ma'ariv. The Magen Avraham (299, fn. 15) quotes the Avudraham that women customarily did not perform *melachah* during the entire Motza'ei Shabbos. Hence, for them, the *kedushah* of Shabbos continued for a longer time than it did for men, so they would not drink from the Havdalah cup.

This concept is already mentioned in *Parshas Chayei Sarah* (24:67) where Rashi, explaining the word *"ha'ohelah"* (to her tent), teaches that the candle in Sarah's and Rivkah's tents remained lit from one Erev Shabbos to the next. We see from this that they drew the *kedushah* of Shabbos from one Shabbos to the next. Therefore, women would not drink from the wine of the Havdalah to demonstrate that for them, the *kedushah* of Shabbos continues even after Shabbos.
(Reb Yosef Chaim Sonnenfeld, in his *haskamah* of the *sefer Mishneh Sachir*)

In earlier generations, we find that women did not have this custom, and would drink from the Havdalah cup just like the men. The Leket Yosher writes that his *rebbi*, the author of *Terumas Hadeshen*, would give his wife some of the Havdalah wine to drink. This is also what it seems like from the Tur, who writes that *he drinks a cheekful* (melo lugmav) *and gives some wine to his household members to taste.*

(*Tur* 299; *Machzor Vitri*, p. 116; *Shu"t Maharshdam, Even Ha'ezer* 155)

Water in the Havdalah Cup

The Tur quotes Rav Amram Gaon that it is the custom to add (throw) some water into the Havdalah cup after one drinks from it to "wash" the cup and then drink the water. Our Rabbis, too, taught that it is a mitzvah to do so (*Pirkei D'Rabi Eliezer* 20), because the leftovers of a mitzvah prevent harm. The remaining water is then spilled over the hands and passed over the eyes, to demonstrate the preciousness of the mitzvos. (*Tur* 299; *Rema* 296:1)

Once, the chassidim were pushing to receive some of the Havdalah wine to drink, which caused the chair of Reb Yissachar Dov of Belz to be pushed back. The Rebbe said, "Why push? The water with which we will wash the cup of the Havdalah is just as important as the Havdalah wine itself!" This is indeed what the Tur says in *hilchos Havdalah*, although many people are not aware of this.

(*Hachassidim V'hayesharim*, part II, p. 850)

Water from the Well of Miriam

Women had a custom to draw water on Motza'ei Shabbos immediately after they heard *Barchu*. Aggadah teaches us that Miriam's well is somewhere inside the lake of Teveriah. Every Motza'ei Shabbos, the well's water reaches all the other wells and springs. If a sick person drinks some of its waters, even if his entire body is filled with boils, the water will immediately heal him.

There is a story told about a man whose body was filled with boils. One Motza'ei Shabbos, this man's wife went out to draw water from the well and succeeded in drawing water from Miriam's well. However, the man was upset that his wife did not return home quickly enough, and when she came home, his angry response caused the pitcher to fall off his wife's shoulders and break. As the water flew out of the pitcher, some of the drops touched the man's skin. The patches of skin which were touched by the water were immediately healed. Our *chachamim* would say about this story, "One who is angry gains only his anger!"

This hope of drawing water from Miriam's well is the reason for the custom to draw water on Motza'ei Shabbos. The Rema concludes his statement regarding this topic with the words, *I myself did not see this custom*.

(*Beis Yosef*, quoting the *Kol Bo*; *Rema* 299:10)

Before Havdalah, the Chasam Sofer would make sure that a cup of water drawn for this purpose would first be placed on the table. After he would drink the cup of wine, he would pour some of this water into the cup and drink from it. Then he would pour the rest of the water over his hands and pass them over his eyes and head. (*Minhagei Chasam Sofer*, ch. 6, *hagahos* 11)

Havdalah Wine on Back of Neck

After Havdalah, some people have a custom to apply some of the Havdalah wine onto the back of the neck as a *segulah* for better memory. The Ramban in *Parshas Bo* writes that at the back of the head are the sinews which are responsible for the memory.

(*Yafeh Nidreshes, Sukkos*, p. 79)

Chapter 21
Escorting the Queen—Melaveh Malkah

Importance of Melaveh Malkah

A person should always set his table for a meal on Motza'ei Shabbos, to accompany Shabbos, even if he only intends to eat a *kezayis*. *(Tur* and *Shulchan Aruch* 300)

The Tur wrote the halachah of the *seudas melaveh malkah* in its own separate *siman*; the same is true for *siman* 419, which discusses the *halachos* of the *seudah* of Rosh Chodesh. He put them into individual sections because people are generally not careful with these *seudos,* and he wanted people to become more aware of their importance. *(Avnei Zikaron* 694)

One allusion to the importance of *melaveh malkah* can be found in the number of the section where it appears in the Tur—*siman* 300. The number 300 is represented by the letter *shin*, which is an acronym *(shin, yud, nun)* for the words *shulchano ya'aseh na'eh* and *shemimenu yehaneh naschoy*— "He should make his table beautiful, so the *'naschoy'* will take pleasure from it." The *naschoy*, the Beis Yosef teaches, is a small part of the body that derives pleasure only from *melaveh malkah*. *(Yalkut HaGershuni, Orach Chaim* 419 and 300)

The *pasuk* in *Melachim I* (18:21) states, *Until when will you skip both* se'ifim? The word *"se'ifim"* is generally translated as "opinions," but in this case, the *sefarim* play on the words and refer to it as sections in a *sefer*. "Until when," they ask, "will you skip both *se'ifim* in the Tur, the one about *melaveh malkah*, and the one discussing the *halachos* of Rosh Chodesh (419)?"

The *poskim* explain that when the Gemara states that *a person must always set his table for a meal,* they mean this literally; he should spread a white tablecloth over the table and do everything that he generally does when preparing for a respectable meal, even if he is only about to eat a small *kezayis*.

(*Poskim*)

The Gemara (*Shabbos* 119b) states: *Rabbi Elazar said: A person should always set his table on Erev Shabbos, even if he only wants to eat a* kezayis. *And Rabbi Chanina said: A person should always set his table on Motza'ei Shabbos, even if he only wants to eat a* kezayis. Both were saying that even if one is still satiated, and if eating more would constitute overeating (*achilah gassah*), he should set his table with different cooked foods for a full *seudah*. This is despite the fact that all he needs to eat is a *kezayis* to fulfill the mitzvah of *seudas Shabbos* or *melaveh malkah*. This is why the Tur (300) writes that a person should set "***his*** *table*," i.e. a complete *seudah* according to his individual custom when conducting a meal, even if he has no need for so much food.

(*Bach* 300, s.v. *L'olam yesader adam*)

The Chazon Ish said that one who does not eat a *kezayis* of bread on Motza'ei Shabbos will regret it in the Next World.

(*Teshuvos and Hanhagos*, part II, 166)

A person who does not eat *melaveh malkah* is considered as though he has not fulfilled the mitzvah of the third meal, either. Since he eats nothing at night, it is like the third meal that he ate on Shabbos was instead of his night meal, and not in honor of Shabbos.

(*Chessed L'Avraham, Ben Ish Chai, Parshas Vayeitzei*)

The words *"Shabbos oneg"* (delighting in Shabbos) have the same numerical value as the words *"zeh arba seudos"* (these are four meals). The fourth meal is to welcome Dovid Hamelech. We can see an allusion to this in the fact that the words *Dovid melach Yisrael chai v'kayam*—"Dovid, king of Yisrael, lives on" have the same numerical value as *"arba seudos"* (four meals). That is why we are taught that when one spends his time trying to recite the *brachah* recited over the new moon on Motza'ei Shabbos instead of eating the fourth meal, he has said *"Dovid Melech Yisrael chai v'kayam,"* but he is not conducting Dovid Hamelech's special meal! The best option, therefore, is to do each in its proper time.

(*Kaf Hachaim*, Palagi, 36:77)

The Vilna Gaon's wife once accepted upon herself a fast. She stopped eating at *shalosh seudos* and went to sleep immediately after Havdalah. When her husband heard this, he sent her a message telling her that all the fasts that she could possibly fast would not be able to rectify missing *seudas melaveh malkah* even one time. When she heard this, she immediately got up and went to eat *melaveh malkah*.

(*Tosafos Ma'aseh Rav* 38)

One must rejoice during *melaveh malkah* just like at the *seudos* on Shabbos itself, for it is a *seudas mitzvah*.

(*Siddur Rash*)

Reb Itzikel of Pshevorsk heard from the holy Rav of Tziechnov, that he was once given a message from Heaven (whether in a dream or otherwise), that on the week of a person's *yahrtzeit*, his *neshamah* receives a tremendous *tikkun* (rectification) through others providing the *melaveh malkah* meal in his merit.

(*Tiferes Naftali*, stories, 100)

It is quoted in the name of Reb Elimelech of Lizhensk that if a person decides to fast during the weeks of *Shovavim* and skips *melaveh malkah*, his fast is only considered to have begun on Tuesday. Reb Chaim Uri, the son of Reb Yozif

Nanisher added, "How much more so is one who eats *melaveh malkah* on Motza'ei Shabbos considered as though he fasted all the days of the week!"

(*Otzar Yisrael*, section on Reb Elimelech, 54)

After Shabbos, chassidim would eat a *melaveh malkah* meal together, telling over stories of *tzaddikim*.

Reb Yochanan of Stolin said that "chassidim" are those who sit together to eat *seudas melaveh malkah*. He also instructed the chassidim of his brother, Reb Yaakov Chaim of Stolin, to make sure to eat this meal, for the benefits of eating *melaveh malkah* are everlasting. (*Yalkut Ma'amarim, Shabbos Kodesh*, p. 206)

Reasons for Melaveh Malkah

One reason for the meal on Motza'ei Shabbos is that the entire week receives its blessing from the blessing of the Shabbos, and a mitzvah is considered to belong to one who concludes it (*Tanchuma, Eikev* 6). Therefore, after one concludes the mitzvah of Shabbos properly, we say "Blessed are you when [Shabbos] arrives, and when you leave"—it is blessed as it leaves, too. However, the blessing of Shabbos needs something upon which to take effect (*Zohar*, part I, 88), and that is why one should set his table on Motza'ei Shabbos—to provide a place for the blessing to rest. This will create a connection with Shabbos in whatever he will do throughout the week.

This is why the meal is called *melaveh malkah*. The word "*melaveh*" means *mechaber*, connect (we see this from *hapa'am yilaveh ishi eilai*—"this time my husband will **become attached** to me" [*Bereishis* 29:34]). The *melaveh malkah* meal allows us to connect to the Shabbos Queen all week long.

(*Chasam Sofer*, end of *Maseches Shabbos*)

Another reason for the *melaveh malkah* meal is that it revives one's soul, similar to the *brachah* on the *besamim*.

(Ibid.)

Eating on Shabbos is like eating *korbanos*. One may eat a *korban* on the day that it is sacrificed and that night. Hence, we eat the Shabbos meals during the day and also that night.
(*Chamishah Ma'amaros, Parshas Re'eh*)

The *sefarim* explain that by eating *melaveh malkah,* one can draw down holiness into all of the other meals of the week. It is well known that Hashem created everything in opposites, and if one wants to connect the two opposites, he needs an intermediary. Thus, the *melaveh malkah* meal—a combination of *kodesh* and *chol,* the holy and the mundane—connects the weekday meals to the *seudos* of Shabbos. (*Ach Pri Tevuah, Massei*)

Through the *melaveh malkah* meal we draw down the holiness of Shabbos to all the other meals that will be eaten throughout the week. (*Sha'ar Hakavanos*)

Another reason for eating *melaveh malkah* is because Dovid Hamelech realized how precious, beloved, and longed-for every Jew is, even those who seem simple. On Motza'ei Shabbos, many people become disheartened by their own feelings of lowliness and inadequacy, after falling down from the great levels attained on Shabbos. On Shabbos, there is unlimited joy and happiness, but on Motza'ei Shabbos, that comes to an end.

Chazal (*Beitzah* 16a) say that the word "*vayinafash*" (and He rested) is comprised of the words *vey, avdah nefesh*—"woe, a soul has been lost." The Maggid of Kozhnitz was quoted to say "like the Kiddush is the *chiddush* (renewal)..." and "like the Havdalah—is the *mapalah* (downfall)." To strengthen us after Havdalah, Dovid Hamelech instituted *seudas melaveh malkah* on Motza'ei Shabbos. (*Avodas Yissachar, Likutim*, section 11)

An additional reason for eating *melaveh malkah* is that the burials of Yosef, Moshe, and Dovid were all on Motza'ei Shabbos, for all three passed away on Shabbos. Immediately after Shabbos on those weeks, Bnei Yisrael needed encouragement so as not to be disheartened by the loss of their leaders. They all made a *seudas havra'ah* (the customary meal given to mourners after the funeral) on Motza'ei Shabbos as the *seudah* of *melaveh malkah*. This was a *"seudas chizuk,"* which consoled them by reminding them that their leaders' merits will continue to live on.

From this, we can understand the Arizal's ruling that one should not study Torah before eating this *seudah*. Until the *seudah*, Bnei Yisrael were considered *onenim* (mourners before burial), who are forbidden to perform mitzvos and learn Torah. The Tosafos (*Menachos* 30a, s.v. *Mikan*) quotes Rav Sar Shalom Gaon's words: *One should not study Torah on Shabbos afternoon, because of the passing of Moshe and Dovid. And when a chacham dies—the batei midrash cease* (see there). Accordingly, we can say that this continues until after *melaveh malkah*.   (*Sever Naftali* 14 and 20)

The Seudah of the Naschoy Bone

Reb Mendel Shapira of Dragmiresht (author of the *Moznei V'hin Tzedek*) said that when he was a young child, he was at the home of his grandfather, Reb Avraham Yitzchak Weinberger of Kleinvordein (author of *Pnei Yitzchak* and *Milel L'Avraham*), when his grandfather, the Kol Aryeh, came to visit.

Among those who came to greet the important guest was the wealthy Reb Moshe Chaim Weiss of Kleinvordein (author of *Bris Moshe*, a commentary on the Smag). During the conversation, the Kol Aryeh asked Reb Moshe, "Did you heed my words regarding the *seudah* of *melaveh malkah*?" Reb Moshe remained silent and did not respond. The Kol Aryeh then turned to the Pnei Yitzchak and told him that he had promised Reb Moshe that if he will be careful to conduct the *melaveh malkah* meal with 10 men, he will be blessed with children.

The Kol Aryeh said to Reb Moshe, "Reb Moshe, why do you not heed my instructions? You will be sorry!" The Pnei Yitzchak turned to the Kol Aryeh and whispered to him, "Medically, he cannot have any children!" The Kol Aryeh shook his head as if to say, "He should just comply with my instructions."

Relating the story, Reb Mendel concluded, "I was a child, and as I stood there, I thought to myself, 'My grandfather certainly knows what he is saying. He is the *rav* here and he knows all of Reb Moshe's secrets!' But I was proven wrong—the Kol Aryeh was right, and in his old age, Reb Moshe had a baby girl, continuing his legacy."

Chazal say that whoever makes Havdalah over wine on Motza'ei Shabbos will merit sons, as it says, *to differentiate between holiness and mundane* (*Shavuos* 18b). In the same place, it also says, *to differentiate between the impure and the pure* and close to it, *when a woman conceives and gives birth to a male* (*Vayikra* 12:2).

Yet, this requires further explanation. According to the above, it does not show us that one needs to make the Havdalah specifically over wine—just, "to differentiate between holiness and mundane." If one has recited the Havdalah during Ma'ariv, his reward should also be to have sons.

Clearly, there is more to this statement. The Mateh Moshe (513) explains that there is a certain part of the body named, "*naschoy*" which only experiences pleasure from food on Motza'ei Shabbos. This bone is also called the *luz* bone, and it is the very foundation and essence of a person. When a person dies, the bone does not disintegrate and cannot be destroyed in any way; it is eternal. When Mashiach comes, a person will be resurrected from this bone, and this is the bone through which one receives pleasure and punishment after death.

The midrash in *Vayikra Rabbah* says: *From what was man created? From the* luz *of the spine. And when the person dies, this bone does not disintegrate. Even if one places it in fire, it cannot be burned. In grinding stones, it is not crushed.*

With a hammer, it is not shattered... At the time of techiyas [hameisim], *this bone will be wetted with the* tal hatechiyah *and become like yeast. It will spread out, and from it, all the person's limbs and tendons and flesh...will extend...* (see *Chessed L'Avraham* 4:52; *Siddur Hemdin* at length).

This bone only receives pleasure from food (and drinks) on Motza'ei Shabbos, so when one makes Havdalah over wine, this provides the bone with vitality and strength, and also helps him merit children. (*Toldos Kol Aryeh*)

The Gemara states that there is a bone in the spine called the *naschoy,* from which *techiyas hameisim* will occur (*Vayikra Rabbah* 18). The *sefarim* state that this bone does not take pleasure in anything other than *seudas melaveh malkah* (quoted in *Taz, Orach Chaim* 300).

Eating *seudos* on Shabbos is a semblance of *Olam Haba,* and is a mitzvah, as the *pasuk* says, *and you shall proclaim the Shabbos a delight.* The meals that we eat during the week, on the other hand, are not holy, but merely permissible. Hence, the *seudah* of *melaveh malkah* is an intermediary between that which is permissible and that which is a mitzvah, since it is referred to as a mitzvah in the Gemara and the *Shulchan Aruch* (*Orach Chaim* 300), where *Chazal* say that a person should set his table on Motza'ei Shabbos, even if he is only planning on eating a *kezayis*.

The *naschoy* bone is the only part of the body that is eternal; it does not disintegrate and cannot be destroyed, yet it is physical. Hence, it serves as the intermediary between the eternal and the physical body, which disintegrates and returns to dust.

This is why the resurrection, combining the two worlds— *Olam Hazeh,* which is physical, and *Olam Haba,* which is eternal—will take place through the *naschoy* bone. This is also the reason why this bone enjoys the *melaveh malkah* meal, which is also an intermediary. (*Ohr Ganuz LaShabbos* 14)

In the future, *techiyas hameisim* will take place through the *naschoy* bone, as explained in the *Midrash Rabbah* (*Bereishis* 28:3; *Zohar, Bereishis* 137 and *Vayikra* 222; see also the *Mateh Moshe*).

There are opinions that this bone takes no pleasure in any weekday meal. Since the sin of the *Eitz Hada'as* took place on a Friday, this bone did not take any pleasure in it. Therefore, this particular bone was not part of the punishment of death, and it cannot be broken or destroyed. It is holy and eternal, and *techiyas hameisim* will begin from it.

It is possible that we say, "*Dovid Melech Yisrael chai v'kayam*—Dovid, king of Yisrael, lives forever," because Dovid Hamelech never enjoyed any meal other than the *seudah* of Motza'ei Shabbos, which he instituted. His entire body was like the *naschoy* bone. The reason that this bone enjoys only the *seudah* of Motza'ei Shabbos and not the *seudos* of Shabbos, which is a greater mitzvah, is possibly because on Motza'ei Shabbos one is satiated, and if not for this mitzvah, he would not have eaten. During *melaveh malkah,* a person is only eating for the sake of accompanying the King and it is therefore entirely for the sake of the mitzvah. On Shabbos, even without having a mitzvah to eat, one would eat simply because he is hungry. (*Ohr Ganuz, Shabbos* 17)

One must also drink during *melaveh malkah*, since the part of the body that receives pleasure from this *seudah*, and from which the resurrection will begin, is a bone. Bones benefit from drinks, as *Chazal* teach that one can see on the bones whether wine was of good quality or not. One can exempt himself by drinking Havdalah wine. (*Eishel Avraham, Tanyana*, 300)

The First Melaveh Malkah

The *pasuk* states, *So Hashem banished him from Gan Eden... And having driven out Man...* (*Bereishis* 3:23-24) The midrash (*Tanna D'vei Eliyahu Rabbah* 1) says that this teaches us that Hakadosh Baruch Hu "divorced" Adam, as one divorces a wife. Elsewhere, the midrash (*Bereishis Rabbah* 12:46) says that Adam Harishon was sent out of Gan Eden on Motza'ei Shabbos. Even though his sin was on Erev Shabbos, and that was when he was cursed with the punishments and lost all his lofty spiritual levels, for the sake of the Shabbos's honor, he remained in Gan Eden over Shabbos and was only expelled on Motza'ei Shabbos.

A person is never sent away without some provisions. We know that in doing the mitzvah of *eglah arufah*, the *beis din* says, "*Our eyes did not see that we allowed him to go with no food and no accompaniment*" (*Sotah* 45b). We also find that when Shaul did not give Dovid a piece of bread to take with him as he took leave of him, it brought about the killing of the entire city of Nov (*Yevamos* 78b). It would also seem that Adam was not sent out empty-handed, from the word "*vayegaresh*"—like a woman receiving *gerushin*, a divorce, who is entitled to compensation. Adam Harishon must have received a cup of wine for Havdalah and bread, fruits, and water—enough for at least one meal.

Adam's world became darkened after his terrible spiritual fall. But even in great sadness and darkness, Adam fortified himself and said, "Whatever was, was!" With thoughts of *teshuvah*, he accepted upon himself to serve Hashem from the depths of his heart with joy. He did not give up; he strengthened himself even in this new lowly state within the physical world that he fell into, just like *tzaddikim* and chassidim would do. All this is explained in the *sefarim* of the *talmidim* of the Ba'al Shem Tov.

When Adam discovered how to create a fire on Motza'ei Shabbos, he made the very first Havdalah over the wine, differentiating between light and darkness. He said, "Now comes a different kind of service of Hashem!" This filled him with joy, as the *pasuk* in *Mishlei* (31:6) states: *Give strong drink to the woebegone and wine to those of embittered soul;* and in *Tehillim* (104:15) it states: *Wine gladdens man's heart.*

When Adam drank wine, the illumination of Shabbos that was drawn onto him from Gan Eden grew very strong inside him. Adam felt great joy, and he then prepared a *seudah* of warm bread and cooked food from the fruits of Gan Eden.

This was so good in Hashem's eyes that Adam was allowed to continue to draw upon himself this "accompaniment" of the illumination of Shabbos from then on, and this provided relief to him and Chavah (*Bereishis* 3:20).

Since their sin had been through eating a fruit named, "*da'as*," the rectification was therefore in the first meal that they ate after being expelled from Gan Eden, which drew down the *da'as* of Shabbos. (Shabbos is called "*da'as*," as the *pasuk* in *Shemos* (31:13) says about Shabbos: ...*lada'as ki Ani Hashem makdishchem*—"to know that I am Hashem, Who makes you holy.") From then on, all of his descendants were given this gift. Whoever observes the Shabbos will also be able to draw down the illumination of Shabbos on Motza'ei Shabbos, which is similar to *Olam Haba* (*Brachos* 57b), to provide him with strength to serve Hashem anew. The Shabbos Queen remains with the person until he conducts the special meal to honor and accompany her.

Thus, Shabbos accompanies us, and we accompany her. This *seudah* can also be called *Seudas Hischazkus*—a *seudah* of strengthening oneself—and one must be exceedingly careful with this *seudah* and have great *kavanah* and joy, just like Adam Harishon. (*Sever Naftali* 14 and 20)

The Seudah of Dovid, Melech Hamashiach

The *seudah* of *melaveh malkah* is called, "the *seudah* of Dovid, *Malka Meshicha*" (the Melech Hamashiach).

The Gemara in *Shabbos* (30a) quotes Rav Yehudah, who quotes Rav Mai referring to the *pasuk*: *Let me know my end, Hashem, and the measure of my days, what it is; that I may know when I will cease* (*Tehillim* 39:5). Dovid Hamelech asked Hashem when he would die, but Hashem told him "This is something that is hidden from every living being." Dovid Hamelech then asked, "On what day of the week will I die?" Hashem told him, "On Shabbos." Rav Mai says: *Thus, Shabbos day[s], he would study Torah [and fast]... The Angel of Death came to him, but he could not [bring him to die], since his mouth did not stop uttering Torah. He said, "What should I do to him?" [Dovid Hamelech] had a garden behind his home. The Angel of Death went and stirred the trees. He went to see what was happening, and [the Angel of Death] removed one stair. [Dovid Hamelech] fell, [and in that moment, he fell silent] and he died.*

This seems difficult to understand. How could Dovid Hamelech fast every Shabbos? The Gemara in *Pesachim* (68b) explicitly rules that everyone agrees that on Shabbos one must eat (*Magen Avraham* 242). We can explain this based on what the *poskim* ruled (*Orach Chaim* 278) that if one receives pleasure from fasting, he is allowed to fast on Shabbos. Since Dovid Hamelech was told that he was going to die on Shabbos, and his learning was saving him from the Angel of Death, he certainly enjoyed his fasting far more than he would have enjoyed eating. Possibly, this was a matter of life and death.

On Motza'ei Shabbos, Dovid would eat to make up for the *seudos* of Shabbos, since on Motza'ei Shabbos some of the *kedushah* of the Shabbos still remains. We commemorate this with our *seudah* of *melaveh malkah*.

(*Peirush Radal* to *Pirkei D'Rabbi Eliezer Hagadol* 1:22)

On every Motza'ei Shabbos, after Shabbos had passed and he found himself still alive, Dovid Hamelech knew that he would live to serve Hashem at least six more days. To express his gratitude, he would conduct a meal. That is why it is called a *seudas hoda'ah*—a thanksgiving meal. This is also why it is called "*seudas Dovid Malka Meshicha*"—because Dovid

Hamelech and his entire household were joyful and would make a great feast, and all of Klal Yisrael joined him in joy and feasts. *(Likutei Mahariach, part II; Yalkut Me'orei Ohr)*

Segulos of Melaveh Malkah

The Gra would be extremely careful to observe the *seudah* of *melaveh malkah* properly, for this brings many blessings and *yeshuos*; it can save a person from diseases and provide him with good livelihood.

(Ma'aseh Rav, Teshuvos and Hanhagos, part II, 166)

Dovid Hamelech said in *Tehillim* (119:117): *Se'adeini v'ivasheia*—"Sustain me and I will be saved." This means that one should eat the *melaveh malkah* meal and he will be saved. *(Avkas Rochlim)*

It is told in the name of the Ba'al Shem Tov that one who eats bread at *melaveh malkah* and lights four candles each Motza'ei Shabbos in honor of *melaveh malkah*, is promised that Dovid Hamelech will be with him at his *seudah*, and that he will not leave the world without seeing Dovid Hamelech. If he is in need of a specific salvation, such as if one of the members of his household is sick or he is suffering from any other difficulty, he should make sure to enjoy the *melaveh malkah* and say, "Ribono Shel Olam, may the merit of Dovid Hamelech protect me that I may be answered regarding this particular request," and he is promised that Hashem will help him. He must observe the *seudah* of *melaveh malkah* to the greatest extent possible every single week.

(Imrei Eish, quoting the Ba'al Shem Tov)

Reb Elazar of Lizhensk says that through the *seudah* of *melaveh malkah* it is possible to bring salvation to Bnei Yisrael, even more than through the *seudos* of Shabbos and Yamim Tovim. He explained this with a parable: There was once a king who levied heavy taxes on his country. Once, the citizens heard that the king was going to visit their province for a few days. They all put on festive clothes and went out to greet the king with joyous singing. Throughout the king's stay, they conducted great feasts with music and song. Finally, when the king was about to leave, the people gathered and fell before his feet, pleading, "Your Highness! All the days that you were with us, we rejoiced with you and did not share our pain, because we did not want to dampen your spirits. Now that you are about to leave, we must tell you that we simply can no longer bear the burden of the taxes that we are forced to pay. We beg you to remove this great burden!" Their request, presented in this fashion, found favor in the king's eyes and he granted them their request.

We, Am Yisrael, are like this nation. Every Jew suffers from various hardships, whether in livelihood or in other areas. Yet, when Shabbos arrives, we put on festive clothing and honor the Shabbos with three meals, songs, and praises. We say nothing about our own needs, as *Chazal* forbade us from making personal requests on Shabbos. However, when the *seudah* of *melaveh malkah* arrives, as we take leave of the holy day, a wise person takes this opportunity to approach the King of kings and pour his heart out with his requests. Certainly, Hashem will fulfill all his desires.

(*Chamra Tava, Shabbos Chazon* 127)

The *pasuk* in *Shemos* (22:24) states: *Im kesef talveh es ami*— "When you lend money to My people." The words *im kesef talveh* allude to *parnassah*. If you want to receive money, then "*talveh*"—make a *seudas melaveh malkah*.

(*Segulas Yisrael*)

Make your Shabbos weekday (*Shabbos* 118a) [generally instructing that it is preferable to make the Shabbos look like weekday and not buy special foods, rather than to ask others for financial help]—i.e. the *seudas melaveh malkah*, which takes place when it is already weekday, yet it still belongs with the Shabbos meals—is a *segulah* for the continuation of the statement: *...you will not need [the financial help of] other people*. (*Tzemach Dovid*)

The Rebbe of Ruzhin, quoting his grandfather Reb Avraham, "the *Malach*," said that one who observes the *seudas melaveh malkah* is ensured to always have food. This is alluded to in the words *Se'adeni v'ivasheia v'esha b'chukecha samid*—"sustain me that I may be saved and I will always be engrossed in Your statutes" (*Tehillim* 119:117). "*Se'adeni*"—whoever observes my *seudah*, "*v'ivasheia*"—I will save him and be of help to him. And what will be his salvation? "I will always be engrossed in Your statutes." The word, "*chok*" can refer to food and physical needs (*Beitzah* 16a). (*Mashmia Shalom, likutim* 196)

Setting the table for *melaveh malkah* is a *segulah* for livelihood. *Sifrei chassidus* teach that on Shabbos, one may not request any personal requests. Therefore, on Motza'ei Shabbos we conduct a meal, so that the blessing will have something on which to take effect, and we ask Hashem to provide us with livelihood for the coming week. It is generally not fitting for blessing to rest on that which is physical, but since the *melaveh malkah* is also a *seudas mitzvah* and is eaten in honor of the Shabbos and its departure, it is appropriate for *brachah* to rest upon it.

Additionally, it is said that this *seudah* is named after Dovid Hamelech, and he would bring livelihood to Bnei Yisrael, as the Gemara (*Brachos* 3b) teaches: *Said Rav Acha bar Bizna, said Rabi Shimon Chasida: A violin was hung above Dovid's bed, and when midnight would arrive, a Northern wind would come and blow on it, and it would play on its own. Immediately, [Dovid] would rise and study Torah until daybreak. Once the day broke, the* chachmei Yisrael *entered and told him, "Our master, the king! Your nation Yisrael needs livelihood!" He said to them, "Go and receive livelihood one from another. They told him, ["There is not enough for everyone to be sustained!"]*

He told them, "Go and send your hands to the troops [i.e. fight the enemy and take the spoils]." Immediately, they consulted with Achitofel and with the Sanhedrin and asked the Urim V'tumim *whether it was a good time for them to go out to war, so that all Yisrael will have plentiful livelihood.*
(See the Shem Mishmuel and Chasam Sofer)

When the Rebbe of Stropkov was in Krenitz, he would be very careful to eat bread made of grains during the *melaveh malkah* meal, in addition to the challos. He said that it is a *segulah* for wealth. (*Zemiros Shabbos Shalom Umevorach*, p. 163)

The *seudas melaveh malkah* is a *segulah* for a long life.
(Likutei Divrei Dovid, Lelov)

It is told in the name of Reb Elimelech, that a *segulah* for women to have an easy labor is to eat something every Motza'ei Shabbos in honor of *melaveh malkah*. They should explicitly say aloud: *L'shem mitzvas seudas melaveh malkah*.
(*Divrei Yitzchak*, sec. 32; *Ta'amei Haminhagim*, *Eser Tzachtzachos* 1:66)

The reason for this *segulah* is that the *naschoy* bone is only nourished from the *seudas melaveh malkah* (see above). Therefore, it did not partake in the sin of the *Eitz Hada'as*, which was eaten on Erev Shabbos, and was not part of the punishment of, *"in pain shall you bear children"* (*Bereishis* 3:16). (*She'eiris Yisrael*, p. 152; *Aleph Ksav*, part II, 598)

The Rebbe of Kolshitz instructed those who were summoned to enlist in the army to help prepare the foods for the *melaveh malkah* meal, as a merit to receive an exemption from the army. (*Divrei Chanah Hashalem*, p. 293)

One who eats the *seudas melaveh malkah* is guaranteed not to be harmed all week from the food. It is also said that if one eats fish during the meal, he is promised that no inadvertent transgression will come about during the meal.
(*Sifsei Tzaddikim*, writings of Reb Tzvi Dovid Glazer, p. 76, sec. 3)

One should eat *melaveh malkah* within four hours of the end of Shabbos, even if one feels satiated and it is difficult for him to eat and drink, he should push himself. This will protect him, and he will never need to take bitter food and drink for healing purposes. (*Orchos Yosher*, end of ch. 10)

Reb Itzikel of Pshevorsk said that he once saw in the writings of Reb Eliezer of Dzhikov, in the name of Reb Elazar of Lizhensk, that there are three times that are an *eis ratzon*, an opportune time, for having one's requests fulfilled: the *seudah* of *melaveh malkah*, Shemini Atzeres, and the last day of Chanukah. (*Mei Zahav*, p. 269)

The fourth meal, *melaveh malkah*, corresponds to Dovid Hamelech, the fourth "*regel*" of the *Merkavah* (Kabbalistic concepts). Dovid Hamelech also saves a person from *chibut hakever* (torment in the grave), in the merit of *melaveh malkah*. (*Pri Eitz Chaim, Sha'ar HaShabbos*; Rema of Pano)

Since one of the *segulos* of the *seudas melaveh malkah* is that it saves one from torment in the grave, women are also obligated in it. (*Damesek Eliezer* 60:107)

During the days of the Ba'al Shem Tov, there was a person who became a heretic. The Ba'al Shem Tov sent someone to convince him to continue eating *melaveh malkah*. Since this person had always been careful to conduct a *seudas melaveh malkah* in the past, he allowed himself to be persuaded to continue. When he tasted the food of *melaveh malkah*, his opinions changed, and he was saved from heresy.
(*Minchas Shabbos* 96)

Many people have a custom to eat some cake on Motza'ei Shabbos before *melaveh malkah* as a *segulah* for *simchah*, and then wash their hands for *melaveh malkah*.
(As heard from elderly chassidim)

Timing of the Seudah

As soon as one has concluded reciting Havdalah, it is proper for him not to do any work that is not *ochel nefesh* (something that he personally needs, such as preparing a meal), or even learn Torah, until he fulfills the mitzvah of *melaveh malkah*.
(*Pri Eitz Chaim, Sha'ar HaShabbos*, ch. 24; *Chessed La'alafim* 300:1)

Preferably, a person should eat *melaveh malkah* as soon as possible after Shabbos, since after an hour has passed it can no longer be considered Shabbos (and *melaveh malkah* is considered the fourth Shabbos meal). (*Ya'avetz, Nusach HaShabbos, Beis Dovid* 4)

One should make sure to eat *melaveh malkah* less than four hours after Shabbos. Even if he is still satiated and it is difficult for him, he should push himself and, in that merit, he will be saved from having to eat and drink bitter remedies.

It seems that even though one is told to eat the meal within four hours, that is in order to perform the mitzvah in the best possible manner. However, if one has no choice, he can fulfill the mitzvah until *chatzos* (halachic midnight), as it is written in *Sha'ar Hakavanos* that the holiness of Shabbos remains for the first half of the night. That is the reason that one is warned not to say *viduy* on Motza'ei Shabbos before half the night has passed. (*Kaf Hachaim*, year 2, *Parshas Vayeitzei* 26)

It is preferable not to begin the meal after one-third of the night has passed. (*Chessed La'alafim* 300)

For those who are careful to eat *melaveh malkah*, there is no obligation for it to be specifically with bread and it can be fulfilled even many hours after Havdalah. Perhaps it is even possible to fulfill it the following day, since the person's intent is to honor Shabbos by accompanying its departure. There were *gedolim* who did so. (*Eishel Avraham* 174:4)

Reb Shimon of Yaroslav (a *talmid* of Reb Elimelech of Lizhensk) would eat his *melaveh malkah* meal on Sunday morning with other people, wearing Shabbos clothes.

Once, he quoted a story about the Maharam Sofer of Pshevorsk, who was visited on a Motza'ei Shabbos by two *neshamos* of people who had died and were now asking him to do a favor for them. The Maharam asked them how they were treated in *Shamayim*, and one of the *neshamos* responded that since he had not been careful to eat the *seudah* of *melaveh malkah*, as soon as Motza'ei Shabbos is over he is returned to Gehinnom. The second *neshamah* responded that since he was careful to eat *melaveh malkah*, he was allowed to remain outside of Gehinnom as long as there is still a Jew in the world who did not yet eat his *melaveh malkah* meal.

Now, Reb Shimon's listeners understood why he would eat his *melaveh malkah* on Sunday morning.

(*Levushei Michlol* 4; *Ohel Shimon Hashalem*, end of the *sefer*, p. 73)

The Sanzer Rav would eat the *melaveh malkah* meal on Sunday morning, and he would not write anything before the meal. Sometimes, they would sing the *zemer* "*Ish Chassid*" during that Sunday morning meal. (*Darkei Chaim, Minhagim* 75)

Reb Aharon Leib of Premishlan would not say *Tachanun* on Sunday, since he held that the time for the *seudah* of *melaveh malkah* is until *chatzos* on Sunday afternoon.

(*Gedolim Tzaddikim*, p. 15; *Divrei Meir Hachadash*, p. 174)

The custom is to continue the great *seudah*, *melaveh malkah*, until close to daylight. Even in the winter, this meal continues until after midnight, and it definitely does in the summer when it doesn't start until very late.

(*Eishel Avraham*, end of 299)

The Saraf of Strelisk once told someone, "Look! As long as I did not yet eat the *seudah* of *melaveh malkah*, the key to the Gehinnom was in my hands!" What he meant was that until he ate *melaveh malkah*, the *resha'im* were allowed to remain outside Gehinnom.

Therefore, some *tzaddikim* would not conduct their *melaveh malkah* meals at the time explicitly prescribed in the Gemara, the *Shulchan Aruch*, and the Arizal, to help the souls of Klal Yisrael suffering in Gehinnom.

The Rebbe of Ropshitz would say wittily: "Each person, according to his level of *chassidus*, extends the time of *melaveh malkah* further. I, then, will extend mine until next Motza'ei Shabbos…"

(*Hilula D'Rabi*, p. 20, sec. 48; see also *Ohel Naftali*, sec. 272)

Fresh Food

It is good to prepare something fresh for *melaveh malkah* and not just eat leftovers. One should eat the *seudah* with the intention of accompanying the Shabbos and having its *brachah* remain on the weekday meals. (*Maharsha, Shabbos* 119b)

The Gemara (*Shabbos* 119b) relates that Rabbi Avahu would have a fine calf slaughtered for *melaveh malkah* every week, and he would then eat only the kidney. When Rav Avimai, his son, grew up, he asked his father, "Why should you waste so much meat? Let us leave some kidney from Erev Shabbos and eat that!" Rabbi Avahu followed his son's advice, but then a lion came and devoured the calf that they had spared.

The Maharsha explains that one should make a beautiful *seudah* to accompany the Queen on Motza'ei Shabbos. It is not respectful to merely have a kidney left over from the Shabbos *seudah*. A person should make a proper *seudah* for *melaveh malkah*, as *Chazal* say, *A person should always set his table on Motza'ei Shabbos, even if he only wants to eat a* kezayis.

The Magen Avraham (300, fn. 1) also notes that from the words of the Gemara it seems that it is proper to cook meat or a different, fresh dish on Motza'ei Shabbos.

(*Shabbos* 119b; and in the *Maharsha* there, s.v. *V'asah aryeh v'achlaya*)

From the aforementioned Gemara about Rabbi Avahu, we learn that it is preferable to prepare a new dish especially for Motza'ei Shabbos and not use leftovers. This was alluded to by Shlomo Hamelech in *Koheles* (11:2): *Distribute portions to seven*, that refers to Shabbos, *and also to eight*, which refers to Motza'ei Shabbos. One must prepare a special, new portion for *melaveh malkah*, and not just leave some over from Erev Shabbos. He gives a reason for this, *for you never know what calamity will strike the land*. Indeed, in Rabbi Avahu's story, a lion came and consumed the calf. (*Maranan V'Rabbanan*, part I, 217)

The entire week is blessed from the blessing of Shabbos, and a mitzvah is considered as belonging to the one who completed it. That is why once a person has completed the mitzvah of Shabbos properly, we say *"Blessed are you when you come,"* when the week arrives, and *"Blessed are you when you leave,"* when the Shabbos leaves. Every blessing needs something on which it can take effect. Therefore, a person must set his table on Motza'ei Shabbos in order to create a place for the *brachah* to rest. In that way, he will maintain a connection to Shabbos throughout the week.

Thus, it is not proper for one to serve food that was prepared the week before. It must all be from the new week, after he was blessed with the *brachah* of the past Shabbos in everything that he will do, for each week is blessed individually. Therefore, it is clear why Rabbi Avahu used a new calf on Motza'ei Shabbos —so that the first thing that he would do during the new week would be a mitzvah on which the blessing could rest.

(*Drashos Chasam Sofer*)

Some people try to have something fresh served at *melaveh malkah*—fruit or jam or sweets that were not eaten at any of the three Shabbos meals.

(*Ben Ish Chai*, year 2; *Parshas Vayeitzei*, sec. 26)

In the home of Reb Yeshayah Kerestirer, they would quickly slaughter, cook, and prepare delicacies immediately after

Shabbos. They would cook meat and fish, and bake large loaves of challah, along with soup, borscht, potatoes, legumes, kugel and wine. They would prepare a truly lavish feast.

(Mei Be'er Yeshayah, p. 58)

Shabbos Leftovers

The Shabbos leftovers are extremely important, and they chase away all kinds of coarseness and heresy, and contain many types of holiness.

(See the sefer Divrei Yisrael, Kuzmir, Mikeitz, p. 63)

Each week, the Maharam Sofer of Pshevorsk would put away leftovers from Shabbos, such as biscuits and cookies. When a distinguished visitor would visit him during the week, he would serve him some of these leftovers, and he would say they were like "*shayarei menachos,*" remainders of the *Korban Minchah*. (*Bnei Yissaschar, Ma'amarei Chadshei Tammuz-Av* 41:10)

Generally, if a person has both a whole loaf bread and a slice of bread, he should use the whole one. However, if the slice was left over from Shabbos, while the whole loaf is a new one, he should use the slice. Since it received the holiness of Shabbos, it is more important than the whole loaf.

(Machzor Vitri)

On Motza'ei Shabbos, for the *melaveh malkah* meal, the Chiddushei Harim would not use a whole loaf of challah but rather a piece of leftover challah from Shabbos. We can explain this based on the Gemara (*Brachos* 39b): *Since it was used for a mitzvah, it is used for a mitzvah again.* The Chiddushei Harim explains that we learn from *korbanos* that *shirayim* (leftovers) contain *kedushah*. We learn this also from *terumos* and *ma'asros* and other food used for mitzvos.

(Sifsei Tzaddik, Parshas Vayeira)

Some have the custom to eat warmed-up leftovers from Shabbos during *melaveh malkah*, because leftovers from a mitzvah are important. It is even written in the Torah: *Their leftovers bound up in their garments upon their shoulders* (*Shemos* 12:34). Rashi explains there that this is because *leftovers from the mitzvah of matzah and maror are important, and even though they had many animals with them [who could have carried it], they carried it on their shoulders to show their affection for the mitzvos.* The leftovers of the Shabbos meals are also precious and appropriate to be used for a mitzvah, i.e. *seudas melaveh malkah*.

(*Responsa Teshuvos and Hanhagos,* part II, 166)

If there are pieces of challah left over from the Shabbos *seudos*, it is perhaps not appropriate to give them to animals or to a gentile, since they are leftovers of a mitzvah.

(*Zichru Toras Moshe, Shemini*)

The *kedushah* of Shabbos in all the foods continues after Shabbos. For this reason, people are careful not to give the Shabbos foods to a gentile even after Shabbos.

(*Vayedaber Moshe*, p. 84)

Reb Elyah Rosen of Ushpitzin noted a hint in the Torah for the *seudah* of *melaveh malkah* and the custom to use leftovers from the Shabbos food for it. The *Yerushalmi*, quoted in the Tosafos (*Bava Kamma* 16b, s.v. *V'hu*), states that the resurrection will begin from the *luz* bone. The *Zohar* (*Toldos* 137a) calls the *luz* bone "*Besuel Ha'arami*." We know that this bone does not receive pleasure from any meal except *melaveh malkah*. In the Torah, before the *pasuk* which contains the word "*hayom*" three times, teaching us about the three meals of Shabbos, it says (*Shemos* 16:23): *Bake what you wish to bake and cook what you wish to cook; and whatever is left over* (i.e. the leftovers from the three Shabbos *seudos*) *put away for yourselves as a safekeeping*—i.e. set aside to eat for *melaveh malkah*, which gives pleasure to this bone which is *a safekeeping until the morning*—until *Olam Haba*, when the resurrection will take place. *They put it away until morning...and it did not stink and there was no infestation in it.* As the Tosafos above writes, this bone is not damaged by worms. In fact, the words, *v'rimah lo haysah bo*— "there was no infestation in it" (ibid. 16:24), contain exactly the same letters as the words *"Besuel Ha'arami."*

(*Melitzei Eish*, 24 Shevat)

Hot Food

It says in the Gemara: *Hot bread* (i.e. a hot dish) *on Motza'ei Shabbos is therapeutic* (*Shabbos* 119b). One should eat something hot and fresh for the *melaveh malkah* meal. This is particularly enjoyable since freshly cooked or heated food and drinks were prohibited over Shabbos. This is similar to the reason that we make a *brachah* over fire on Motza'ei Shabbos and Motza'ei Yom Kippur, because fire is something that one is not permitted to enjoy on Shabbos and Yom Kippur. Since most of the foods and drinks on Shabbos are cold and not beneficial for those who are ill, *Chazal* say that the hot food of the *melaveh malkah* meal on Motza'ei Shabbos is therapeutic.

(*Maharsha, Shabbos* 119b, s.v. *Pas chamah*)

Some people have a custom to dip a piece of bread in a hot drink in order to fulfill having "warm bread" during this meal. (*Zemiros Shabbos Shalom Umevorach*, p. 165)

The Gemara in *Shabbos* (119b) states, *Hot [food or drink] on Motza'ei Shabbos is therapeutic.* Yet, the Gemara does not explain what it heals. Reb Meshulam Zusha would say that it heals depression. This is alluded to in the *pasuk* in *Tehillim* (147:3): *He is...the One Who binds up their sorrows*, since the word *"mechabesh"* (binds up) is acronym for *"chamin b'Motza'ei Shabbos m'lugma,"* and the following word is *"l'atzvosam –* their sorrows,"* to teach us that it is a healing for depression.

(*Devash Hasadeh* 71; *Divrei Yitzchak* 33)

Rebbetzin Rosa Bluma, the daughter of Reb Moshe Yosef Teitelbaum of Uhel, said in the name of *tzaddikim* that if hot food on Motza'ei Shabbos is therapeutic, then cholent (*chamin,* used both in this statement of *Chazal* as well as the term for cholent) eaten on Shabbos is surely therapeutic. (*Rabbi Dovid Meisels*)

On Motza'ei Shabbos, the *neshamah yeseirah* leaves the person's body, but the body naturally resists its departure. *Chazal* therefore instructed us to shock the body with a hot drink or hot water in order to weaken its resistance, so that the *neshamah yeseirah* can depart. (*Imrei Da'as*, p. 9)

Lechem Mishneh

A person should always set his table with two loaves on Motza'ei Shabbos, even if he can only eat a *kezayis*, in order to properly accompany Shabbos on its way out.
(*Ben Ish Chai, Vayeitzei*, sec. 26)

On Motza'ei Shabbos, one should set his table with two loaves, then take one in his hand and say, "This is the *seudah* of Dovid Hamelech." In this merit, he will be spared from torment in the grave.
(*Shelah, Shabbos, Ner Mitzvah*, quoting the *Kanfei Yonah,* part II, 3)

It is possible that one who takes *lechem mishneh* for *seudas melaveh malkah* is transgressing the prohibition of *bal tosif* (adding to a mitzvah beyond the required amount).
(*Likutei Chaver Ben Chaim*, part II, p. 31)

One should make the *brachah* over one whole challah and then cut it into small slices, rather than large slices as is done on Shabbos. The *Shulchan Aruch* rules that one should not cut a slice larger than a *kebeitzah*, since doing so appears gluttonous. (*Magen Avos*, p. 525)

One should prepare four loaves of bread, each bigger than the other. The smallest should be used for the *lechem mishnah* for *shalosh seudos* and then as the bread for *melaveh malkah*.
(*Mekor Chaim, Kitzur Halachos* 274)

Fish

Rebbes had a custom to serve sweet fish and gefilte fish at their holy tables. *(Magen Avos, p. 525)*

Dovid Hamelech dressed in non-Jewish garb and came with his sack filled with live fish to the home of the Noam Elimelech and asked him to buy the fish from him. The Rav sent him to his wife, who told him that she had already completed her preparations for Shabbos earlier in the afternoon and no longer needed fish.

Dovid Hamelech then went back to the Noam Elimelech who once again sent him to the Rebbetzin, yet again she told him the same thing. Once again, he went over to the Rav and told him what the Rebbetzin had said. He took the live fish from his sack and threw them to the ground, saying, "It would be good for you to take them for the *melaveh malkah* meal!"

At that point, the Rebbe realized this is Dovid Hamelech with a message that he should begin eating *melaveh malkah*. He told him, "We don't have the strength to eat your *seudah* because we are already old, but I will tell my children to honor your *seudah* from now on..." *(Divrei Areivim, p. 46)*

During the *seudah* of *melaveh malkah*, the Sadigura Rebbe would ask that herring should be served, and he would say, "*Shmu'os tovos!*" *(Adir Bamarom, p. 404)*

Reb Elazar of Reisha was accustomed to eating herring in honor of *melaveh malkah* and would cut it with his own hands. He would also cut the fat and the onions and give them out to the chosen few who merited being with him during *melaveh malkah*.

During the last year of his life, it was once impossible to obtain herring, and the Rav said that if there is no herring, he would not go to the *seudas melaveh malkah*.

It was winter, snowy and extremely cold, and it was late. Two chassidim accepted upon themselves to look for herring in the villages around Reisha. One of the chassidim, Reb Leibish Tzwibel, reached the village of Drobininke near Titshin and found two pieces of herring there. He returned close to midnight and joyously told the Rebbe, "I tried hard, and I found, *baruch Hashem*!" The Rebbe was extremely happy that he would be able to fulfill his *minhag* and eat the *melaveh malkah* meal in the correct manner.

This chassid had no children. For a few years, he had been repeatedly asking the Rebbe to promise him children, yet it didn't help. Now, he saw that the timing was right. Immediately after *Birkas Hamazon*, Reb Leibish planted himself by the door and told the Rebbe, "Rebbe, I was *moser nefesh* to bring herring!" The Rebbe asked him to please leave him alone, since he had no strength. Yet Reb Leibish felt that this was the time that he could receive what he most desired. He stubbornly continued to beg the Rebbe to bless him with children, until the Rebbe finally acquiesced and told him, "Give 40 *reinish* (a large sum of money) and you will be answered." Reb Leibish asked the Rebbe to give him time to bring the money, since he did not have that much on him, and the Rebbe allowed him until the next evening at Minchah time.

The following evening, Reb Leibish came to the Rebbe with the bag of money. The Rebbe took all the money from him and counted it. Then, he turned to Reb Leibish and said, "Leibish, I see that bringing the money was very difficult for you. You will have two children for the sum of money that you brought." Indeed, a year later, Reb Leibish's wife gave birth to twin boys, just as the Rebbe had foretold. (*Mishneh Lamelech, Toldos,* p. 109)

Drinking Liquor

After eating the fish, we drink liquor and say, *"L'chaim."* Even though, simply explained, the reason for drinking liquor after the fish is to separate between the fish and the meat, there is basis for drinking *"l'chaim"* after eating fish even if no meat will be eaten afterwards, since it is proper to have in mind the combination of the letters of Hashem's name: *Shin, Dalet* and *Yud* with *dagim*, *yayin*, and *saraf* (liquor).

(Magen Avos, p. 525)

Reb Nechemiah Yechiel of Bichovah would eat his *melaveh malkah* meal with many people at his table, many candles, much singing, and telling of stories of *tzaddikim*. He would call it *"ta'anis Baha"b"* (which usually refers to fasting on a Monday, Thursday, and Monday) as an acronym for the words *"Beigel, Herring, Bronfen"* (bread, salted fish, and liquor). He would instruct his chassidim to buy 160 rolls for the meal.

(Toras Hayehudi Hakadosh, p. 44)

Drinking Wine

A number of *tzaddikim*, including the Yismach Moshe, would drink wine during *melaveh malkah*.   (Likutei Mahariach)

The reason for this is because the root of the house of Dovid Hamelech was through the story of Lot and his daughters, when they found wine from Gan Eden. This eventually brought about the birth of Dovid Hamelech through Rus, a descendent of Moav (Rashi, Bereishis 19:34; Bereishis Rabbah 51:10).

(Tiferes Yaakov)

Soup

The Beis Aharon of Karlin drank a cup of wine and ate some chicken soup for *melaveh malkah*.

For *melaveh malkah*, Belzer Chassidim would prepare a meal, wash their hands, and cook *gritz* (vegetable soup).

(Kovetz Beis Aharon and Yisrael, year 19, issue 6, 114)

Once, a wealthy man invited Reb Tzvi Elimelech, the Rebbe of Bluzhov, to come and eat the *melaveh malkah* meal with his chassidim in his home. That same day was also the *yahrtzeit* of a famous *tzaddik*, a *talmid* of the Ba'al Shem Tov.

The *tzaddik* accepted the invitation and sat down to lead the meal. During the meal, beef soup was served. The *tzaddik* took a full spoon and was about to put it in his mouth when he suddenly put the spoon down and returned it to the bowl. This happened a few times, until he decided not to eat the soup. The host took this personally, especially since, when the Rebbe put the spoon down and refused to eat, some of the other chassidim at the table refused to eat it as well. While he was trying to find out what had caused the Rebbe to refrain from eating the soup, a scream was suddenly heard from the kitchen. Soon afterwards, the host's wife appeared and loudly yelled for them not to eat the soup. A great commotion ensued, and it was discovered that the maid had mixed up the pots and the beef soup was cooked in a *milchig* pot that had been used to cook dairy in the past 24 hours.

This created an even greater commotion, with the chassidim discussing the great wonders of the Rebbe. They were astonished that he knew what had happened to the soup even before it was discovered, thereby preventing others from sinning. The Rebbe tried to belittle his astounding greatness that was evident and said, "*Narishe chassidim*! I really wanted the soup, and so I understood that the *yetzer hara* was hiding in there…" (*Ivdei D'Aharon* chapter 11)

Borscht

The Ohr Yisrael of Stolin was very careful to eat borscht during *melaveh malkah*. (*Divrei Aharon, Minhagei Karlin*, p. 219)

The holy Reb Yochanan of Stolin did not want any person who did not eat borscht during *melaveh malkah* to lead the prayers. He said that the word "*borscht*" is an acronym for the words "***sh**omreim, **b**archeim, **t**ahareim, **r**achameim*" (protect them, bless them, purify them, have mercy on them). (*Yesha Aharon*, p. 105)

One reason for eating borscht is based on the Gemara's teaching (*Shabbos* 118a) that one who eats three meals on

Shabbos is saved from three difficulties: suffering before Mashiach's arrival, Gehinnom, and the war of Gog and Magog. The Tana D'vei Eliyahu (ch. 3) says that during the war of Gog and Magog, there will be blood and flesh [of the *goyim*] on Yisrael's mountains and borscht looks like blood.

(*Shomer Emunim*)

Reb Yaakov of Pshevorsk says, quoting the Rebbe of Tziechnov, that there is a custom to eat borscht at *melaveh malkah* because the word "*brischt*" is an acronym for the words "***Rabbi Yisrael Ba'al Shem Tov***."

(*Divrei Yissachar Dov*, p. 15, sec. 48)

It is said that the Maharim of Kotzk once asked the Rebbe of Aleksander what brings him pleasure in *Olam Hazeh*. The Rebbe responded, "Borscht and a good *pilpul* (Talmudic analysis and dispute)." The Rebbe of Kotzk responded, "For over 20 years, I have derived no pleasure from anything in This World, only from Torah and prayer."

(*Ohr Pnei Yitzchak*)

Meat

There are those who are stringent to eat meat during this meal. In the Gemara it seems that it is appropriate to cook fish or something else on Motza'ei Shabbos for this meal.

(*Magen Avraham* 301:1; *Shulchan Aruch Harav* 301:3)

According to this Gemara, which teaches that it is appropriate to cook meat, it would seem to mean specifically beef.

(*Ha'eshel, Likutei Shoshanim* 40:17)

Kugel

In Reb Aharon of Belz's household, they would serve kugel on Motza'ei Shabbos in honor of *melaveh malkah*, and on Motza'ei Yom Tov they would also serve kugel for the *seudas melaveh malkah* of Yom Tov, which is called *Seudas Shlomo*.

(*Ish Chassid*, p. 51)

Garlic

Eating garlic on Motza'ei Shabbos is a *segulah* for *parnassah*. (*Zemiros Nitei Aharon*, quoting the *Derech Tzaddikim*)

Wherever garlic is mentioned as a *segulah*, it is referring to at least three cloves. One should eat three cloves of garlic at *melaveh malkah* as a *segulah* for having many children.

(*Osri Lagefen Milei d'Chassidusa*, part IV, p. 568)

It was a chassidic custom to eat garlic during *melaveh malkah*, as explained in the *sefer Ba'al Shem Tov* on the Torah (*Yisro*, sec. 51) that it is a *segulah*.

This is based on the fact that the numerical value of the word *shum* (garlic) is the seventh name in *Ana B'koach*—*shin-kuf-vav-yud-tzaddi-yud-tav* (since a *mem* at the end of a word is equivalent to 600). This is also alluded to in the *pasuk* in (*Bereishis* 27:28), ***V'yitein lecha ha'Elokim mital hashamayim umishmanei** ha'aretz*—"And may Hashem give you of the dew of the heavens and of the fatness of the earth." The word "*mishmanei*" (fatness) is derived from the word *shum*.

(*Yafeh Sichasan*, p. 175)

Another reason is based on *Chazal's* words that *garlic imbues love and removes jealousy* (*Bava Kamma* 82a). Rashi explains that this is because it gladdens the heart. The reason that Ezra Hasofer instituted that garlic should be eaten on Friday night is to show that we must remove hatred and jealousy from our hearts and bring love in instead. (*Zemiros Vayedaber Moshe*, p. 581)

Another reason for eating garlic is because just as a little bit of spice is enough to make a large amount of food taste good, the *melaveh malkah* meal rectifies all the Shabbos meals so they are more desirable to Hashem.

The author of the *Pardes* says that with this *seudah*, one draws the holiness of the Shabbos *seudah* into all the meals of the week. Perhaps this is the reason that we add sharp seasoning—to demonstrate the drawing forth of the holiness.

(*Teshuvos and Hanhagos*, part II, 166)

Chassidim would commonly say that there is a *segulah* to eat garlic during the *melaveh malkah* meal, and the word *shum* (garlic) backwards is an acronym for "Motza'ei Shabbos." Garlic is eaten on Motza'ei Shabbos for the same reason that Ezra Hasofer instituted eating it on Friday night.

(*Ma'aseh Yechiel, Parshas Lech Lecha*)

Reb Mordechai of Nadvorna would give out garlic on every occasion, especially during the *melaveh malkah* meal. He gave a few reasons for this; one was that the word *shum* is the has the same numerical value as the word *ratzon* (will). By eating garlic, Hashem's *ratzon* and abundance are poured into Bnei Yisrael through Hashem's holy name. He would also say that garlic has 80 ways of healing and many *segulos,* as long as it is not cut with a knife.

(*Tiferes Mordechai*, sec. 105; *Ro'eh Even Yisrael*, p. 173)

Radishes

The Gra would have a custom to eat a radish during *melaveh malkah*, probably because it is a sharp food. Some say that it is a *segulah* for *parnassah*. We are not certain of the reason for this, but if Bnei Yisrael are not *nevi'im themselves*, they are sons of *nevi'im*, and every custom has a source, especially since this was a custom of the Gra.

(*Teshuvos and Hanhagos, Orach Chaim*, 267)

Dairy Foods

Although there are those who express wonder about those who do not eat meat during *melaveh malkah*, and dairy foods are not as respectful for accompanying the King, there is no obligation to specifically eat meat during *melaveh malkah*. If someone desires dairy food, it renders it as important as meat.

(*Eishel Avraham*, 3rd ed., 300)

The Rebbe of Sanz did not wash his hands for *melaveh malkah*; he only had cheese and coffee on Motza'ei Shabbos, and he would eat the *melaveh malkah* meal on Sunday morning. *(Darkei Chaim*, sec. 75)

They would bring fried eggs with butter to Reb Shlomo of Bobov's table. Sometimes he would taste some of it and distribute it to those present. *(Magen Avos*, p. 526)

Once, on Motza'ei Shabbos, Rebbe Meir of Ostrovtza came into the *beis midrash* and saw the chassidim eating a dairy *melaveh malkah*. As soon as he entered, they covered the food, ashamed. The Rebbe saw this and told them, "Do not be ashamed. When Bnei Yisrael were in the desert they also ate only dairy on Motza'ei Shabbos. After all, they were forbidden to eat meat that they desired, and could only eat the meat of the *Shelamim* (Chullin 16b). Since *Shelamim* could only be eaten for two days and one night, they never had meat to eat on Motza'ei Shabbos, since the *Shelamim* slaughtered on Erev Shabbos would be eaten until sunset on Friday, and then on Shabbos itself. On Motza'ei Shabbos, no *Shelamim* were offered and they had no choice but to eat dairy…"
(B'shishim Chachmah, Temidim K'sidram, p. 1254)

In the Gemara in *Chullin* (17a) it says that while Hakadosh Baruch Hu forbade Bnei Yisrael from eating any domestic animal that could otherwise be offered as a *Shelamim*, they were allowed to eat kosher beasts (deer, ram, etc.) which could not be offered as *Shelamim*. According to this, it is not definite that Bnei Yisrael ate dairy for *melaveh malkah* in the desert.

Perhaps we can explain this by noting that *melaveh malkah* atones for our sins, as we find described in many of the verses sung during the meal. Since a person's meal provides atonement, it is possible that Bnei Yisrael preferred to eat milk from a kosher domestic animal that was sacrificed on Friday, to serve as an additional atonement for them, rather than eating a beast that could not be offered as a *korban* at all.
(Olam Hachassidus, issue 37)

Another reason for eating dairy during *melaveh malkah* is that all the *seudos* of Shabbos include meat. Since we want to also include dairy in the *kedushah* of the Shabbos foods, we eat dairy on Motza'ei Shabbos. *(Magen Avos, p. 527)*

No Eggs

One should refrain from eating eggs, even those leftover from the Shabbos meal, since eggs are traditionally eaten by mourners. Motza'ei Shabbos is an auspicious time that has the power to effect happiness and joy, so it would be inappropriate to partake in a meal fit for mourning. *(Pekudas Elazar, Kaf Hachaim)*

Coffee or Tea

In extenuating circumstances, one who is weak can fulfill the obligation of *melaveh malkah* by drinking tea or coffee.
(Siddur HaYa'avetz, Seder Motza'ei Shabbos, mechitzah 4, sec. 4)

In regard to drinking a hot drink on Motza'ei Shabbos, the Vayechi Yosef would say that tea has an advantage over coffee since coffee (in Yiddish, *kave*) refers to the future, as the *pasuk* says, *Kavei el Hashem*—"Hope to Hashem" which refers to the *Geulah*. Tea, on the other hand, (in Yiddish, *tei*) refers to "*Tehei hasha'ah hazos sha'as rachamim*—"May this hour be a time of compassion," which refers to the present. The Shatzer Rebbe of London offered a similar explanation. *(Tiferes Sheb'tiferes, p. 430)*

Reb Elimelech of Lizhensk would drink tea with sugar every Motza'ei Shabbos. Each week, Dovid Hamelech would appear to him with a golden crown on his head. One week, there was no sugar to be found in the house, and the Rebbe drank the tea without sugar. That week Dovid Hamelech appeared without his crown.

When Reb Elimelech questioned him about the crown, Dovid Hamelech replied by asking him where the sugar was. He explained that this was the reason that he appeared without a crown. *(Beis Shlomo, Noach, Darkei Chaim V'shalom, p. 153)*

Although Reb Zusha of Anipoli lived in extreme poverty throughout his life, he was always happy with his lot. One Motza'ei Shabbos, his wife apologized to him that she did not have sugar to put into his tea. Reb Zusha then told Hashem, "Hashem, when You wish for us to lack sweetness, that too is sweet. However, one thing I ask of You, allow us to feel the sweetness in whatever You bring our way."

(Tiferes Banim al Kitzur Shulchan Aruch, Orach Chaim, p. 355)

Kos shel Brachah

Reb Itzikel of Pshevorsk said that he had an accepted practice from his ancestors that drinking *kos shel brachah* after *melaveh malkah* is a *segulah* in many areas.

(Rabbi Dovid Meisels)

Not Eating Melaveh Malkah

The Ostrovtza Rebbe comments that many don't make elaborate *melaveh malkah seudos*. *Seudas melaveh malkah* is referred to as *Seudas Dovid Malkasa*—the meal in honor of Dovid Hamelech. King Dovid was wont to minimize the expense of his meals and instead, use the money saved for the Beis Hamikdash. Thus, it is fitting to follow his example and keep the meal in his memory to a bare minimum.

(Remazei Shabbos)

Melaveh malkah honors the Shabbos Queen as she takes leave. Reb Chanina rules that one is not obligated to make Havdalah over wine, and being *mavdil* during *davening* is sufficient, but he therefore holds it is necessary to conduct a festive *melaveh malkah* to accompany the Shabbos Queen. However, most people disagree and have the custom to recite Havdalah over a cup of wine. Wine is an honorable beverage that can be considered *melaveh malkah*. Thus, they have fulfilled their obligation of *melaveh malkah* simply by reciting Havdalah.

(Shu"t Zecher Yehosef)

Chapter 22
Yom Tov, Shabbos Yom Tov, and Other Special Shabbasos—an Added Dimension

The Difference between Shabbos and Yom Tov Meals

Eating a meal on Yom Tov is compared to welcoming the *Shechinah* to our table, as the *pasuk* says, *Vayechzu es ha'Elokim vayochlu vayishtu* —"and they envisioned G-d and they ate and drank" (*Shemos* 24:11). It is also in place of "seeing" Hashem in the *Azarah* in the Beis Hamikdash, so one who delights in a Yom Tov meal is like one who sacrificed a *korban*.

Yom Tov is called *"ushpiza"* (a guest) and is thus welcomed happily like a guest. It says in *Nechemiah* (8:10): *Chedvas Hashem hi ma'uzchem*—"The enjoyment of Hashem is your strength." Hashem said to Bnei Yisrael: *"Lovi alai* - 'Borrow for My sake,'" and be joyous and fulfill the mitzvah of *chedvah*, as it says, *v'samachta b'chagecha*—"and you should rejoice in your festival," and trust Me that I will remunerate with *brachah* for you" (*Beitzah* 15b).

(*Beis Simchah, Hilchos Yom Tov*, chap. 1)

Rabbeinu Yonah writes that we eat a *seudah* on Yom Tov to express our happiness with the mitzvah. We eat a *seudah* on Erev Yom Kippur since we want to demonstrates how happy we are that Hashem will forgive our sins (*Sha'arei Teshuvah, sha'ar* 4, sec. 9).

We can see from the words of the Rabbeinu Yonah that eating a *seudah* on Yom Tov is because of the *simchah shel mitzvah*. It appears that this *simchah* is not because of a mitzvah like shaking the four *minim* or sitting in the sukkah, because on Shavuos, or the last days of Sukkos, we do not have any specific mitzvos that we were commanded to fulfill, yet we still are commanded to eat a *seudah*. Thus, it must mean that the *simchah shel mitzvah* on Yom Tov refers to resting, and refraining from *melachah*. It is possible that this applies to Shabbos as well. (*Davkeinu B'mitzvosecha*, p. 45)

On Yom Tov there is a concept of "*chatzi laHashem*"— half the time is dedicated to Hashem. While on Shabbos, if one desires, he may dedicate the Shabbos totally "*lachem*" for his own pleasure, as long as he does not miss the proper time for *davening*, as the *pasuk* in *Yeshayah* (58:13) tells us, *V'karasa laShabbos oneg*—"And you should call the Shabbos a delight." (*Magen Avraham* 242: 1)

It seems from the *Gemara Yerushalmi* (*Shabbos* 15:3) that Shabbos was given to us in order that we involve ourselves in Torah learning and not in pleasures, and that we should only devote a little bit of time to pleasures. From the Gemara (*Pesachim* ibid.) it also seems that since we are taught that *all agree that Shabbos is partly for you* and not that *half should be for you*, it is inferred that only a little bit of time should be devoted to personal pleasure. This is understood from the Rambam as well, and that is how it is ruled halachically.

(*Bach*, sec. 242)

It is clear that on Shabbos one must fulfill the obligation of "*oneg*," but one is not obligated to eat. Therefore, if one derives pleasure from fasting, he has still fulfilled his obligation. Regarding Yom Tov, however, there is an obligation of *simchah*, and the Gemara in *Moed Kattan* (9:1) states: *There is no joy without eating*. Even if we don't have meat from the *korbanos*, we must still eat and drink, and even pleasurable fasting is forbidden (unless one is fasting a *ta'anis chalom*). However, it is not explicit that the eating must be pleasurable, and one may therefore fulfill his obligation even if he does not enjoy his food.

Hence, is not clear that one should abstain from eating on Erev Yom Tov from the time of Minchah (in order to have an appetite for the Yom Tov meal) as on Erev Shabbos. We derive from the Rambam's teachings (*Hilchos Yom Tov*, chap. 6, halachah 16; *Shulchan Aruch, Orach Chaim*, sec. 529) that this halachah is not as clear-cut for Yom Tov as it is for Shabbos, since Yom Tov does not carry the same obligation of *oneg* as Shabbos, and it is not as definite that one must eat with an appetite.

(*She'eilos Uteshuvos Chasam Sofer, Ohr Hachaim*, sec. 168)

The difference between the obligation to eat a Shabbos meal and the obligation to eat on Yom Tov is that eating on Shabbos is derived from *oneg*—pleasure, as explained in the *Shulchan Aruch HaRav*. Two concepts about Shabbos were taught by the *nevi'im*: honor and pleasure. The *pasuk* in *Yeshayah* (58:13) states, *V'karasa l'Shabbos oneg likdosh Hashem mechubad*— "and [if] you proclaim the Shabbos a delight, the holy one [day] of Hashem an honored one." Shabbos is included in the principle of *"mikra'ei kodesh"* as the *pasuk* (*Vayikra* 23:3) tells us, *U'vayom hashvi'i Shabbos Shabbason mikra kodesh...*—"and the seventh day is a Shabbos of resting, a holy assembly..." Our Sages teach that *"mikra kodesh"* denotes sanctifying and honoring Shabbos with clean clothing, and delighting in it with the pleasures of food and drink (*Shulchan Aruch Harav* 242:1).

It can therefore be deduced that *oneg Shabbos* is an integral part of the sanctity of Shabbos, because sanctifying it obligates one to eat and delight in it.

Eating on Yom Tov, however, is based on the principle of *simchah*, joy, and is not an inherent part of the sanctity of Yom Tov. On the contrary, there are many allowances on Yom Tov because of *simchas Yom Tov* (*Rambam, Hilchos Yom Tov* 3:4). It follows that there are two opposite principles regarding Yom Tov: the principle of *"mikra kodesh,"* which forbids *melachah*, and the principle of *simchah,* which allows for *melachos* necessary for food preparation.

Rashi *(Beitzah* 2, s.v. *V'ein),* however, writes in regard to preparing the Yom Tov *seudah,* that Yom Tov is also called, "Shabbos." Hence, it seems that the principle of a Yom Tov meal is based on the concept of Shabbos, and this *kedushah* of Shabbos is an inherent part of the Yom Tov.

(Kovetz He'aros Ubi'urim, sec. 819)

Yom Tov that Falls Out on Shabbos

The Tevuas Shor *(Bechor Shor, Ta'anis* 20) contends that the obligation for Shabbos meals is based on the principle of *oneg,* and the obligation for Yom Tov meals is based on the principle of *simchah*. It therefore follows that when Yom Tov falls on Shabbos, we fulfill both *oneg* and *simchah*—which equal the numerical value of *tzafon* (north) and *darom* (south). By fulfilling both *oneg* and *simchah* we merit a double benefit. *Tzafon* and *darom* also refer to the left and right sides, which symbolize long life and wealth as the *pasuk* in *Mishlei* (3:17) tells us, *Orech yamim b'yeminah uv'smolah osher v'chavod*— "long days at her right, and wealth and honor at her left." By fulfilling both *oneg* and *simchah* on Yom Tov which occurs on Shabbos, we merit long life, wealth, and honor.

(Ateres Yeshuah, Moadim, vol. II, 44:4)

One should increase delicacies and fruit when Yom Tov falls out on Shabbos, as well as on Shabbos Chol Hamoed, so that the holiness of both Shabbos and Yom Tov is apparent.

(Kaf Hachaim, 529: 37)

The order of foods served on a Yom Tov which falls out on Shabbos is similar to that of every other Shabbos of the year.

(Magen Avos, p. 222)

Shabbos Yom Tov—Three Seudos

On a Shabbos which falls on an Erev Yom Tov or the first day of Yom Tov, it is best to eat *shalosh seudos* before *Minchah ketanah* (the tenth hour of the day). If a person did not do so, he may eat afterwards. However, he should not eat too much, only a bit more than a *kezayis* of bread, so as not to ruin his appetite for the Yom Tov meal that night.

(*Shulchan Aruch* 529; *Rema* 1; as well as *Shulchan Aruch Harav* there)

For this reason, many people have a custom to divide the morning meal into two, in order to fulfill their obligation of *shalosh seudos* earlier in the day. When doing so, one should make sure to take a short break between the two "meals," by sharing *divrei Torah* or taking a short walk. Some also have the custom to *daven* Minchah between the two meals; this is a good practice, as *shalosh seudos* should take place after Minchah. (*Shulchan Aruch, Orach Chaim; Rema* 291:2)

A person should also be careful not to divide his meal and begin the second part before *Minchah gedolah,* which is half hour after *chatzos* (midday) and the beginning of the time that one may eat *shalosh seudos*. (*Shulchan Aruch, Orach Chaim*, 291:2)

In Ropshitz, whenever Yom Tov would fall out on Shabbos, they would make *shalosh seudos* brief. The Rav of Ropshitz would say; "Shabbos, Shabbos! You are a very important and precious guest, but there is another guest that is even more respected than you are, for it only comes three times a year (i.e. Yom Tov)!" With that, he would take the cup of wine and proceed to recite *Birkas Hamazon*. (*Ohel Naftali* 348)

Minhagim for Special Shabbasos

The *minhag* is to add an additional Shabbos dish on special Shabbasos in honor of the third *sefer Torah* that is taken out.

(*Darkei Chaim V'shalom*, sec. 455)

During special Shabbasos (such as Shabbos *Parshas Bo*, when we read about *Yetzias Mitzrayim*, or *Beshalach*, when we read about *Krias Yam Suf*, or *Shabbos Shekalim* or *Zachor*, etc.), *kneidlach* are added to the soup. *(Nezer Hakodesh)*

People provide "*tikkun*" (*l'chaim* and cake) on the day of a *yahrtzeit*. On the Shabbos before, some people would provide *shalosh seudos* in shul, but they would not provide the morning kiddush on that Shabbos. *(Minhagei Komarno, Simchos, p. 34)*

Chapter 23
In Honor of a New Month— Shabbos Mevarchim or Rosh Chodesh

Shabbos Mevarchim

On Shabbos Mevarchim, an additional kugel is added. Belzer chassidim would make sweet lokshen kugel every week. On Shabbos Mevarchim, they would add a challah kugel.

(Kuntris Dibburei Kodesh, p. 36)

Eating Shalosh Seudos on Shabbos Erev Rosh Chodesh

There are several opinions regarding reciting *Retzei* and *Ya'aleh V'yavo* in *Birkas Hamazon* at *shalosh seudos* on Shabbos Erev Rosh Chodesh.

The Magen Avraham writes in the name of the Shelah that one should only recite *Ya'aleh V'yavo* and not *Retzei*, even if he did not eat a *kezayis* of challah after nightfall.

The Magen Avraham is of the opinion that if one did not eat a *kezayis* after nightfall, he should only recite *Retzei*. If he did eat a *kezayis* after nightfall, he should only recite *Ya'aleh V'yavo* and not *Retzei*.

The *Shulchan Aruch Harav* states that if one did not eat a *kezayis* of challah after nightfall he should only recite *Retzei*. If he did eat a *kezayis* after nightfall he should recite both *Retzei* and *Ya'aleh V'yavo*, as mentioned by the Taz.

Many people are accustomed to eating another *kezayis* of challah after nightfall and then reciting both *Retzei* and *Ya'aleh V'yavo*. The Yismach Moshe and the Belzer chassidim were among those who did this. (*Darchei Hayashar V'hatov*, p. 23)

The Sanzer Rav would refrain from eating after nightfall and would not recite *Ya'aleh V'yavo*. (See *Tamar Yifrach*, sec. 127)

Shabbos Rosh Chodesh

There are those who add a dish to the usual menu in honor of Rosh Chodesh, whether during the week or on Shabbos, so that it is noticeable that it is Rosh Chodesh. One should announce that the food is in honor of Rosh Chodesh.

(*Shiyarei Knesses Hagedolah*, sec. 419)

The *hagahos* on the *Pesikta* state that if Rosh Chodesh comes out on Shabbos, one should remember both Shabbos and Rosh Chodesh with food. (*Otzar Yad Hachaim*, p. 16)

If Rosh Chodesh falls out on Shabbos, one should add an additional dish in honor of Rosh Chodesh, so that he will not forget to say *Ya'aleh V'yavo*. (*Kaf Hachaim* 242:9)

It is a mitzvah to eat a *seudah* on Rosh Chodesh. If Rosh Chodesh is on Shabbos, some have the custom to serve an additional kugel in honor of Rosh Chodesh, to make it apparent that it is Rosh Chodesh.

The *Yerushalmi* states that on Shabbos Rosh Chodesh, one should eat a *seudah* on Sunday, as is done with Purim that falls on Shabbos. The Magen Avraham writes (419:1) that one should continue *shalosh seudos* until after nightfall in honor of Rosh Chodesh. (While it is still Shabbos, the *seudah* is in honor of Shabbos, but after nightfall it is clear that it is being eaten in honor of Rosh Chodesh).

If one usually continues *shalosh seudos* after nightfall, he should serve a special dish at the Shabbos day *seudah*. If one did not serve an additional dish on Shabbos, he should add a special dish at *melaveh malkah* in honor of Rosh Chodesh.

(*Be'er Heitev*, sec. 419; *Sha'ar Hatzion* ibid.:5; *Mishmeres Shalom* 30:4)

When one adds an extra dish to his Shabbos menu in honor of Rosh Chodesh, it should be recognizable. One may add a Shabbos food that he does not usually eat. However, one should not add a weekday food in honor of Rosh Chodesh, because this detracts from the honor of Shabbos.

(*Naharos Eisan, Hilchos Rosh Chodesh* 24:4)

The *Sefer Chug Ha'aretz* states that just as there is a difference of opinion as to when to eat the Purim *seudah* when Purim falls out on Shabbos, similar views exist as to when to eat the Rosh Chodesh *seudah* when Rosh Chodesh falls on Shabbos (see the *Magen Avraham* and the *Taz*). If so, it is a wonder that those who follow the *Yerushalmi* that the Purim *seudah* should be eaten on Sunday do the opposite with the *seudas Rosh Chodesh* that falls on Shabbos (i.e. they don't push it off), even though the mitzvah of Rosh Chodesh is clearly stated in the Torah. (*Chug Ha'aretz*)

Chapter 24
Shabbasos in Elul/Tishrei

Shabbos before Rosh Hashanah

One year, during the morning *seudah* on the Shabbos before Rosh Hashanah, Reb Yechezkel of Kuzmir turned to the people at his table and said, "Make sure to eat for the sake of Heaven, because our food is capable of chasing away worldliness and heresy from those who eat it. Our food also contains all types of holiness. In this *seudah,* on the Shabbos that is before Rosh Hashanah, the food contains the power of all the *Selichos*, from *Zechor Bris*, all the *piyutim* that will be said during Shacharis and *Mussaf* of Rosh Hashanah, the *Kol Nidrei*, Shacharis, *Mussaf* and *Ne'ilah* of Yom Kippur, and the days of Sukkos, Shemini Atzeres, and Simchas Torah up until Isru Chag. It is as the *pasuk* (Shmuel I 1:9-10) teaches about Chanah: *And Chanah rose after she ate in Shiloh and after she drank...and she prayed*. How is this possible? *Chazal* say that one may not eat before praying, could Chana have transgressed *Chazal's* words? She should have prayed before eating! However, she partook of the meal of her holy husband, Elakanah, an *ish Elokim* (a G-dly man), that contained the power of all the prayers that she prayed afterwards. By eating and drinking at this meal with her holy husband in such a holy place, Chanah reached extremely lofty levels and thus was able to pray. That is the meaning of the words, '*And Chanah rose*.' Specifically after she ate and drank, she was able to pray. The *seudah* on the Shabbos before Rosh Hashanah also contains the power of all the *tefillos* up until Isru Chag, so eat *l'shem Shamayim*!"

(*Divrei Yisrael, Parshas Mikeitz*, p. 63)

Shabbos Rosh Hashanah

Rosh Hashanah which falls out on Shabbos is a most opportune time to merit *"ohr ki tov"* (a type of spiritual light), and to feel the sweet taste and pleasure in the words of the Torah. It is also the time during which one feels the good that is in every food. *(Pri Tzaddik, Rosh Hashanah 5)*

When Rosh Hashanah falls out on Shabbos, the shofar is not blown, in order to prevent carrying the shofar outside the permissible area on Shabbos *(Rosh Hashanah 29b)*. The same is true for the mitzvah of *lulav* on Sukkos. When this occurs, the mitzvos of eating and *oneg Shabbos* compensate for loss of the mitzvos of blowing the shofar and shaking the *lulav*, which were not performed.

This is alluded to in the words from the *zemer*, *"Shabbos Hayom."* *Mei'avor derech ugevulim*—"from passing ways and borders," because of the prohibition against "passing" something to a public domain, *mei'asos hayom pe'alim*—"from performing the day's actions," we are obligated to avoid various "actions of the day," such as blowing the shofar and shaking the *lulav*. The compensation for the missing mitzvos is then *le'echol v'lishtos b'hilulim*—"to eat and to drink with praises." *(Yud-Gimmel Oros, part I)*

Mekubalim write that if one does not eat fish on Shabbos, he is punished and sent back to the world as a *gilgul*. For this reason, when Rosh Hashanah falls out on Shabbos, one should not change his usual custom of eating fish because, in any case, there is a mitzvah of *oneg* on Shabbos. He should do as he does on all other Shabbasos. *(Ketzei Hamateh 583:16)*

On regular Shabbasos, one should first eat *compote-tzimmes* with a *brachah* of *Ha'eitz*, then the *mehren-tzimmes*, and then the *farfel*. The *compote-tzimmes* is eaten first because of the *brachah* recited over it, while the *mehren-tzimmes* and *farfel* are eaten as part of the meal, without a *brachah*.

When Rosh Hashanah falls out on Shabbos, during the night meal, after eating the meat, the custom is to first eat the *mehren-tzimmes* (cooked carrots), then the *compote-tzimmes*, and then the *farfel-tzimmes*. During this meal, there is no new *brachah* of *Ha'eitz* made on compote, since it was already made in the beginning of the meal on the apple and honey. We first eat the *mehren*, because of its importance as one of the *simanim* of the Yom Tov, and we recite "*Yehi ratzon sheyirbu zechuyoseinu.*" *(Zachreinu L'chaim,* p. 120)

Reb Aharon of Karlin would say that according to *tzaddikim*, the kugel eaten on Shabbos is good for sweetening the *din* (Divine judgment). Aba Chaim, the *badchan*, once asked him, "If that is the case, why do we blow the shofar to sweeten the *din*? We can do that by simply eating kugel!" The Rebbe cleverly responded, "When Rosh Hashanah falls out on Shabbos and we do not blow the shofar, one can sweeten the *din* by eating kugel! *A minhag brecht avek ale dinim* (A *minhag* breaks all the difficult judgments, turning them into blessings)!"

(Noam Siach Salka, quoting the *tzaddik* of Kashenov)

Reb Itzikel of Pshevorsk would say, "When Rosh Hashanah falls out on Shabbos and we cannot blow the shofar, kugel should be eaten..." *(Hamelech B'mesibo*, Pshevorsk, p. 41)

It is said that once, when Rosh Hashanah fell out on Thursday and Friday and was immediately followed by Shabbos, the Beis Aharon of Karlin turned to people who were grabbing kugel and asked them, "Is this how Jews look after three days of *tefillos*?!" *(Shulchan Menachem, Parshas Ki Savo)*

Shalosh Seudos

In order to fulfill the mitzvah of *shalosh seudos* on a Shabbos Rosh Hashanah we divide the morning meal into two, ending the first before we eat the cholent.

(Darkei Chaim 98; *Zachreinu L'chaim,* p. 124)

Shabbos Shuvah

Some people use long challos on this Shabbos, instead of round ones. *(Minhag Satmar, Bobov; Zachreinu L'chaim, p. 142)*

One Shabbos Shuvah, older chassidim sitting at the table of the Rav of Kalashitz stated that the *minhag* is to dip challah into honey also on Shabbos Shuvah. The Rav told them, "When my grandfather, the holy Rav of Shiniva, was *niftar*, I was fourteen and a half years old, and I do not remember that he ever dipped the challah into honey on Shabbos Shuvah." During that meal, the Rav indeed did not dip the challah into the honey. However, the next year he began to do so, although he never stated the reason. *(Divrei Chanah)*

On Shabbos Shuvah, Bobover Rebbes had a custom to eat two types of fish, including sour fish, just like on all other Shabbasos of the year, because the main ruling of the *poskim* (*Magen Avraham*, beginning of *siman* 583) is that we only avoid eating sour foods on Rosh Hashanah. *(Zachreinu L'chaim, p. 142)*

If one does not eat fish on Rosh Hashanah and he has fish on Shabbos Shuvah or on any other night during the Aseres Yemei Teshuvah, he should recite, *"Shenifreh v'nirbeh k'dagim"* and *"Shenehiyeh l'rosh v'lo l'zanav"* (on the head). *(Mo'ed L'chol Chai 14:19)*

In truth, one should fast on Shabbos Shuvah. Indeed, the *sefer Maggid Meisharim* writes that meat should not be eaten on this Shabbos, yet this is not something that our fathers and Rebbes did since honoring Shabbos with food and drink is also a mitzvah, especially if one's purpose in eating is so that he will have strength to serve Hashem.

This is how we can explain the *pasuk* in *Yeshayah* (58:13): *If you proclaim the Shabbos a delight, and the holy [day] of Hashem honored....* The words *"the holy day of Hashem honored"* are referring to Yom Kippur. From this *pasuk*, *Chazal* derive the halachah that one must "honor it with clean clothing." (After all, how else can one honor it if there is no food?) The *pasuk* teaches us that *"if you proclaim the Shabbos a delight,"* if you honor Shabbos Shuvah with food and drink, that is just as great as *"the holy day of Hashem, honored,"* i.e. fasting on Yom Kippur. (*Seder Shanah Acharonah,* Munkatch, p. 156)

Even if one does not do so on every other Motza'ei Shabbos of the year, he should exercise extra effort to set his table properly with a white tablecloth for *seudas melaveh malkah* following Shabbos Shuvah. (*Mateh Ephraim*)

The Shabbos between Yom Kippur and Sukkos

The midrash states that on Motza'ei Yom Kippur, a *bas kol* announces, "Go and eat your bread in joy, for Hashem has already desired your deeds." This is even truer for the Shabbos *seudah* which takes place during the days between Yom Kippur and Sukkos. When a person is unsure whether a particular business deal was successful, he has no appetite to enjoy his food. However, when one knows that his business is doing well and he is earning a lot of money, he has the presence of mind to enjoy his meal to the fullest. The same is true for Klal Yisrael when they look at their actions to see whether they are good in Hashem's eyes. At first, they are confused and saddened, because every person knows his faults and how much *siyata d'Shmaya* he requires every step of the way, so how can they eat and enjoy food? However, after Yom Kippur, when Hashem promises that He has cleansed them with an explicit promise in the Torah, *For on this day, atonement will be made for you* (*Vayikra* 16:30), every Jewish heart fills with joy, secure in the knowledge that Hashem forgave him for all his misdeeds.

We learn from this *pasuk* that Yom Kippur will bring atonement in every generation, no matter what state we may be in. The reasons for all other Yamim Tovim is always something that occurred in the past. Pesach is because we left Mitzrayim,

Sukkos is a commemoration of the *ananei hakavod*, Shavuos is because of *Kabbalas HaTorah*. A person may conclude that since these events occurred in the past, the same power is no longer valid in the same way. However, with regard to the sanctity of Yom Kippur, the *pasuk* clearly states, *for on this day atonement will be made for you...you will be purified*. This purification is something that will be in the future and will never change. The sanctity of Yom Kippur will always come to atone for us and make our deeds desirable before Hashem. Thus, we can find the courage to eat our bread in joy after Yom Kippur, because all our past deeds were reconciled, and we can now begin anew and correct our actions before Hashem.

(*Toras Emes*, Shabbos Bein Yom Kippur L'Sukkos, s.v. Echol b'simchah)

When Yom Kippur falls on Shabbos, the meal on Motza'ei Yom Kippur is not *melaveh malkah,* but rather a fulfillment of the *pasuk* (Koheles 9:7): *Go eat your bread in happiness.*

The Arizal states that there are two ways to add to the holiness of Shabbos; either by concentrating on the meaning of the prayers or by conducting meaningful Shabbos meals. *Seudas melaveh malkah* is a conduit to empower the following week's meals with the light and holiness of Shabbos. On Motza'ei Yom Kippur which is also Motza'ei Shabbos, this would not apply because there were no Shabbos *seudos*. Thus, the meal concluding Yom Kippur is not considered *melaveh malkah*. (*She'eilos Uteshuvos Torah Lishmah*)

Shabbos Chol Hamoed

The custom is to bake regular, long challahs in honor of Shabbos Chol Hamoed just like for every other Shabbos.

(*Satmar*)

Some people bake round challahs for all *seudos* from Rosh Hashanah until Simchas Torah.

During the Friday night *seudah*, all the regular Shabbos foods are eaten, just like on every other Shabbos. The same is true for the morning *seudah*, although there are some who add cooked carrots and compote. *(Ma'agal Hashanah)*

On a Shabbos that is also Yom Tov, as well as on Shabbos Chol Hamoed, one should prepare plenty of foods, as well as fruits, to show that there are two sanctities present.
(Kaf Hachaim 529, fn. 37)

Shabbos Bereishis

During the *seudah* of Shabbos Bereishis, some have a custom to dip a piece of challah into honey (the word *devash*, honey, is an acronym for the words *devash*, **Sh**abbos, **B**ereishis). Side dishes and pickled vegetables are eaten as well.
(Ropshitz, Dzikov, Belz)

Shabbos Bereishis is still part of the Yamim Nora'im, so *tzaddikim* would continue certain customs, such as dipping challah into honey, saying, "*Yehi ratzon sheyirbu zechuyoseinu,*" eating cooked carrots, saying, "*HaRachaman Hu yechadesh aleinu hashanah hazos...*" etc. in *Birkas Hamazon*, as well as keeping the white *paroches* over the *aron kodesh* and the special coverings on the *amudim* in shul.
(Halichos Tzaddik, p. 175)

On Shabbos Bereishis, Reb Aharon of Belz would eat the *simanim* of *karti* (leek) and *rubya* (black-eyed peas) along with the meat, as well as pickled vegetables. *(Temidim K'sidram)*

Many people have a custom to serve two additional kugels—one just like every Shabbos in which we bless the new month, and one in honor of Shabbos Bereishis. *(Temidim K'sidram)*

Belzer chassidim would eat an extra compote made with the fruits used to decorate the sukkah, besides for the compote served every Friday night. They would cook an apple and pomegranate in honey for this Shabbos, as well as for the Shabbasos of *Parshas Noach* and *Parshas Lech-Lecha*.
(Temidim K'sidram)

It is customary for the *Chassan Bereishis* to provide the kiddush in shul on this Shabbos.

Eating oil on Shabbos Bereishis is especially appropriate. The topic of the *parshah* following the discussion of the Yamim Tovim is: *They shall take for you pure olive oil* (Vayikra 24:2). Olive oil is the source of *chachmah* (Menachos 85b).

Shemini Atzeres is the final "connector" of Sukkos, it contains and connects all the Yamim Tovim, which are sometimes referred to as *"chachmah"* (wisdom). (The numerical equivalent of *Yom Tov* is the same as that of *chachmah*.) After all of the Yamim Tovim, we conclude with Shemini Atzeres, which is called, "Shlomo's *chachmah*" (the Ushpizin of Shemini Atzeres is Shlomo). This is the greatest form of *chachmah* since Shlomo Hamelech was the wisest of all men.

After all of the Yamim Tovim comes the light of the first Shabbos, called, "Shabbos Bereishis," for it is the *reishis chachmah*, "the beginning of wisdom." Targum Yonasan translates the word, *"Bereishis"* as, *"b'chachmah"* (with wisdom). We also know that *Reishis chachmah yiras Hashem*—"The beginning of wisdom is awe of Hashem" (Tehillim 111:10) is alluded to in the word *"Bereishis,"* and the *Tikkunei Zohar* (12:1) says that the letters in the word, *"Bereishis"* comprise the words, *"yarei Shabbos"* (awe on Shabbos).

In other words, on Shabbos, every Jew receives *reishis chachmah—yirah*. This is true even for someone who is considered to be an *am ha'aretz* and is not very wise or well-versed in Torah (Yerushalmi, Demai 4:1). Deep inside, he receives an abundance of *chachmah* on Shabbos, a *chachmah* whose "beginning is awe." This is especially true on Shabbos Bereishis, which contains both *chachmah* and *yarei Shabbos*, as explained above.

The main *chachmah*, which begins with *yirah*, is the *yirah* which burns away a person's negative desires. This is the *kedushah* of Isru Chag, about which *Chazal* said (*Sukkah* 45b): *Every person who "ties up"* (isru) *the Yom Tov by eating and drinking is considered as though he erected a* mizbe'ach *and offered a* korban *on it*. This is because by doing so he creates a permanent "tie" to all the other eating and drinking that he will do for the remainder of the year. They will now all be with *chachmah*—coming from the side of his wise soul *(nefesh hamaskeles)* instead of his animalistic soul. Because olive oil is the source of *chachmah*, it is eaten on this Shabbos.

(*Shevet Mi'Yehudah, Parshas Bereishis*, p. 36b)

During the Friday night *seudah* of Shabbos Bereishis, the *flammen-tzimmes* (plum compote) would once again be eaten. Plum compote was eaten on every Shabbos until Shavuos, and avoided during the summer months due to concerns of infestation. During those months, they would eat *baren tzimmes* (cooked pears). (*Halichos Tzaddik*, p. 176)

Shabbos Bereishis is also the *Shabbos Mevarchim* for Chodesh Cheshvan, which, according to Kabbala, is equivalent to the words, "*Udevash hayom hazeh Hashem*" (letters which comprise Hashem's name). The Ateres Tzvi explains that this was the reason that *mead* (wine with honey) would be drunk on Shabbos Bereishis. Reb Itzikel of Pshevorsk, as well, as other *tzaddikim* said the same.

Some people have a custom to dip a piece of challah or bread into honey on Motza'ei Shabbos Bereishis, because *melaveh malkah* is still part of Shabbos. (*Halichos Tzaddik*, p. 175)

Chapter 25
Shabbos Chanukah

Additions and Changes to the Seudos

Reb Eliezer, *av beis din* of Dzikov, speaking on a Shabbos Chanukah which was Rosh Chodesh, said that the Tosafos in *Brachos* (51a) speaks about the "left assisting the right." When Rosh Chodesh Teves falls on Shabbos Chanukah, this is a case in which, "the left assists the right."

Simply explained, this means that the *seudos* on Chanukah are not obligatory, the *seudos* on Rosh Chodesh are a mitzvah, and the *seudos* of Shabbos are obligatory, a person must eat at least a piece of bread on Shabbos, as explained in the *Shas* and the *poskim*. Our main service is to take something that is *reshus* (non-obligatory) and elevate it to a status of *chovah* (obligatory) and a mitzvah. Thus, on this Shabbos when the *seudos* are for Shabbos, Rosh Chodesh, and Chanukah, all three—*reshus*, mitzvah, and *chovah*—are elevated. The *reshus*, which on its own is considered the "left," is elevated to become "right." We know that this is the greatest form of perfection in our service of Hashem, to elevate something from *reshus* to a higher status. *(Sha'ar Yissachar)*

During the Friday night *seudah* on Chanukah, after singing the usual *zemiros Shabbos*, *Ma'oz Tzur* would be sung and wine would be served. *(Halichos Tzaddik, p. 97)*

During the *seudos* on Shabbos Chanukah, more food is served than on other Shabbasos, in honor of Shabbos Chanukah and in order to publicize the miracle. *(Ben Ish Chai, part I, Vayeishev 24)*

One should make the *seudah* on Shabbos Chanukah more lavish than usual, especially if it is also Rosh Chodesh. Even if Rosh Chodesh Teves is not on Shabbos, he should make a *seudah* to further publicize the miracle. *(Ben Ish Chai)*

During *shalosh seudos*, Belzer chassidim have a custom not to give out the *lechtige fish* (fish eaten after nightfall, but before Havdalah) so that they can hurry to light the Chanukah candles.

On Motza'ei Shabbos Chanukah, it is customary not to drink mead after lighting the menorah, unlike other nights of Chanukah. Perhaps, it is because many are scrupulous not to eat or drink before *melaveh malkah*. Similarly, those who customarily eat *esrog* compote following *Kiddush Levanah* refrain from doing so on this Motza'ei Shabbos.

(Halichos Tzaddik)

The Shem Mishmuel's father explained the statement in *Sukkah* (47b), *Is there a cup every day [of Chol Hamoed]?* based on the *Zohar's* words, that wine arouses the *yetzer hara*. However, on Shabbos and Yom Tov, since there is an elevation of the worlds, the wine is elevated too, and does not cause damage. On Chol Hamoed, on the other hand, there is no prohibition against *melachah,* and no elevation of the worlds, so the wine continues to cause spiritual damage. For this reason, there can be no mitzvah to drink wine on Chol Hamoed.

According to this explanation, we can understand the opinion of those who say that on Shabbos Chanukah, if one forgot to recite *Al Hanissim* during *Birkas Hamazon*, he must repeat the entire *brachah* again. During the week, a person is not obligated to repeat the *brachah* since there is no *chiyuv seudah* (obligation to eat a *seudah*) on Chanukah. The reason for this is because a *seudah* consists of wine, as Rashi explains in a number of places. Since wine is not drunk on Chanukah during the week, there is no obligation to eat a *seudah*. However, on Shabbos Chanukah, when the wine is elevated due to Shabbos, the *seudah* is a mitzvah also in regard to Chanukah and one must repeat *Birkas Hamazon* if he forgot *Al Hanissim*.

(*Shem Mishmuel, Mikeitz* 681)

Eating Olive Oil on Shabbos Chanukah

In many communities of chassidim, they would mix the onion and eggs with the olive oil used to light the Chanukah candles to show that they are lighting the candles with oil that is edible (as some rule is halachically required).

In his *She'eilos Uteshuvos*, the Maharsham quotes many different opinions and then rules that it is permissible to use oil that is not edible. However, he concludes by saying that for the mitzvah of Chanukah candles, it is appropriate for someone who has fear of Heaven to be stringent and purchase oil that is not questionable.

(*She'eilos Uteshuvos Maharsham*, part I, *siman* 39)

Eating olive oil on Shabbos Chanukah is especially appropriate, since oil has the power *"to make the face glow"* (*Tehillim* 104:15), so that no matter what spiritual or physical state a person may be in, sadness will not show on his face. This is the power of oil, which is called *"chachmah"* (*Menachos* 85b), as we see in the *shemen mishchas hakodesh* (holy oil of anointment) (*Shemos* 30:25), and from the words, *the wise man— his concern is in his heart, and his glow is on his face* (*Chovos Halevavos*). We also know that a person must greet Shabbos with a shining, glowing face. Even if the week was filled with many worries, physical or spiritual, he must forget all his concerns and make sure that his face glows so that he welcomes the Shabbos properly. He must greet it with joy, like a wise son greeting his father, who makes sure that his face will not display any concern or sadness, even if his father is aware of his concerns, so as not to cause him any pain. As a result, his father's heart is filled with love for him. This is what the *pasuk* means with the words: *And Yisrael loved*

Yosef more than all his sons, for he was a ben zekunim *for him* (Bereishis 37:3). Targum Onkelos translates the words *"ben zekunim"* as *bar chakim hu leih*—"he is a wise son for him." In other words, Yosef had the *chachmah* of putting a glow on his face. *(Shevet Mi'Yehduah)*

To explain the reason that we use olive oil on Chanukah, the Gemara *(Horiyus* 13b) states: *Rabbi Yochanan said: Just as oil causes one to forget seventy years' worth of study, olive oil restores seventy years' worth of study.* Since the *Yevanim* tried to make Bnei Yisrael forget the Torah, we eat olive oil, which restores Torah study. *(Rabbi Dovid Meisels)*

During the morning *seudah* on Shabbos Chanukah, the Sanzer Rav would eat garlic dipped into the same olive oil he used to light the Chanukah candles.

The reason for this is probably that the Rav wanted to eat from the olive oil used to light the Chanukah candles. In order to make it a special food, he chose to add garlic, because garlic is good for a person's health, as taught by *Chazal (Bava Kamma* 82a). *(Magen Avos,* p. 424)

Another reason for this is to demonstrate the importance and preciousness that we attribute to the olive oil used to light the Chanukah candles, by using it as another food for our *oneg* on Shabbos. (Ibid.)

During the Shabbos morning *seudah*, after eating the eggs with the onions, garlic is eaten as well, cut into small pieces and mixed with the olive oil used to light the menorah. It is sprinkled three times with salt and once with pepper, and eaten with a slice of challah.

The eggs with onions are eaten before the garlic, based on *Chazal's* teaching *(Zevachim* 89a) that what is frequent takes precedence over something which is not.

(Yemei HaChanukah, p. 128)

An additional explanation for eating olive oil mixed with garlic is that oil symbolizes *chachmah*, wisdom, as the Bnei Yissaschar says (*Ma'amarei Chadshei Kislev*, Teves, essay 2): The words *lerei'ach shemanecha tovim*—"your oils have a good scent" (*Shir Hashirim* 1:3) are an acronym for the numerical equivalent of the words "*ner Chanukah*." Furthermore, Chazal say that *choshech* (darkness) refers to Yavan, who wanted to strengthen external wisdoms and destroy the true wisdom, Torah wisdom (section 12). That is why Yavan's rule is called *choshech* (*Koheles* 2:14), while *chachmah* is called light (ibid. 8:1).

Hashem made the miracle of Chanukah come about with the Menorah, which is on the southern side of the Beis Hamikdash, symbolizing *chachmah*, as it says, *One who wishes to become wise should turn southward* (*Bava Basra* 25b). This is because light is *chachmah,* and the south is always lit up, even during the shorter days. The power of Yavan is on the northern side, which is always dark, even during the longer days, symbolizing that their wisdom is really darkness. Hakadosh Baruch Hu performed the Chanukah miracle specifically with oil, which alludes to *chachmah*. Wherever there is olive oil, there is *chachmah*, as *Chazal* (*Menachos* 85b) explain the *pasuk* in *Shmuel II* (14:2): *And Yoav sent a wise woman [specifically] to Tekoa.* "Tekoa" alludes to oil (since it was a place with a large quantity of oil).

In the above *pasuk*, *lerei'ach shemanecha tovim*, the last letters of the words comprise the word "*chacham*," the middle letters share the same numerical equivalent as "*choshech*," and the first letters are numerically equivalent to "*ner Chanukah*."

Garlic alludes to *emunah* without understanding the reasons. The numerical equivalent of the word "*shum*" (garlic) is the same as that of the word "*ratzon*." "*Ratzon*" means doing something without reason, without understanding, as we know the wise teaching that "there is no reason in *ratzon.*" Even after a person merits reaching high levels of understanding through *chachmah*, he still must observe the mitzvos through *emunah*—which is greater than *chachmah*.

(*Likutei Imrei Kodesh, Chanukah*)

Another reason for eating garlic with olive oil is because oil alludes to *chachmah* (wisdom), while garlic alludes to *ratzon* (desire). The Targum Yonasan translates *Bereishis bara Elokim* as "With wisdom, Hashem created..." In another place, the *pasuk* states: *Hashem b'chachmah yasad aretz*, "Hashem founded the earth with wisdom" (*Mishlei* 3:19).

Quoting *Chazal's* words, which explain the word "*Bereishis*" as "for the Torah, which is called '*reishis*,'" Rashi explains this *pasuk* to mean the same; "With wisdom," means with the Torah. Thus, *reishis* is wisdom, which is the Torah, the foundation into which Hashem looked to create the world. Hashem's **ratzon** (desire) is *reishis* (the Torah), forever. This is the *chachmah* through which the world was created, and that is what the word *bereishis* means, with *chachmah*.

In the same place (*Bereishis* 1:1), Rashi also explains why the Torah begins with "*Bereishis*." It is written in *Tehillim* (111:7), *The strength of His deeds He declared to His people, to give them the heritage of the nations*. If the nations of the world will come to Bnei Yisrael and claim that they robbed the lands of the seven nations, Bnei Yisrael will be able to tell them, "The entire world belongs to Hashem; He is the One Who created it, and He can decide to give any part of it to whomever He wishes. With His will, He gave it to [the seven nations], and with His will, He took it from them and gave it to us." In fact, it is all part of the same *ratzon*. From the time when Hashem gave Eretz Yisrael to Canaan, it was the beginning of the process of the land being given to Klal Yisrael, since Klal Yisrael was to receive the land through war. When they received it, it was called Eretz Cana'an. That is why the Torah always refers to it with that name. Klal Yisrael are the ones who make it into Eretz Yisrael. Externally, however, it seems as though these are two separate desires.

Therefore, we eat garlic mixed with olive oil to allude to the fact that there is no "change of desire," it is all part of the same *ratzon Hashem*. Hashem's desire in creating the world was solely for the sake of the Torah. Eretz Yisrael, too, was given to us only on the condition that we will use it to observe the Torah and its mitzvos, as the *pasuk* in *Tehillim* (105:44) says: *And He gave them the lands of nations, and they inherited the toil of regimes.* It is in the merit of our observance of the Torah and mitzvos that we deserved the miracle of Chanukah.

(*Rabbi Dovid Meisels*)

Extra Kugels

Every Shabbos, three types of kugel would be served; one made of potatoes, and two other kugel*s*, including one sweet one. On a Shabbos in which two *sifrei Torah* would be taken out in *shul*, such as a Shabbos Rosh Chodesh, a fourth kugel would be served. And on Shabbos Chanukah which was also Rosh Chodesh, when three *sifrei Torah* would be taken out, yet another kugel would be served, totaling five kugel*s*.

(*Minhagei Komarno* 235)

During the morning *seudah* on Shabbos Chanukah, another kugel made of fresh potatoes was served in honor of Chanukah. When Rosh Chodesh Teves would come out on Shabbos, yet another kugel would be served, this one made of cooked potatoes. (*Zemiros Divrei Yoel, Shabbos Chanukah*)

There are some who add another kugel in honor of Shabbos Chanukah, and if it is also Rosh Chodesh Teves, they add another kugel in honor of Rosh Chodesh.(*Halichos Tzaddik*, p. 97)

Chapter 26
Shabbos Shirah and Tu B'Shevat

Shabbos Shirah

While eating the fish on Shabbos Shirah, it is fitting for one to recite the Gemara in *Pesachim* 118b, which begins with the words: *Reb Nassan omeir v'emes Hashem l'olam* until the words ...*b'osah sha'ah paschu dagim shel yam v'amru v'emes Hashem l'olam*. *(Davar B'ito)*

At *Krias Yam Suf*, Hashem removed the wheels of the Egyptians' chariots. The Toldos Yitzchak writes that Hashem removed only one wheel from each chariot, which caused the wagons to wobble. This shaking of the wagons caused the Egyptians to break their bones.

Accordingly, there are those who eat a round dish, alluding to the wheels. This dish is eaten warm and is also referred to as *chamin*, to allude to the hot water of the Yam Suf which punished the Egyptians, and to the fact that Hashem heated the seabed of the Yam Suf when the Egyptians passed through it, causing the horses' horseshoes to fall off, and agitating the horses, inflicting greater pain to the Egyptians.

The word *Beshalach* is an acronym for *B'Shabbos Shirah le'echol chamin*, on Shabbos Shirah one should eat *chamin*, which refers to this dish. *(Zecher Dovid)*

An allusion to eating *kneidlach* on Shabbos Shirah is found in a *pasuk* in *Tehillim* (33:7) regarding *Shiras Hayam*: *Kones kaneid mei hayam*—"Hashem gathered the water of the sea as a mound." The word *"kaneid"* is similar to *kneidel*.

The Kedushas Tzion of Bobov, in the name of the Zera Kodesh, explains that *kones kaneid* symbolizes gathering together many small parts into one whole, as Rashi states that *neid* in this case means, "like a pile." To allude to this we make *kneidlach,* which consist of many small crumbs which come together. This idea also alludes to unity among Klal Yisrael.

The Kedushas Tzion adds that *kneidlach* also signify unity because they are round, and a circle has no beginning or end (see *Bnei Yissaschar, Av, ma'amar* 4). Indeed, at the End of Days there will be a dance for *tzaddikim,* which symbolizes unity, since a circle dance has no beginning or end.

(Haggadah Beis Tzaddikim Bobov)

The *minhag* is to add an additional kugel in honor of Shabbos Shirah. <div align="right">(<i>Rabbi Dovid Meisels</i>)</div>

Eating Wheat

There are those who eat whole cooked wheat kernels on Shabbos Shirah. One should be careful to eat them only during a *seudah* [because it is not clear which *brachah acharonah* should be recited over them]. <div align="right">(<i>Bach, Orach Chaim</i> 208)</div>

The Chasam Sofer was accustomed to eating wheat kernels on Shabbos Shirah, in remembrance of the *mann,* which is discussed in *Parshas Beshalach.* (Wheat symbolizes a person's sustenance, and the *mann* provided the Jews with sustenance in the desert.)

The *minhag* in Mattersdorf was to eat a special cooked dish consisting of wheat in honor of Shabbos Shirah.

The word *Beshalach* is an acronym for **B'Shabbos Shirah** *le'echol chitim*—on Shabbos Shirah one should eat wheat.

(Olelos Ephraim, vol. 3, p. 11, ma'amar 377)

The Gemara in *Kesubos* states that we can gain knowledge of different remedies from the words of *Chazal. Chazal* state that one is forbidden to put chewed up wheat on a wound on Shabbos because it is used as a remedy. This teaches us that wheat contains healing properties.

In *Parshas Beshalach* we read the *pasuk, Ani Hashem rofecha*—"I, Hashem, am your healer" (*Shemos* 15:26). Therefore, on this Shabbos we eat wheat, which is associated with healing and reminds us that the words of *Chazal* encompass many different areas of knowledge, including science of medicine.
(*She'eilos Uteshuvos Siach Yitzchak, Orach Chaim* 294)

Throwing Food to the Birds

Since the birds sang praises to Hashem at the Yam Suf, we feed them food on Shabbos Shirah. (*Tosafos Shabbos* 324:17)

There are those who take off a portion of the cooked wheat that was prepared in honor of Shabbos Shirah and feed it to the birds on Shabbos itself. This practice is not correct because one is only allowed to feed animals on Shabbos if they are his responsibility. Since birds are wild, one is not permitted to feed them. (*Magen Avraham, Orach Chaim* 324:7; *Likutei Maharich*)

The Magen Avraham disapproves of throwing food to the birds on Shabbos. However, some authorities are of the opinion that it could be done, since the main reason for not feeding animals on Shabbos is that one is not allowed to exert himself on Shabbos for the sake of the animals. In this case, we are not doing it specifically to feed the animals but for our own sake, so that we should remember the *shirah* that was sung at the Yam Suf. Therefore, feeding the birds on Shabbos Shirah is permitted. (*Aruch Hashulchan* 324:3, *Tosafos Shabbos* ibid.:17)

The main reason for not feeding animals on Shabbos is because of the prohibition of *torach* on Shabbos, so that one should not exert himself on behalf of the animals. However, if one has in mind to perform a mitzvah, the exertion is not for the animals but for himself. (*Da'as Torah* 324:11; *Minchas Shabbos*)

Since one is not actually feeding the birds but only placing the food on the window, and the birds only eat it at a later time, it is not considered as if he is feeding the birds. Therefore, it is permissible to do so on Shabbos. (*Mekor Chaim* 324:11)

Since the birds are only being fed the remains of food that would otherwise be discarded, it is permissible to give it to the birds. If the person is taking the food off his table to discard it anyway, he is not exerting himself more by giving the food to the birds than by discarding it in a different place.

(*Eishel Avraham*)

Birds are associated with *shirah*, song. Music and song can only be produced using air. A person uses air to sing and instruments need air to produce music. Birds also have a connection to song because they fly in the air. (Similarly, *Az Yashir* is written with "air" between the words, i.e. larger spaces than usual. The entire Torah, which is called *shirah*, also has air, more space than usual, between each *parshah*.) Since Shabbos Shirah has a connection to birds, we give them food on this Shabbos.

(*Imrei Pinchas L'Shabbos Shirah*, sec. 223, 224)

The reason we throw bread to the birds on Shabbos Shirah can be explained with a parable. There was a king who had a large palace in which he had his own special wing. No one was allowed into the king's private quarters besides a bird who sang for him. The bird enchanted the king with its sweet chirping and singing. All the musical instruments could not compare to the beautiful song produced by this small creature.

Knesses Yisrael is compared to a bird, as the *pasuk* in *Tehillim* (84:4) states, *Even a bird found a house,* referring to Bnei Yisrael. During *Yetzias Mitzrayim* and *Krias Yam Suf,* all the angels sang *shirah* before Hashem, but Hashem had the most pleasure from the *shirah* of the Jews, who are compared to the king's special bird. Therefore, we feed the birds on Shabbos Shirah to remind us how beloved we are to Hashem.

(*Ner Yisrael*)

The Ruzhiner Rebbe explained that the reason for giving kasha to the birds is so that they should take the *dina kashya*, the strict justice, and we should remain with the favorable judgment.

(*Tiferes Yisrael*)

In *Parshas Beshalach* we find that we are instructed to store a small flask of *mann* for future generations. The reason for this is so that future generations will know that if one has true trust in Hashem, Hashem will provide for him just as He provided for the Jews in the *midbar*.

Today, we no longer have this flask of *mann* and this commemoration. Instead, we throw bread to the birds on Shabbos Shirah, when we read about the *mann*. By doing so, we demonstrate that Bnei Yisrael should trust in Hashem and not invest so much time earning a livelihood. They will then have more time to occupy themselves with Torah and mitzvos, and Hashem will provide their sustenance without toil and difficulty, just as the birds receive the bread being thrown to them on this Shabbos, without having to search for it.

(*Ohr Pnei Moshe*; *Ta'amei Haminhagim, Likutim*, sec. 97)

Another reason for throwing bread to the birds is repeated in the name of Reb Meir of Premishlan. The *pasuk* states that Moshe Rabbeinu instructed the nation that on Shabbos there would be no *mann* and they should not go out to gather it on Shabbos. The *pasuk* then states that some people went out on Shabbos to gather *mann* and they did not find any. Why does the *pasuk* uses the word *find*, which is generally used when something is lost, and not simply state *and there was nothing there*?

The answer is that Dasan and Aviram wanted to disprove the words of Moshe Rabbeinu, so they took the remaining *mann* (of the double portion received on Friday which was intended for Shabbos day) and spread it out on the ground so that it would appear to have fallen on Friday night. The birds came and ate it before dawn, so when Dasan and Aviram wanted to show the nation that the *mann* fell, "*they did not find it.*" Therefore, on Shabbos *Parshas Beshalach*, when we read *Parshas Hamann,* we throw some of the Shabbos food to the birds, in remembrance of this miracle. (*Marganita D'Rabbi Meir*; *Nimukei Orach Chaim* 324, p. 76)

The *Zohar* states that our actions in This World have an effect in Heaven. On Shabbos Shirah, we throw wheat to the birds because by feeding birds that are not our responsibility, we invoke mercy on High. Accordingly, although we are not worthy of being sustained, Hashem, in His tremendous compassion and kindness, gives us livelihood.
(*Yismach Yisrael, Beshalach*, s.v *Ub'devareinu*)

The Ba'al HaTanya related that on Shabbos Shirah, the Maharal of Prague would gather all the children in the courtyard of the *beis midrash*. The Maharal would announce that it was Shabbos Shirah and instruct the teachers to relate the story of *Krias Yam Suf* to the children, how the birds sang and danced as Moshe Rabbeinu and the entire Klal Yisrael sang *Az Yashir,* and the little children picked fruits from the trees that had miraculously sprouted at sea and fed the birds.

The Maharal instructed that the children be given kasha to distribute to the birds and chickens as a remembrance of the children feeding fruit to the birds. He would then bless the children and their parents that they merit raising their children to be occupied with Torah and good deeds, and marrying them off at the right time. (*Sichos Tzemach Tzedek*, p. 95)

Shabbos Tu B'Shevat

Since people eat fruit every Shabbos, when Tu B'Shevat occurs on Shabbos it may not be noticeable that the fruit is being eaten specifically in honor of Tu B'Shevat. One may think that he is required to eat fruits on Motza'ei Shabbos as well, as is mentioned in the *Magen Avraham* (419) regarding Rosh Chodesh which falls on Shabbos. However, the two are not comparable since the *Shulchan Aruch* states that it is a mitzvah to eat a *seudah* on Rosh Chodesh (see *Sha'ar Hatzion* 419:1). Eating fruits on Tu B'Shevat does not carry the same stringency, since it not mentioned in the *Shulchan Aruch*. Therefore, in practice, eating fruits on Shabbos is sufficient. Additionally, if one eats more fruits on Tu B'Shevat than on any other Shabbos, it will be noticeable that it is in honor of Tu B'Shevat. (*She'eilos Uteshuvos Be'er Sarim*, vol. 3, sec. 75)

When Tu B'Shevat occurs on Shabbos, one might think that one should eat the fruits at the day *seudah*, since the honor of the day *seudah* takes precedence over the honor of the night *seudah*. However, the fruits are not being eaten in honor of Shabbos, but rather in honor of Tu B'Shevat, and can be eaten at either *seudah*.

(*Shevet Mi'Yehudah, Beshalach, Seudas Yom Shabbos* 5669)

Shabbos Aseres Hadibros

Reb Aharon of Belz once said that on Shabbos *Parshas Yisro*, one should add a kugel in honor of "*Shabbos Aseres Hadibros*." (*B'kedushaso Shel Aharon*, p. 459)

Chapter 27
Shabbasos in Adar

Shabbos Zachor

Many add a kugel in honor of *Parshas Zachor*.

(*Temidim K'sidram*)

Some are accustomed to eating a special kugel on Shabbos Zachor which they call *Mechiyas Amalek* kugel. The word *Amalek* is an acronym for *epel* (apple), *mehl* (flour) *lokshen* (noodles), and *kartafel* (potato) and this has all four or those ingredients.

There are those who bake four kugels for Shabbos Zachor, because on this Shabbos we are obligated by the Torah to erase Amalek. Amalek did not bring doubts into the hearts of Jews regarding *halachos* which are clearly spelled out; they began with *minhagim*. Therefore, we eat several kugels to strengthen our *minhagim* and erase Amalek.

(*Kuntris Imros Noam*)

Shabbos Erev Purim

The *minhag* of the Chasam Sofer when Purim fell on Sunday was that on the Shabbos before Purim, he *davened* Minchah immediately after the morning *seudah*. He ate *shalosh seudos* before the tenth hour of the day.

(Intro. to *Sifsei Chachamim, Megillah*, 9:22)

Seudas Purim on Erev Shabbos

When Purim falls on Erev Shabbos, if one eats the main *seudah* of the day after *chatzos*, it is a lack of honor to *seudas*

Shabbos, which is *d'Oraisa.* Therefore, it seems that one should eat the *seudah* in the morning, before *chatzos.*

(*Yosef Ometz*)

The Rema states that if Purim falls on Friday, one should eat the Purim *seudah* in the morning. The Yad Ephraim explains that this refers to eating it before the tenth hour of the day. The *Mishnah Berurah* states that some authorities are of the opinion that this means that ideally one should eat the *seudah* before *chatzos.* One should not eat the *seudah* after the time of Minchah, so as not to spoil his appetite for the Shabbos *seudah.*

(*Sefer Haminhagim*)

One should begin the Purim *seudah* on Erev Shabbos before the tenth hour of the day. It is mentioned in one of the *Rishonim* that if one will not finish before the tenth hour, he is still permitted to eat, as long as he began eating earlier.

(*She'eilos Uteshuvos Maharil,* sec. 56)

If one did not eat the Purim *seudah* before the tenth hour of the day he can eat the Purim *seudah* afterward, even if he will no longer have an appetite for the Friday night *seudah* and will not be able to eat it. (See *Shulchan Aruch Harav* 249:6 that if one is at a *seudas mitzvah* on Friday, he is permitted to eat even if he might not be able to eat the Shabbos *seudah* later. This is because one can fulfill a current obligation and does not need to take into account the *seudah* that he needs to eat later. If necessary, he may fulfill the obligation of eating three *seudos* during Shabbos day.)

One may eat the Purim *seudah,* even if he might not be able to eat the Friday night *seudah,* since the Taz (693:2) states that *seudas Purim* fulfills an obligation placed upon us by our *nevi'im* and *chachamim* to feast and rejoice, and is therefore more significant than Shabbasos and Yamim Tovim.

(See *Shulchan Aruch Harav* 249:6)

Some authorities are of the opinion that when Purim in Yerushalayim is a *Purim meshulash* (Purim that is spread over Friday, Shabbos, and Sunday), one should also eat a small meal on Friday (which is the day that the *Megillah* is read). However, one should be careful not to eat too late in the day, so that he has an appetite for the Shabbos *seudah*.

(*Seder Purim Meshulash Al Pi Shitas HaMeiri*, pp. 2b, 5b)

The Shevet Mi'Yehudah is of the opinion that one should eat the Purim *seudah* on Erev Shabbos after the time of Minchah, because that was the time that the sin of the *Eitz Hada'as* was performed and eating the Purim *seudah* rectifies this sin.

(See *Shevet M'Yehudah*)

Reb Mordechai Dov of Hornesteipel, the son-in-law of the Sanzer Rav, once drank a large amount of wine on Purim that fell on Erev Shabbos. When it was almost candle lighting time, he exclaimed that he needed to hurry to greet the Shabbos. He continued by saying, "*Chazal* state that, '[The effect of] A strong wine can be removed by fear' and the *sefarim* state that a person should fear the holiness of Shabbos."

Indeed, it was not possible to tell that he had drunk a large amount of wine. (*Tehillos Chaim*)

Shabbos of Purim Hameshulash

Purim Hameshulash occurs in Yerushalayim when the 15th of Adar is on Shabbos. On Friday, the *megillah* is read and *matanos l'evyonim* distributed. On Shabbos, *Al Hanisim* is recited and the *parshah* of *Vayavo Amalek* is read. On Sunday, the *seudah* is eaten and *mishloach manos* are given. Some authorities are of the opinion that on *Purim Hameshulash*, one should eat a Purim *seudah* on Shabbos as well.

(*Pri Chadash* 688:6; *Sefer Chug Ha'aretz*, sec.6)

There are those who say that in order to fulfill all opinions, one should cook a special dish for Shabbos of a *Purim Meshulash* and drink several cups of wine. (*Kaf Hachaim* 688:45)

The Kaf Hachaim states, in the name of the *Sefer Tikkun Yissaschar,* that one should make an additional *seudah* on Shabbos in honor of Purim. If he was unable to do so, he should eat a special dish during *shalosh seudos* in honor of *seudas Purim.* (Ibid.:46)

The Magen Avraham cites the Maharalbach that the Purim *seudah* should not be eaten on Sunday, but on Shabbos. The Pri Chadash states that one should eat *seudos* on Shabbos and Sunday. (See *Sha'ar Hatziyun* 688:30)

The Chug Ha'aretz would eat a more lavish *seudah* on the Shabbos of *Purim Meshulash* than any other Shabbos of the year. Prior to eating he would say, "If Shabbos is the proper time to fulfill the mitzvah of *seudas Purim,* then this *seudah* should be eaten in the honor of Purim as well." When eating the Purim *seudah* on Sunday, he would say, "If the proper time to fulfill the mitzvah of *seudas Purim* is today, then I am fulfilling this mitzvah now."

The Birkei Yosef agrees with the abovementioned practice of the Chug Ha'aretz. He writes that although, according to halachah, the Purim *seudah* should be eaten on Sunday, one who eats a *seudah* on Shabbos as well should be blessed.

(*Chug Ha'aretz,* sec. 6)

It is a mitzvah to eat additional dishes and to drink wine on Shabbos of *Purim Hameshulash* to fulfill the mitzvah of *seudas Purim.* It is also a mitzvah to send a small amount of *mishloach manos* in an area where one is permitted to carry.

(*Purim Hameshulash of Reb Yosef Chaim Sonnenfeld*)

The Knesses Hagedolah cites the Ralbach that *seudas Purim* should be eaten on Shabbos of *Purim Hameshulash.* Additionally, *mishloach manos* should be sent on Shabbos, since they are part of the *seudah.*

(See *Radvaz,* vol. 5, sec. 2105; vol., 1 sec. 508)

The Radvaz cites the Bartenura who writes that *seudas Purim* and *mishloach manos* are fulfilled on Sunday. Since the Bartenura resided in Yerushalayim, it can be assumed that he was familiar with the *minhag* there.

The Ralbach, of the great rabbis of Yerushalayim, held that the *seudah* should be eaten on Shabbos, and since he was the *rav* of the city it would seem that it would obligate all of Yerushalayim to follow his ruling. However, since the *Talmud Yerushalmi*, which was definitely written in Yerushalayim, states that it should be eaten on Sunday, the ruling of the Ralbach is not binding. (*Radvaz*, ibid.)

If Purim falls on Shabbos, one who eats a *seudah* late at night is technically eating *melaveh malkah* as he does every other week, and it is not considered to be *seudas Purim*.

(*Temidim K'sidram*)

Parshas Parah

There is a *minhag* to add a kugel in honor of *Shabbos Parah*. (*Temidim K'sidram*, p. 146)

Shabbos Hachodesh

The custom is to add another kugel in honor of *Shabbos Hachodesh*; some add a third kugel when *Shabbos Mevarchim* occurs on *Shabbos Hachodesh*.

Chapter 28
Shabbos Hagadol, Pesach, and the Shabbos after Pesach

Shabbos Hagadol

It is interesting that specifically on Shabbos Hagadol, which is greater than other Shabbasos of the year, people crowd into the corners of their homes to eat their meals, minimize their Shabbos menu, and wear worn-out clothing. It would seem that it would be fitting to honor and delight in this particular Shabbos with finer clothing and delicacies, according to one's means.

Conversely, since the great light of the *Geulah* can be drawn from this holy Shabbos, it is fitting that we demonstrate that all physical matters and human desires are futile and pale in comparison to the spiritual light that can be derived from this particular Shabbos. *(Ohel Moed, Lelov)*

It is customary that every *rav* lectures on Shabbos Hagadol before *Mussaf*, and that a Kiddush with the *rav* follows *davening*. Sweets and treats are prepared and provided by the congregation. *(Kisvei Ri Shov, pg. 130)*

Challos for Shabbos Hagadol

Some had the *minhag* to bake bread on Erev Shabbos Hagadol. They called these loaves *Challas Ani* and *Lechem Beis Haknesses* and would distribute them to the poor.

One reason for this *minhag* was because they baked this bread from flour which was ground for the matzos for Pesach. This is according to the words of the Maharshal, that one should set aside some flour from the flour that will be used for baking matzos for Pesach. In this way, if there is a question that a portion of that flour might have been *chametz,* one can assume that the questionable portion of the flour was is those challos which were eaten before Pesach, and can consider the problem resolved. (*Mateh Moshe, Se'if Katan* 543)

This *minhag* is also in remembrance of the covenant that Bnei Yisrael made with one another during the exodus from Mitzrayim, that they will perform kindness with each other and help one another. Therefore, on the Shabbos before Pesach, the Yom Tov of *Yetzias Mitzrayim*, we bake challos to distribute to the poor. (*Zecher Dovid*, p. 137; *Yeshuos Yaakov*)

Three Types of Kugels

The *minhag* in Belz is to prepare three extra kugel*s* for Shabbos Hagadol, or the Shabbos preceding it, when Shabbos Hagadol falls out on Erev Pesach. One kugel is in honor of Shabbos Hagadol. The second kugel made from the flour used for baking matzos, based on the Maharshal (as brought by the *Magen Avraham*, sec. 430) quoted above, that one should eat some of the flour used for matzos before Yom Tov. The third kugel is made from challah reserved from that year's Simchas Torah meal. The Belzer Rebbe would customarily repeat on Motza'ei Simchas Torah that it is brought down in the siddur of the Arizal that there is a *yichud* (unification) that is drawn from Shemini Atzeres until Erev Pesach that is reinforced by the idea that if one utilizes his time during the winter days he can activate an inherent *kedushah* and thereby experience the holiness of the Yamim Tovim. (*Temidim K'sidram*, Nissan)

Purim Leftovers

On Shabbos Hagadol, it was customary to eat *mishloach manos* leftovers that were put away. *(Minhagei Beis Alik)*

Kindel (special traditional pastries) that are left over from Purim were eaten as dessert on Shabbos Hagadol or for the last *chametz* meal on Erev Pesach.

(Chodesh B'chadsho, Minhagei Mattersdorf)

Afikoman in the Cholent

There are various practices observed on *Leil Shimurim* (the first night of Pesach) to engender great *shemirah*, protection, for the entire year. It is for this reason that there is a widespread *minhag* to put aside a small piece of the *afikoman* from the first two nights of Pesach to carry in one's pocket all year long until the following Pesach. The author of the *Koach Yehudah*'s father was careful about guarding this piece, and on Shabbos Hagadol he would mix it into the cholent; it seems that this is an old custom. *(Koach Yehudah)*

Erev Pesach that Falls out on Shabbos

The *Sha'arei Teshuvah* cites the Ramaz who states that it is not necessary to prepare *yud-beis* (12) *challos* on Erev Pesach, since we do not eat three meals. However, the *Sha'arei Teshuvah* wonders about this. The *minhag* in Belz was to prepare 12 challos as usual.

(Sha'arei Teshuvah, in the name of the Ramaz)

Eggs

Some follow the *minhag* not to eat eggs during the Shabbos day meal, since the egg is used on the Seder plate on Pesach night to commemorate the *Korban Chagigah*. Others maintain that one may eat eggs on Shabbos morning, since it is unlike eating lettuce or horseradish (which is used for *maror* and is therefore more stringent) on Erev Pesach. One should follow his own *minhag* regarding this matter.

(Ben Ish Chai, Parshas Tzav, sec. 3)

Shalosh Seudos

Since the time for *shalosh seudos* is after Minchah, and one cannot eat matzah or *chametz* at that time, it is best to eat a meal of fruit.
(Tur, sec. 444)

Some follow the custom to fulfill the obligation for a third meal with fruit or meat and fish, since our custom is not to eat *matzah ashirah* (matzah made with juices or eggs) on Erev Pesach.
(Rema 444: 1, 462:4)

Some follow the *minhag* to eat the Shabbos day meal after Shacharis as usual, and conclude before the time at which one may no longer eat *chametz*. Others divide the morning meal into two. They wash their hands for bread and eat two courses, the fish and eggs and onions, and then recite *Birkas Hamazon*. They then wait a while in order to avoid a *brachah she'einah tzrichah* (an unnecessary *brachah*), and then wash their hands for bread again and continue the meal. Some maintain that one can thus fulfill his obligation for the third meal.
(Magen Avraham, sec. 444:1; Chok Yaakov, ibid. 2)

Some never divide the morning meal. *(Mishnah Berurah, sec. 117)*

The Sanzer Rebbe would divide his meal into two, while the rest of the congregation did not. The Rebbe maintained that it was sufficient for him to divide his meal and the others could fulfill their obligation through him.
(Darchei Chaim, Minhagei Sanz, sec. 98)

One should be careful not to eat a lot during the third meal, so that he should have an appetite for the matzah at the Seder.
(Mishnah Berurah 444:8)

It is preferable to eat fruits of the *shivas haminim* (seven species) for *shalosh seudos*, because one is then required to recite the *brachah mei'ein shalosh* (*Al Ha'eitz*) after eating.
(Chag Hamatzos 15:34)

The Magen Avraham writes that meat and fish are preferred over fruit for the third meal on Shabbos Hagadol. The Chok Yaakov (sec. 102) disagrees, and contends that it is preferable to eat fruit, which is not as filling, so that one can eat the matzah with the proper appetite. Additionally, meat and fish are generally eaten with bread, so there is a concern that one may forget and eat it with matzah.

(*Magen Avraham* 444: 2; *Chok Yaakov* ibid.)

The *Shulchan Aruch Harav* (ibid. 3) writes that one should eat meat and fish or other side dishes, since some maintain that one can fulfill the obligation of *shalosh seudos* in this manner on any Shabbos. If he does not have these foods, he may fulfill his obligation with fruit, etc.

The Kaf Hachaim writes that one should eat a *kezayis* of cooked food if he can (as he was told by the *maggid* of Maran, the *malach* that learned with the Beis Yosef). (*Kaf Hachaim*, ibid. 12)

One may choose to eat either meat, fish, or fruit for the third meal, since some authorities rule that one does not fulfill his obligation of *shalosh seudos* by eating any of these foods, therefore they are equally suitable. (*Yosef Ometz*, sec. 670)

Some maintain that one should fulfill the obligation for the third meal with *divrei Torah*, as the *Zohar* relates that Rebbe Shimon bar Yochai would immerse himself in the words of Torah instead of *shalosh seudos*.

(*Magen Avraham* 444:2, in the name of the Shelah)

The *Zohar* on *Parshas Emor* (95) writes that although we generally do not omit *shalosh seudos* when Yom Tov falls on Motza'ei Shabbos out of concern that it is close to Yom Tov and one should have an appetite for the *seudah,* there are a number of reasons for skipping *shalosh seudos* on Erev Pesach. First of all, one must eat the matzah and *maror* at the Seder with proper appetite. Also, since one may not eat bread or matzah then, it may not be considered a meal in any case.

The Ikrei Hadas (*Ohr Hachaim* 17: 33, in the name of the *Eshdas Hapisgah*) therefore writes that a G-d-fearing individual will follow the reasoning of the Shelah in the name of the *Zohar*, who writes that Rebbe Shimon bar Yochai would involve himself in *divrei Torah* instead of eating a meal.

The Kaf Hachaim writes that Rabi Shimon bar Yochai was as familiar with the pathways in Heaven as he was with the pathways on earth, and he knew the specific Torah learning needed in order to engender a *tikkun* in place of a meal. For us, however, it is necessary to eat a meal. It is certainly preferable to have both food and *divrei Torah*.   (*Kaf Hachaim* 444:18)

Shabbos Chol Hamoed Pesach

Some follow the *minhag* to recite *Hamotzi* over a matzah and a half to commemorate the *lechem oni* (bread of affliction) on all the seven days of Pesach (including the meals on the first days and *Shevi'i shel Pesach*, Shabbos Chol Hamoed, and Chol Hamoed). This is based on the teachings of *Chazal* that a poor man eats a broken piece, and also refers to the *pasuk*, *Shivas yamim tochal matzos alav lechem oni*—"For seven days you shall eat matzos because of it, bread of affliction" (*Devarim* 16:3). *Lechem oni* refers to one and half matzos and not *lechem mishnah*—two whole matzos.

(*Minhag Teiman, Haggadah Pri Eitz Chaim*, pg. 354)

Galaretta

Galaretta, a dish made from chicken or beef feet that is generally eaten during the Shabbos day meal, is not served on Pesach if it is cooked from chicken feet, since the feet of the chicken step on the ground and there is a concern of *chametz*. If, however, the dish is cooked from beef feet, then it may be eaten on Pesach because the external parts of the feet are not used.   (*Magen Avos*, pg. 408)

Kugel for Shabbos Chol Hamoed

The *minhag* is to eat an additional kugel made from *charoses* and *maror*, in order to draw the power of the Seder into Shabbos. Additionally, by using bitter herbs to prepare a Shabbos dish, we turn bitter into sweet and, "sweeten the judgment" on this day of *rachamim* (compassion).

(Haggadah Beis Tzaddikim, pg. 210)

In Belz, onion kugel is prepared for Shabbos Chol Hamoed Pesach. Rebbe Aharon of Belz said that there is a side benefit to this custom, because it is known from the Ba'al Shem Tov that eating cooked onions is a great *segulah* for *refuah,* but it is difficult to simply eat cooked onions in a soup. When they are in a kugel they are easier to eat. (*Ohr Hatzafon*, vol. 24)

Shabbos "Gella" (Yellow) Matzos

On the Shabbos after Pesach, the *challos* should be round like matzos, symbolic of the matzos eaten on Pesach Sheini. Additionally, a key is inserted into them, alluding to the gates that remain open until Pesach Sheini. It is an error that people refer to it as *"Gella Matzos;"* it should be referred to as *"Geulah Matzos."* (*Imrei Pinchas, Shabbos Achar Pesach*, sec. 298)

Perhaps the reason for round challos is that Bnei Yisrael were obligated to bring a *Korban Todah* which included round challos when they were redeemed from Mitzrayim. Since one cannot bring a *Korban Todah* on Pesach because it contains *chametz,* they brought it after Pesach.

Additionally, it is to commemorate the *ugos,* pastries, that Bnei Yisrael took with them when they left Mitzrayim that tasted like *mann,* which resembled a white round seed.

The reason the challos are colored yellow is based on a midrash on *Shir Hashirim* (5:10), on the *pasuk, Dodi tzach v'edom*—"My beloved is white and reddish." The midrash explains, *tzach l'Yisrael, v'edom l'Mitzrayim*; white refers to the Jews and red to the Egyptians. Yellow is a combination of white and red, which symbolize *nagof* and *rafo,* based on the *pasuk* in *Yeshayah* (19:22). *Nagof* is punishment for the Mitzrim and *rafo* is salvation for Bnei Yisrael.

Perhaps the *minhag* to insert a key in the challah can be understood based on the commentary of Rebbe Yissachar Dov of Belz regarding the *ugos* that Bnei Yisrael took out of Mitzrayim, which are said to have tasted like *mann*. He asks, if the *mann* had not yet fallen, how could Bnei Yisrael know its taste? The Rebbe explained that the answer is derived from the *pasuk* in *Tehillim* (78:25) regarding the *mann, Lechem abirim achal ish*—"Man ate the bread of angels." The *mann* was the bread of angels. Bnei Yisrael were then on the level of angels and were able to discern the taste of *mann*.

The word *maftei'ach* (key) is derived from the word *pesach* (an opening), alluding to the idea that they tasted the *mann* "at the opening," i.e. even before it fell.

(*Haggadah Kol Yehudah*, pg. 32)

There is a *minhag* to bake round challos, which are similar to matzos, for the Shabbos after Pesach. Perhaps this is based on the Gemara (*Kiddushin* 38) that teaches that the matzos which Bnei Yisrael took out of Egypt lasted until the *mann* fell. Hence, we bake challah that is similar to matzah to commemorate the miracle that they had enough matzah to last after Pesach, as well.

Saffron (a spice derived from the crocus flower) is added to the dough (or, due to *kashrus* concerns with saffron, other spices are added) to color it reddish-yellow, and they are then called *"Gella* (yellow) *matzos."* Perhaps the saffron is added to the dough based on the commentary of the *Hagahos Minhagim,* that eating matzah after Pesach is a transgression of *bal tosif* (one may not add to the mitzvos of the Torah), similar to the concept of eating in the Sukkah on Shemini Atzeres (see *Rosh Hashanah* 28). One must therefore avoid eating bread that resembles matzah because of *maris ayin* (an act that can be interpreted as a transgression). In order to differentiate between the matzah and the round challah, one should add saffron to the dough because matzah for Pesach is never baked with spices (*Magen Avraham*, end of sec. 455). We thereby avoid the issue of *maris ayin* and still have special *challah* to commemorate the miracle of matzah after Pesach. (*Divrei Ya'ir, Chiddushei Chag HaPesach*, pg. 23)

The name, *Shabbos Gella Matzos* can be explained with the idea that Shabbos is the root of all holiness and the conduit for revealing *kedushah*. Therefore, the Shabbos after Pesach is really called *"Giluy Matzos"*—revealing the matzos, because it is the day that the holiness that we achieved from eating the matzos on Pesach is revealed. (*Toras Emes, Shabbos Achar Pesach*)

The Kozhnitzer Maggid said that the Shabbos after Pesach, which people call *Shabbos Gella Matzos*, actually refers to *"Giluy Matzos"*—revealing the matzos.

Perhaps this can be explained with the principle that matzos symbolize *chachmah: Hein yiras Hashem hi chachmah*—"Behold, fear of Hashem is wisdom" (*Iyov* 28:28). This means that when one purifies his thoughts with holiness, his fear of Heaven spreads over the limbs of his body until it becomes clearly visible on his face. The word *"hein"* denotes that which is recognizable and clear (as in the expression *"eilu hein,"* which is used when enumerating a list). Given that every Jew achieves *yiras Hashem* on Shabbos, as it says in the *Yerushalmi* (*Demai* 4:1) that even an *am ha'aretz* senses a fear of Heaven on Shabbos, it follows that the *kedushah* achieved by eating matzah is also revealed on one's countenance on Shabbos. The light of Shabbos brings to the fore the added revelation of *yirah*, which resulted from eating matzah (and performing all the other mitzvos of Pesach).

Perhaps, the *minhag* of inserting a key into the challos for this Shabbos is because of the concept of "keys" representing *yirah*—fear of Heaven (*Shabbos* 31). (*Yismach Yisrael, Tazria*)

There are various *minhagim* for this Shabbos regarding the challah: to insert a key into the challah, to shape the challah like a matzah, to add saffron to the dough, which turns it a reddish color, and to call this Shabbos, *Shabbos Gella Matzos.*

The *din* on Shabbos is harsh, and one who "delights the Shabbos" softens the *din* for the entire week. As the Gemara says (*Shabbos* 118): *Kol hame'aneg es HaShabbos nosnin lo nachalah bli metzarim*—"One who delights in Shabbos is given an endless inheritance." The words, *bli metzarim* connote the concept of, *min hameitzar* (from the straits), but *oneg Shabbos* nullifies this harsh judgment of Shabbos.

Since the *middah* (of *sefiras ha'omer*) for the first week after Pesach is *gevurah*—strength, the *din* on this Shabbos is harsher than all year long. Therefore, we bake round challos that are shaded pink (Yitzchak, whose *middah* is *gevurah* is called, *somek* [reddish]) to engender compassion, and change the *gevurah shebegevurah* to kindness and mercy.

Additionally, the Shabbos before Pesach is called Shabbos Hagadol based on the reason from the Tur, that it was the 10th of Nissan, the day Bnei Yisrael tied the sheep to their beds. We remember the miracle on Shabbos Hagadol every year, even though it does not necessarily fall on the tenth of Nissan. Perhaps the same can be said regarding the Shabbos after Pesach. When Bnei Yisrael left Mitzrayim, the 24th of Nissan and the ninth day of the Sefirah, which is *gevurah shebegevurah*, fell on the first Shabbos after Pesach. We always remember this Shabbos as a day of especially harsh judgment, even when it doesn't fall on the 24th of Nissan. Consequently, based on the principle that an increase in *din* brings *rachamim*, we bake challos with saffron and insert a key to demonstrate that the increase in *din* is like a key that opens up the prison gates. (*Olas Moed*, pg. 9)

During the seven weeks of *sefiras ha'omer* one must work on perfecting his service of Hashem through the seven *middos* (attributes), until one attains the original lofty level of the night of Pesach. Moreover, the Gemara teaches that one who achieves Torah and does not have *yiras Shamayim* is compared to a treasurer who received keys for the inner door of the treasury and did not receive keys for the outer door (*Shabbos* 31). It is also explained that *ahavah* and *yirah* are called "keys."

On the Shabbos after Pesach, we have already gained the two *middos* of *ahavah* and *yirah*. This Shabbos, which always falls during the second week of Sefirah, corresponds to the *middah* of *gevurah* - *yiras Shamayim*, the *middah* of Yitzchak Avinu, while the first week corresponds to *chessed*, the *middah* of Avraham Avinu. We have therefore already acquired a combination of the power of right and the left, *chessed* and *gevurah*—an important component of our *avodas Hashem*.

The round challos shaped like matzah allude to this idea, because matzah symbolizes the "right side," the power of the *yetzer tov*, and *chametz* symbolizes the "left side," the *yetzer hara* (*Zohar* 1:4). Challos that are made of *chametz* and shaped like matzah combine the two powers. Additionally, the idea of coloring the challah yellow is symbolic of the combination of the color red which represents *gevurah*, and the color white, which represents *chessed*. Therefore, we call the Shabbos that falls during the second week of *sefiras ha'omer*, "Shabbos Gella Matzos," referring to the combination of both *middos*—*ahavah* and *yirah*. (*She'eiris L'Pinchas, Shabbos Achar Pesach*)

It is known that the commandment to guard against the smallest amount of *chametz* is alluded to in the Hebrew spelling of the words *chametz* and *matzah*. When comparing them, it appears that they have the same letters (*mem, tzaddi, ches* or *heh*), the only difference being a little part missing in the shape of the letter *heh*.

This is alluded to in the *pasuk, Es Chag hamatzos tishmor* —"You shall guard the festival of matzah" (*Shemos* 23:15). It is incumbent upon us to guard the letter *heh* in the word matzah so that the half-line from the letter doesn't move upward and turn it into the letter *ches*. In addition, there is a difference in the numerical value of the letters: the numerical value of the letter *ches* is three more than *heh*. The *pasuk* thus says *Es Chag hamatzos tishmor.* Guard the word "*Chag,*" the *ches* and *gimmel*, which refers to guarding the matzah, so that the *heh* shouldn't turn into a "longer line," and thus read as a *ches*, and that it doesn't catch up with the *gimmel*, the numerical value of the difference between *chametz* and *matzah*.

Accordingly, it can be said that the reason this Shabbos is called *Gella Matzos* is that *chametz* is already permitted at that time. Since we don't want to call it *"chametz,"* which alludes to the *sitra achra* (the side of impurity), we call it *Gella Matzos*, *gimmel al hamatzos*—referring to the extra value of *gimmel* (three) that is added to the matzah when we eat *chametz*, since there is an obligation to eat bread on Shabbos.

(*Tzvi Latzaddik, Ma'amarei Chodesh Nissan* 104)

The Rambam enumerated 20 mitzvos associated with Pesach. Twelve of them are related to the *Korban Pesach*, and the remaining eight are related to *chametz* and matzah. These eight mitzvos include three positive commandments and five negative commandments, because the mitzvah of *sippur Yetzias Mitzrayim* is included in the mitzvah of matzah, as it says, *B'sha'ah sheyeish matzah u'maror...*—"[One should relate the story] at the time [the] matzah and *maror* [are before him]." Hence, the matzah is called, *lechem oni*—bread upon which we ask and answer many things, i.e. the matzah should be on the table while we tell the story of *Yetzias Mitzrayim*.

Furthermore, the Shabbos is called, *"Gella Matzos,"* and the Yiddish word *gehl* (yellow), spelled *gimmel, ayin, heh, lamed,* is an acronym for *gimmel essin, heh lavin*—three positive commandments and five negative commandments. This is also the reason for the *shlissel challah,* as alluded to in the word *maftei'ach* (key): *pas ches mitzvos*—there are eight mitzvos related to bread. *(Tzvi Latzaddik, Nissan)*

An additional reason for the *shlissel challah* can be based on the *pasuk* that Bnei Yisrael left with the dough, *"on their shoulders"* (Shemos 12:34). Rashi comments that it was the leftovers of the matzah and *maror* that they took with them in order to demonstrate that the inspiration from these mitzvos continues even after Yom Tov *(Sefer Vayageid Moshe).*

Therefore, we put a key in the challah, alluding to the idea that Pesach is the key to the entire year and we must remember to take with us the inspiration that we merited on Pesach. The *minhag* to call the Shabbos, *Gella Matzos* or *Geulah Matzos* suggests that we desire the continued influence of the *Geulah,* symbolized by matzah. *(Vayechi Yosef, Shemini)*

In the times of the Chiddushei Harim and Rebbe Bunim of Peshischa, the Shabbos after Pesach was called *Shabbos Gella Matzos*. Many reasons are given for this; the simple reason is that at the Shabbos meal they would smear the yellow eggs on the matzah (as opposed to on Pesach when *gebrokts* was not allowed).

Perhaps it can be suggested that the color yellow is a sign of impurity, as it is with regards to a *nesek* (a sign of *tzara'as*). The Torah teaches that if the affliction spread and was enlarged, *Lo yivaker hakohen lasei'ar hatzahov, tamei hu*—"the *kohen* should not even look for yellow hair, it is impure" (Vayikra 13:36). If, however, it turned white, it is a sign of purity, as the *pasuk* says, *Kulo hafach lavan, tahor hu*—"it is turned completely white, he is pure" (ibid. 13:13). It follows that the color white represents Pesach, which is pure and clean. *Gella matzos* are a reminder for us to be careful not to allow the spread of negativity, represented by the aspect of yellow and a sign of *tzara'as*. As we say in the *tefillah* after counting *sefiras ha'omer*: *May we be purified and sanctified with a Heavenly holiness*, in preparation for *Kabbalas HaTorah*.

(*Pnei Shabbos*, pg. 285)

Shlissel Challah

Shlissel challah is the *minhag* to insert a key in the challah, or form the shape of a key over the challah, for the Shabbos after Pesach.

Others follow the custom to sprinkle sesame seeds in the shape of a key, add a piece of dough in the shape of a key, or insert a key into the challah, making an indentation, to commemorate the *mann* and to remind us that Hashem provides us with the "keys" to livelihood. (*Kol Bo* 49:52)

The *minhag* in Belz was to prepare round challos colored yellow with saffron, and to make indentations in the dough with a key. Rebbe Aharon of Belz would say that one should place the key into fire before inserting it into the dough.

(*Leket Imrei Kodesh*, eighth edition, pg. 22)

Rav Moshe Aryeh Freund, the Yerushlayimer Rav, would puncture the dough with a key and then insert the key lengthwise so that an indentation in the shape of the key formed in the dough. He would then say, "May all the *kavanos* of the Oheiv Yisrael (the Apter Rav) take effect on these challos."

(*Zemiros Ateres Yeshuos*, pg. 22)

The *Mechilta* explains that a slave could not escape from Mitzrayim because it was closed off, and Bnei Yisrael were locked into the country. Suddenly, all 600,000 Jews were redeemed. Hence, the key symbolizes the concept that Hashem opened the "gates" of Mitzrayim and led us into the desert.

Rav Aharon of Belz suggests that the *minhag* to insert a key into the challos after Pesach is a demonstration of our fulfillment of the will of Hashem with the mitzvah of eating matzah. It is in these merits that Hashem will open his treasury in Heaven for us *(Beiso Na'avah Kodesh*, Nissan, vol. 2, pg. 665).

With this commentary, however, the question arises why we insert the key into challah which is *chametz* and denotes the opposite of redemption. The real question is then, why we should go back to eating *chametz* at all, after we've eaten matzah and nullified the *yetzer hara* and, moreover, why is *chametz* included in the *korbanos*?

This can be understood with the analogy of a king's son who fell ill and was ordered to refrain from eating various foods. When the son was distraught about not receiving the foods he desired, the doctor explained that this was only temporary. As soon as he would recover from his disease, his body would have the capacity to digest the foods again

Similarly, matzah is referred to as the "food of *refuah*." After the weeklong ingestion of matzah, we are spiritually healed, and ready to eat and process *chametz* once again.

(Ohr Malei, Shabbos Achar Pesach)

Perhaps a simple reason for the *shlissel challah* is that Bnei Yisrael initially ate the leftover *mann* from the desert from the tenth of Nissan, when they entered Eretz Yisrael, until the *Korban Omer* was sacrificed, on the second day of Pesach. As soon as they began eating from the grains of Eretz Yisrael and the *mann* no longer fell, they needed their own livelihood. Every earthly aspect has a corresponding gate in *Shamayim*, and the *shlissel challah* alludes to the idea that Hashem should open the gates of livelihood for us.

(Oheiv Yisrael, Likutim, Shabbos Acharei Pesach)

After Pesach is the time of year that we count *sefirah*, which corresponds to the 50 gates of *binah*, understanding.

Our *avodah* is to climb from one gate to the other with the corresponding key, so we bake key-shaped challah after Pesach.

(Ibid.)

There are many reasons for inserting a key in the challos in honor of this Shabbos, and *minhag Yisrael Torah hi*—"Jewish custom has the status of Torah."

The *pasuk* in *Shir Hashirim* (5:2) states, *Pischi li achosi…*—"Open for me, my sister," and the midrash (*Shir Hashirim Rabbah* 5:3) states, *Pischu li pesach kichudo shel machat v'ani eftach lachem pesach k'pischo shel ulam.* Hashem asks us to open up in our hearts a small opening no bigger than the tip of a needle, and He will open it for us an opening like the door of the Beis Hamikdash.

All the exalted gates (levels of *kedushah*) that are open on Pesach are closed after Pesach. We need to invest our own efforts to reopen them during Sefirah.

On this Shabbos Mevarchim of Chodesh Iyar, we indent the challos with keys to symbolize that when we open the gates of our hearts after Pesach even a small amount through the mitzvos of Shabbos, Hashem will open the Heavenly gates and His great treasury for us, in the same way that He gave our forefathers *mann,* beginning in Chodesh Iyar.

(*Oheiv Yisrael, Shabbos Achar Pesach*)

There is a widespread *minhag* to use a key from the shul to indent the challah on the Shabbos after Pesach. This is alluded to in the words, *al yis'hallel chogeir k'mifateiach*—"The one who girds himself should not praise like one who opens it" (*Melachim I* 20:11), which means that a warrior should not praise himself when going to war before he knows if he will win. The word *chogeir* has the same numerical value as the words *lechem oni* and an additional three, alluding to the three matzos. This can be understood to mean that one should not feel conceited for having fulfilled the mitzvah of matzah (and other mitzvos). Since the word *"maftei'ach"* (key) is in the *pasuk*, we use a key in the challah. *(Ateres Yeshuah, Moadim*, pg. 54)

On the Shabbos after Pesach we read the Torah portion of *Shemini* or *Acharei Mos*, which discuss the prohibitions against forbidden foods and relationships that represent the *sitra achra,* side of impurity. Keeping these mitzvos is the "key" to our hearts, which helps extricate the *sitra achra* from within us.

The last *pasuk* in *Parshas Shemini* tells us, *Ki ani Hashem hama'aleh eschem mei'Eretz Mitzrayim lihiyos lachem l'Elokim v'hiyisem kedoshim ki kadosh Ani*—"For I am Hashem, Who has brought you up from the land of Egypt to be your G-d, thus you shall be holy, because I am holy" *(Vayikra* 11:45). *Lihiyos* **lachem** *l'Elokim* means that even the *"lachem"*—the pleasures of eating and drinking and physical deeds that are "for you," should be done for Hashem's sake and not merely for one's own pleasure. This is the key to purity, and will open one's heart to Hashem and ensure that he is not involved in forbidden relationships or eat forbidden foods. The challah on this Shabbos is indented with a key as a reminder of this concept. *(Rav Tuv, Shemini)*

In his introduction to Mishnayos, the Kol Remez writes that *Chazal* teach that the Jews will gather from their exile in the merit of the Mishnah, to which it is alluded in Avraham Avinu's question in *Bereishis* (15:8), *"Bameh eida ki irashena*—'How will I know that I will inherit the land?'" Hashem replied, *"Know that...they will be afflicted for 400 years."* Why were they exiled specifically for 400 years? Perhaps this suggests that his children will be redeemed in the *zechus* of the Mishnah, because the word *"hamishneh"* has the numerical value of 400.

The Bnei Yissaschar writes that Mishnayos includes 528 chapters, which is the numerical value of *maftei'ach* (key). (There are only 523 chapters, but five *perakim* of *Tosefta* are included in the calculation.)

We therefore bake challos with keys to demonstrate that just as Bnei Yisrael were redeemed from Mitzrayim in the merit of the Mishnah, and its number of chapter equals the word "*maftei'ach*," we should learn it and thereby merit the *Geulah* quickly. (*Divrei Tzaddikim*)

The great light that is present during the Shabbos after Pesach reveals the *yiras Shamayim* that one gained from eating the matzah on Pesach. Keys represent the concept of *yirah* attained by eating matzah, as *Chazal* teach: *One who acquired Torah and has no* yiras Shamayim *is compared to a treasurer who received keys for the inner door of the treasury and did not receive keys for the outer door* (*Shabbos* 31). It follows that *yirah* is the "key" that leads one into the "rooms" of Torah, and envelops him in the embracing light of the Torah to delve into its secrets. When one learns without the "keys" of the fear of Heaven he cannot enter the depths of Torah, and the Torah cannot enter his heart; the two become estranged. Conversely, Torah cleaves and connects to the thoughts of one who learns with *yiras Shamayim,* and protects him, whether he is learning at that moment or not, because it is eternally bound with his heart and soul. (*Yismach Yisrael, Tazria*)

Once Pesach is over, with all of its many mitzvos, stringencies, hard work, expenses, and the abstinence from delicacies which could have increased our *simchas Yom Tov* (because of the concerns of *chametz*), we know that we certainly earned great reward. We thus ask Hashem that all our deeds be accepted on High and stored away in the Heavenly treasury with the *ohr haganuz* (hidden light).

We therefore insert a key into the challos for the Shabbos after Pesach, signifying that all our service to Hashem on Pesach is locked away in the treasury Above.

(*Haggadah Ohr Ganuz*, Shabbos after Pesach)

Another reason for eating *shlissel challah* is that until now, *chametz* was forbidden and, "under lock and key." Now, after Pesach, we can open it with a "key." (*Yad Ephraim*, sec. 30)

The Rebbe of Rozhvadov once visited the city of Klimentov for the Shabbos after Pesach, when dough in the shape of a key is placed on top of the challah. The Rebbe called the key, "the bird on the challah," and when he cut the challah, he removed the "bird," broke it, and said, "Just as I break this bird, so may it be that the Czar falls speedily." Within a day or two it became known that the Czar had died.

(*Hachachmah Mei'ayin*, pg. 117)

Chapter 29
Shabbos Shavuos

Erev Shavuos That Falls out on Shabbos

The morning meal is divided into two *seudos*. In the first, we eat fish and sing *"Az bayom hashvi'i nachta,"* and then recite *Birkas Hamazon* and *daven* Minchah. Then, we wash our hands for *shalosh seudos* and eat fish and the rest of the Shabbos foods.

(*Darkei Chaim V'shalom*)

Second Day of Shavuos on Shabbos

If the second day of Shavuos falls out on Shabbos, one should eat all the regular Shabbos foods and add another kugel in honor of Yom Tov. Dairy foods are not eaten.

(*Ma'agal Hashanah* 5766, p. 249)

Second Day Yom Tov—a Different Type of Kedushah

The author of the *Kovetz Hahakdamos* once visited the holy Reb Aharon of Belz in Eretz Yisrael. For him, it was the second day of Shavuos since he was from *Chutz La'aretz*. That year, Shavuos came out on Erev Shabbos. For those living in Eretz Yisrael, it was a regular Shabbos, *Parshas Naso*. Every Shabbos, after Kiddush, the Rebbe's custom was to eat fruit preserves, called *"eingemachtz,"* and distribute some to those present. As the Rebbe extended the spoon toward him, he said, "I am not giving you *shirayim*, because you now have a different type of *kedushah* than I do. Still, you can eat *eingemachtz*."

His holy words can be somewhat understood based on the Tanya's explanation in his *Shulchan Aruch* (final edition 1:8), which states that the *eis ratzon* and tremendous *yichudim* (unifications) which take place Above as a result of *Krias Shema*, prayer, and the *kedushah* of Shabbos and Yom Tov, are far above time and place (Kabbalistic terms). However, their illumination is cast downwards to wherever and whenever is appropriate. This is why there is tremendous *kedushah* outside Eretz Yisrael during the second day of Yom Tov, even while in Eretz Yisrael there is no Yom Tov and no special *kedushah*. For this reason, individuals who travel abroad from Eretz Yisrael must observe the sanctity of the second day of Yom Tov, even though they are planning to return to Eretz Yisrael and it is not actually Yom Tov for them (as explained in the *halachos* of Yom Tov).

It is written in the *sefarim hakedoshim* (Shelah Hakadosh, Beis Chachmah) that when it comes to *halachos* in the Torah, the revealed and hidden aspects are intertwined and connected. Since the halachah is that a person visiting Eretz Yisrael from abroad must continue to observe the second day of Yom Tov if he is intending to return, it must be that the *kedushah* of the second day of Yom Tov rests on him even while he is in Eretz Yisrael. (*Kovetz Hahakdamos*, p. 12; *Botzina Kaddisha*, 363, p. 112)

Chapter 30
Shabbasos During the Three Weeks

Shabbos Rosh Chodesh Av

It was customary to add another kugel in honor of Shabbos Rosh Chodesh Av, just like every other Shabbos Rosh Chodesh. (Belz)

Shabbos Chazon

On Erev Shabbos Chazon after *chatzos*, one may be lenient and give young children meat to eat. This is true even on an Erev Shabbos that precedes Tishah B'Av which falls out on Shabbos itself, since after *chatzos* on Friday some of the *kedushah* of Shabbos is already present. (*Kaf Hachaim*, fn. 155)

During the days between Shivah Asar B'Tammuz and Tishah B'Av, Reb Pinchas of Koritz would be low-spirited; the clock in his home would stop, and the challah baked for Shabbos Chazon would never come out good. All of this demonstrated how saddened he was by the destruction of the Beis Hamikdash. (*Likutei Imrei Pinchas*, part II, p. 44)

On Shabbos Chazon, the custom is to welcome Shabbos earlier than usual. Some say that the reason for this is because people are hurrying to eat meat. Before the *Churban*, Bnei Yisrael sinned through three aspects: sight, hearing, and speech. When one damages these three senses with sin, his heart becomes hardened. It is no longer a "heart of flesh," but rather a, "heart of stone." *Chazal* prohibited us from eating meat (flesh) during these days (versus a different type of penance) to demonstrate this.

When Mashiach comes, the *pasuk* in *Yechezkel* (36:26) tells us, *I will remove the heart of stone from your flesh, and give you a heart of flesh*. Therefore, when Shabbos arrives and we are allowed to eat meat, we hurry to welcome Shabbos in early, to allude to our desire to very soon merit, "a heart of flesh."

(Kedushas Aharon, Novlos Chachmah)

Some people would be especially stringent on Shabbos Chazon and not eat meat at all. Others would not eat meat from Shivah Asar B'Tammuz, except for on Shabbos, during which they would eat dried meat, which in Arabic was called "*lekhlie*." This was the custom of the families of *kohanim* in Debdou. *(Netivot Hama'arav, p. 114, sec. 7)*

When Tishah B'Av falls out on Shabbos, one must not attend a *shalom zachar*, nor do a *forshpiel* (a celebratory *seudah* for a *chassan* on Motza'ei Shabbos) on that Shabbos.

(Leket Yosher Orach Chaim, Hilchos Tishah B'Av 6)

Shalosh Seudos of Shabbos Chazon

In Poland, on Shabbos Chazon, the congregants would set a table in front of the *beis midrash*, and every person would bring the leftover meat from the previous two Shabbos meals, and they would eat them all as *shalosh seudos* together. They would call this Shabbos, "*Shabbos Tish*," referring to the table. *(Divrei Harav, p. 140)*

One may eat meat and drink wine during *shalosh seudos*. The custom of Belzer chassidim was not to eat meat or drink wine then, since they did not do so during all the other Shabbasos of the year.

After sunset on Shabbos, some people avoid drinking wine and eating meat. From the Pri Megadim's explanation, it seems that this would be true even if they were in middle of the meal.

The *Mishnah Berurah* quotes other *Acharonim* that if a person did not yet *daven* Ma'ariv, he may eat meat and drink wine, because he is still going to say *Retzei* in *Birkas Hamazon*, and it is still Shabbos for him.

(See *Magen Avraham* 551, fn. 26; *Mishnah Berurah* there, fn. 51)

Whenever Tishah B'Av would fall out on Motza'ei Shabbos, the Rav of Ropshitz would eat a very long *shalosh seudos*, with *zemiros* and singing. He would say, "Shabbos is a very dear and important guest. Let us keep it with us a bit longer! You, Tishah B'Av, can wait. We'd far prefer you did not come at all! I do not consider you an important guest. Wait here, and let us honor the Shabbos Queen and sing *zemiros* in her honor…" (*Ohel Naftali*, 348)

The author of the responsa *Aryeh Dvei Ila'i* said that he once sat with his followers at a *shalosh seudos* on Erev Tishah B'Av. *Bein hashmashos* arrived and the people were unsure whether to continue *shalosh seudos*. The Rav said, "Ribono Shel Olam, what are we doing? We are not eating or drinking, we just cannot take leave of the holy Shabbos!"

(*Likutei Maharich, Minhagei Chodesh Av*)

Whenever Tishah B'Av would fall out on Shabbos, Rav Yitzchak Eizik of Ziditchov would eat meat and drink wine during *shalosh seudos* until just before *bein hashmashos*, prolonging *shalosh seudos* with songs, *zemiros*, and words of Torah, just like every other Shabbos. (*Yalkut Mahari*, p. 185)

When Tishah B'Av would fall out on Shabbos, Belzer chassidim would eat dairy foods and sour cream during *shalosh seudos*. Once, when they took the *shirayim* of sour cream, it became tangled in the *gabbai*'s beard. Reb Aharon of Belz turned to the *gabbai* and said, "*Plitzlung hastu bakumen a veisse burd* (Specifically now, you got a white beard)!"

(*B'kedushaso Shel Aharon*, p. 473)

If Tishah B'Av falls out on Sunday, or if it falls out on Shabbos and is pushed off to Sunday, one should eat meat and drink wine during the *seudah hamafsekes*, even setting a lavish meal, *"like the meal of Shlomo Hamelech at the time of his reign"* (Shulchan Aruch, Orach Chaim 552:10).

One can learn from the fact that it says, *"one eats meat"* and not, *"one is permitted to eat meat,"* that if someone is able to eat meat before the fast, he indeed should. It is not merely a "permission" but rather a directive, because when one does not eat meat during this *seudah* it may seem that he is doing so because of *aveilus*, which is prohibited on Shabbos.

Perhaps this is related to what the Chasam Sofer wrote in his *drashos* (p. 326b): *Had I not been unsure, I would have said that the day of Tishah B'Av itself is actually a day of joy. Because for 900 years, [Hashem was angry at Klal Yisrael for their sins]* (Rashi, Yechezkel 20:5), *and on Tishah B'Av they were forgiven for their sins—"your iniquity is expiated, daughter of Tzion, He will not exile you again"* (Eichah 4:22). *We were given the promise that Hashem will never exile us again on Tishah B'Av, so it really should be a day of joy and happiness. However, the mourning and the crying every year is about the new destruction that takes place due to our many sins. Every day, the suffering is greater than the day before, and every year, it is as though the Beis Hamikdash has been destroyed again. And so, though it would be proper to thank Hashem on this day, and that is why it is indeed called a "mo'ed," since our sins have distanced the end and are constantly adding to the suffering, this overrides the basic joy...*

Accordingly, when Tishah B'Av falls out on Shabbos, the fact that we eat meat then is not because we cannot display *aveilus* on Shabbos (which is the case when Shabbos is on any other day from Rosh Chodesh Av until Tishah B'Av), but rather, because it really is a day of joy, and since it is Shabbos, the joy is not overridden.

Therefore, we are taught that one is not merely permitted to "eat and drink his fill," i.e. eat meat and drink wine, rather it is a mitzvah to do so during the *seudah hamafsekes*, to display the joy as Tishah B'Av comes in. The meat that the person ate in the morning is not as much of an indication that it is due to the joy of this specific day, since a person eats meat every Shabbos. It is only during this *shalosh seudos*, when one does not necessarily eat meat and drink wine, that doing so is truly a display of the day's joy.

Chazal even continue and describe one's table at this meal, "*like the meal of Shlomo Hamelech at the time of his reign.*" In *Melachim I* (5:2), the *pasuk* says that Shlomo Hamelech ruled over the entire side of the river and had peace all around, and Yehudah and Yisrael sat in peace and safety, "*each man under his vine and under his fig tree, from Dan to Be'er Sheva.*" Accordingly, when we refer to Shlomo's meals, we also remember the greatness of Shlomo's rule and how peace reigned. This leads us to ask Hashem to bring that kind of peace to us again: *Bring us back to You, Hashem, and we shall return; renew our days as of old* (Eichah 5:21).

The Midrash Rabbah (end of *Eichah*), referring to the *pasuk* in *Mishlei* (3:4), *Then the offering of Yehudah and Yerushalayim will be pleasing to Hashem as in the days of old, and in previous years*, explains that "*the offering of Yehudah... as in the days of old*" refers to Moshe's times, and "*in previous years*" refers to Shlomo's times. The Yefeh Anaf explains that, "Moshe's times" refers to when the fire came down onto the offering on the eighth day of the *milu'im*, and, "Shlomo's times" refers to when Shlomo inaugurated the Beis Hamikdash. The fire that came down in Shlomo's days was shaped like a crouching lion —a symbol of *hashra'as haShechinah*. This brought about the peace that was in his days, and was the catalyst for his great feast.

Therefore, we can say that *Chazal* are alluding to the fact that besides eating meat and drinking wine, a person should also make his meal like the *seudah* of Shlomo in his days. He must think about Shlomo's greatness in the feast that resulted from the fact that there was peace during his rule, all stemming from the *hashra'as haShechinah* that was in his days, and how this is awaiting us in the future, as well. Eating meat and drinking wine should bring one to think about the joy of the future, as the *nevu'ah* describes: *Your iniquity is expiated, daughter of Tzion, He will not exile you again* (Eichah 4:22). Rashi explains that this refers to the time after *Galus Edom*, when the *Shechinah* will once again be revealed. This is what Bnei Yisrael had in Shlomo's days that we hope will be speedily returned to us. (*Ein Yisrael, Yuma* 21a)

One should not sit down with friends for this meal. The Bechor Shor (*Ta'anis* 30a) disagrees with this, claiming that if one is accustomed to sitting down for *shalosh seudos* with friends on every other Shabbos, such as in shuls, where members eat *shalosh seudos* together, avoiding doing so would be considered *aveilus b'farhesia*—displaying signs of mourning in public, which is prohibited on Shabbos.

(*Magen Avraham*)

The Rema (553:2) writes that it was customary to avoid learning Torah on Erev Tishah B'Av from *chatzos* and onward, other than subjects that are permissible on Tishah B'Av. Therefore, when Tishah B'Av falls out on Shabbos, *Pirkei Avos* is not recited. However, the Turei Zahav (102) writes that this perplexes him, *if there is no prohibition to eat meat and wine—on the contrary, it is an obligation to eat meat in honor of Shabbos, as the Tur rules* (end of 552)—*why would we be stringent and not allow a person to study Torah due to* aveilus?

The Yad Ephraim (552) quotes the Bechor Shor (end of *Ta'anis*), who explains that there are two separate *halachos*. One is *simchah* and one is *oneg*. *Oneg* refers to physical pleasure, while *simchah* is mainly the joy that one feels in his heart. (When *Chazal* say that "simchah *is only with meat and wine*" [*Pesachim* 109], they mean that they bring one to *simchah*, not that they are *simchah* in and of themselves.) On Shabbos, we have no mitzvah of *simchah*, as we do on Yom Tov. The mitzvah on Shabbos is *oneg*, as we see in the words, *"V'karasa laShabbos oneg"* (Yeshayah 58:13). Therefore, eating meat and drinking wine, which are *oneg Shabbos* (Rambam, Hilchos Shabbos 30:10), must not be avoided due to *aveilus*, because they are part of the mitzvah of Shabbos. Studying Torah, on the other hand, brings *simchah*, as we see in the *pasuk* (Tehillim 19:9): *The orders of Hashem are upright, gladdening the heart*. There is no prohibition to avoid *simchah* on Shabbos, because it is not part of the mitzvah of Shabbos.

This explanation also further clarifies the words of the Magen Avraham (552, fn. 14), who quotes the Rokeach's statement that even if one eats a meal "like Shlomo," he should sit down to his meal despondently, not in joy. The reason for this is because only *oneg* is permitted, not *simchah*.

(Otzros Yehoshua, p. 398)

The custom in Rheinus was that during the summer months, they would eat *shalosh seudos* before Minchah. Whenever Tishah B'Av would fall out on Sunday or was pushed off to Sunday from Shabbos, the Maharil would first *daven* Minchah, and then they would eat *shalosh seudos*, so that it would also serve as the *seudah hamafsekes*.

When the Mahari Katz began to lead the community, he did not know of this custom, and ordered the *gabbai* to call in the community members for a *seudah* before Minchah, just like every other Shabbos. He was informed about the aforementioned custom of the Maharil, but it was difficult for him to listen. It was found in the *Sefer Harokeach* that, indeed, *"When Tishah B'Av falls out on Motza'ei Shabbos or on Shabbos, Rabbeinu Yitzchak bar Yehudah would eat [shalosh seudos] between Minchah and Ma'ariv as a* seudah hamafsekes..." The same is also written in the Maharak.

(Maharil, Hilchos Tishah B'Av, siman 17)

Motza'ei Shabbos Chazon

The Mechaber rules that one may make Havdalah on wine on Motza'ei Shabbos Chazon, despite the prohibition of drinking wine during the Nine Days. The Rema, among other *poskim*, disagrees and rules that the wine should be given to a child who does not understand the concept of mourning the *Churban*. In practice, many do make Havdalah on wine even during the Nine Days. The Leket Yosher recounts that the Terumas Hadeshen drank the wine of Havdalah on Motza'ei Shabbos Chazon. However, one should not give the leftover wine to his family to drink.

If the fast of Tishah B'Av falls on Motza'ei Shabbos, Havdalah is made following the completion of the fast on Sunday night. An ill person who must eat on Tishah B'Av may make Havdalah on milk. *(Magen Avos)*

Eating leftover meat from the Shabbos *seudah* for *seudas melaveh malkah* is permitted *(Birkei Yosef)*. However, cooking extra meat for Shabbos deliberately so that one will have leftovers for *melaveh malkah* is prohibited. *(Sha'arei Teshuvah)*

There are many opinions that disagree and counter that meat should not be consumed in the Nine Days, even for *melaveh malkah*.

The Sigheter Rav, Reb Yekusiel Yehudah Teitelbaum, recounted that the *melaveh malkah* of his illustrious grandfather, the Yismach Moshe, consisted of a fresh, whole challah, a portion of fish and a cup of wine. On Motza'ei Shabbos Chazon he did not drink wine. *(Likutei Maharich)*

When the Oheiv Yisrael was asked on Motza'ei Shabbos Chazon what they should serve him for *melaveh malkah*, he responded that he had never eaten dairy at *melaveh malkah*. Consequently, a chicken was slaughtered and prepared. The *melaveh malkah* lasted until the wee hours of the morning, when his followers noticed a bird perched on the windowsill of an open window in the room. The chassidim wanted to shoo it away, but the Rebbe motioned to them to refrain from doing so. The Oheiv Yisrael then revealed that the soul of a great person who wasn't stringent to eat seudas *melaveh malkah* during his lifetime was reincarnated in this bird. Now, he was being sent to witness the importance of this meal, where chicken was being consumed even during a week of mourning.

(*Eretz Hachaim*)

Reb Yeshayah Kerestirer had wine and meat as usual for *melaveh malkah* of Motza'ei Shabbos Chazon (despite the late hour due to his many preparations for this holy meal).

Reb Itzikel of Pshevorsk commented that one who regularly eats meat at *melaveh malkah* should do so on Shabbos Chazon. Those who do not have the custom to do so, should begin doing so.

(*Eretz Hachaim*)

Shabbos Nachamu

Rabi Shimon ben Gamliel said: There were never good days for Yisrael like the fifteenth of Av and Yom Hakippurim. Yom Kippur is the day when we were given the second set of luchos and Tu B'Av is when the generation of the midbar knew with certainty that the 40 years during which members of the generation died as a result of their sin were finally over. For this reason, it was customary to make a seudah on the Shabbos after Tishah B'Av.

(*Ritva, Ta'anis* 30b)

Shabbos Nachamu is the Shabbos immediately after Tishah B'Av. The entire nation would rejoice and be secure in the consolation of the coming of Mashiach.

(*Minhagei Maharil*)

The Shabbos following Tishah B'Av is called, "Shabbos Nachamu," named after the *haftorah*. This is the only Shabbos, other than Shabbos Shuvah, that is named after its *haftorah*. Songs and *piyutim* are sung at length, and it is appropriate to invest in more *oneg* than usual on this Shabbos. Ben Shu'ib writes that it is a mitzvah to make this Shabbos similar to a Yom Tov. *(Yosef Ometz)*

Belzer chassidim had a custom to add another kugel in honor of Shabbos Nachamu. *(Temidim K'sidram)*

Some Sephardim make sure to recite a *Shehecheyanu* on a new fruit on every Shabbos of the *Shivah D'nechemta* (the seven weeks following Tishah B'Av). *(Luach Luntz, Davar B'ito)*

The Shabbos Table

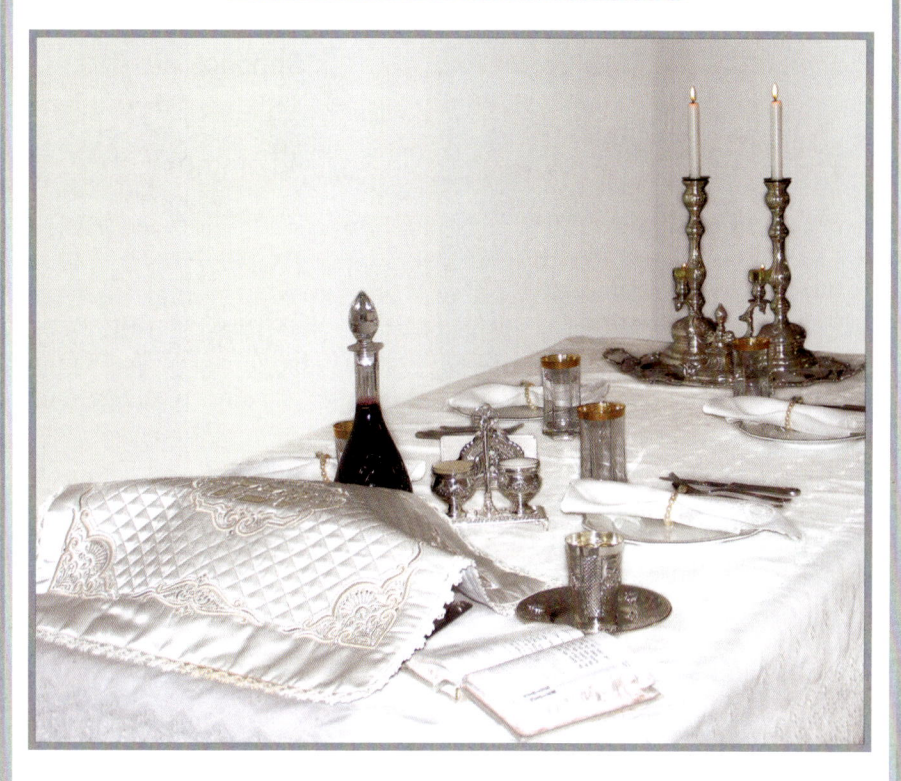

The Shabbos Table

    The *Zohar* (*Pekudei* 252) states that when Shabbos arrives the angels arrange all the Shabbos tables in the one of the heavenly sanctuaries known as the *heichal hazchus*. Thousands upon thousands of angels are appointed over these tables. If the angels see the table set with all types of delicacies they bless the table by saying the *pesukim* of "*Az tisaneg al Hashem*," "*Az tikra vaHashem yaaneh*," "*Az yibaka kashachar orecha*," and "*Hinei ki chein yevorach gaver*," and all the other angels answer amen.

    The *Shechinah* rests above our Shabbos table as is alluded to in the words *Zeh hashulchan asher lifnei Hashem* whose first letters spell the words "*Zeh keili*" which refers to the *pasuk* of "*Zeh keili veanveihu*— This is my G-d and I will adorn Him," from which Chazal learn that we should perform our mitzvos in the best possible manner. Therefore, one should spread a fresh tablecloth on the Shabbos table to honor the presence of the *Shechinah*.   (*Siddur Rebbi Koppel*)

Kiddush Cup

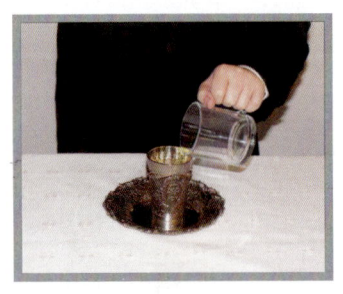

Rinsing the Cup
One should rinse the inside of the Kiddush cup prior to reciting Kiddush. *(Orach Chaim 183)*

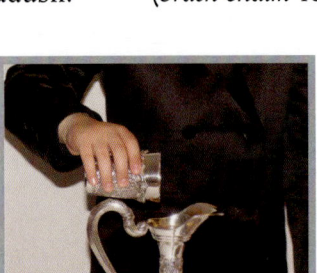

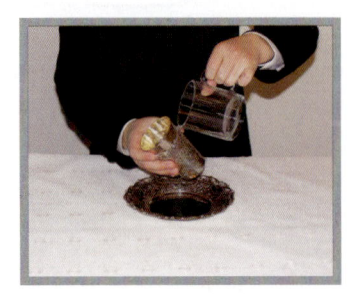

Washing the Cup
One should also wash the outside of the Kiddush cup three times. *(Orach Chaim 183)*

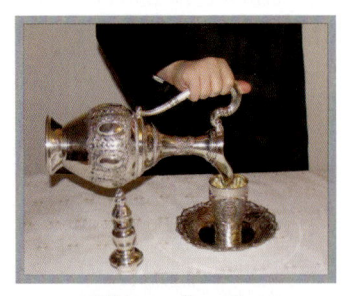

One should pour three drops of water from the Kiddush cup into the bottle of wine. The rest of the water is disposed of. *(Orach Chaim 183)*

Filling the Cup
The one who recites Kiddush fills the cup himself in three steps, pausing twice when pouring. *(Kamarna)*

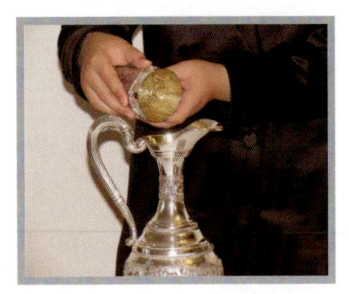

Pouring three drops of water into the wine bottle using both hands, prior to filling the Kiddush cup.

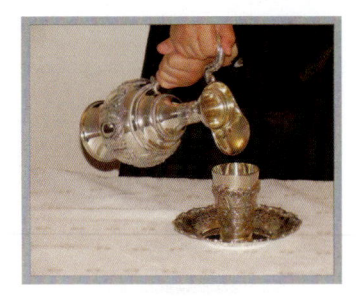

Filling the Kiddush cup using both hands.

Kiddush Cup

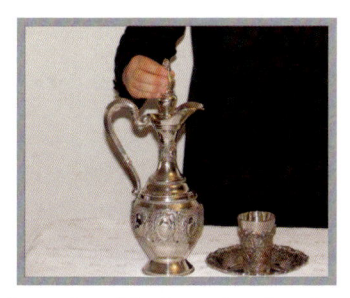

One should close the bottle of wine before Kiddush to allude to the *yayin hameshumar* (wine that Hashem put away at the creation of the world for the End of Days).

(Baal Shem Tov)

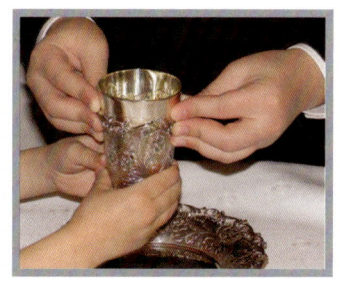

Accepting the Kiddush cup from the person lifting it, using both hands.

(*Shulchan Hatahor* 183:6)

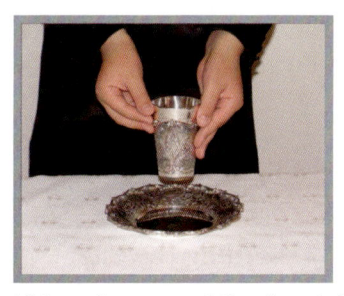

Lifting the cup while the right hand is slightly raised above the left one.

(Ramak, Or Yakar vol. 9, p. 77)

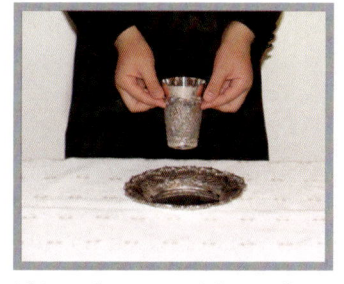

Lifting the cup with ten fingers

(Toldos Yitzchok Nezhchiz, *Likutim*)

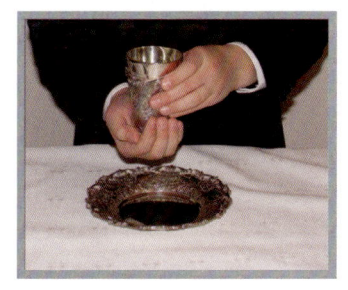

Many lift the cup by themselves using both hands in order to demonstrate their love for the mitzvah.

(*Taz* 183:2)

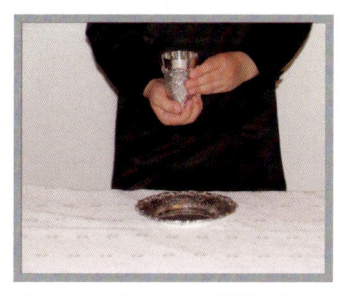

When reciting Kiddush, one should lift the cup a *tefach* above the table so that the cup is visible to all, and they should gaze upon it. (*Shulchan Aruch* 271)

Kiddush Cup

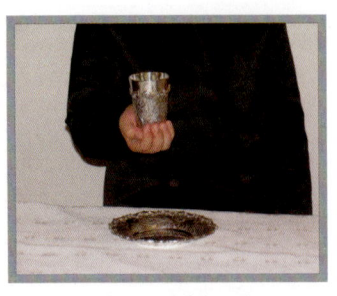

Holding the Kiddush Cup in One's Palm

Holding the cup in one's right palm with the fingers slightly bent, as if to receive something. (*Siddur Tefillah Yesharah*, Berditchev)

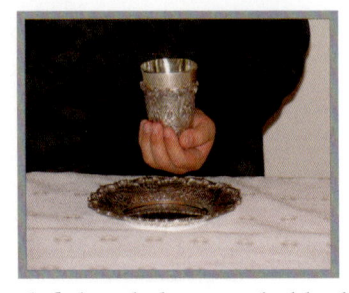

A left-handed person holds the Kiddush cup in the left hand.

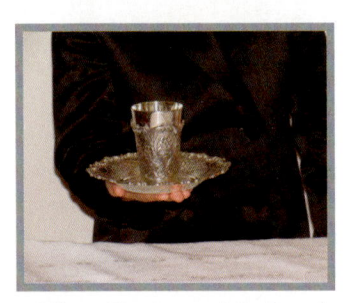

Holding the cup with the plate beneath it.

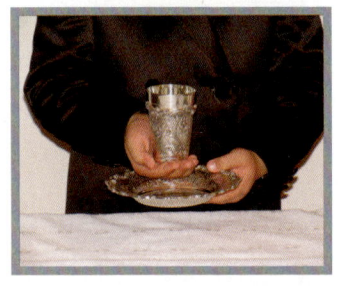

Holding the cup in the right hand and the plate in the left hand.

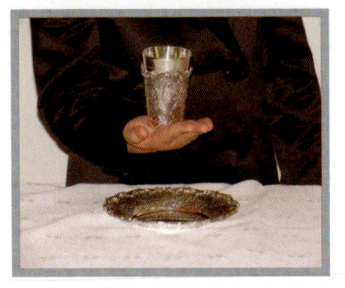

Holding the cup in one's palm. This alludes to the *pasuk* ...*and I placed the cup on Pharaoh's palm* (*Bereishis* 40:11).

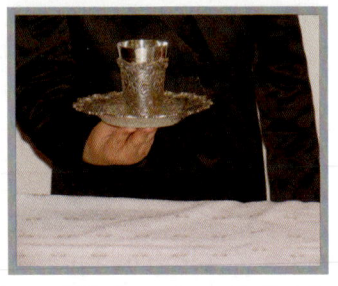

Some lift the cup and the plate together.

Kiddush Cup

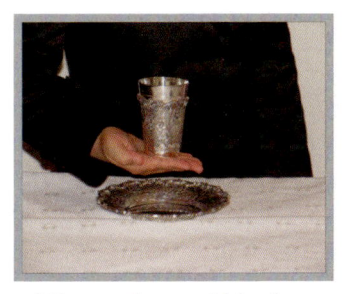

Holding the Kiddush cup partially on one's fingers and partially on one's palm.

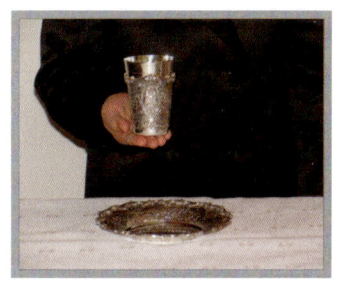

Holding the cup on five outstretched fingers.

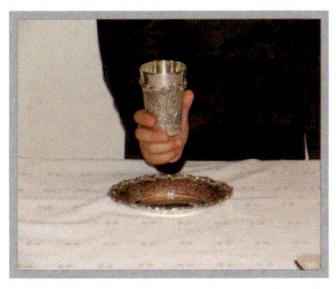

Grasping the cup with four fingers around it and the thumb on the top.

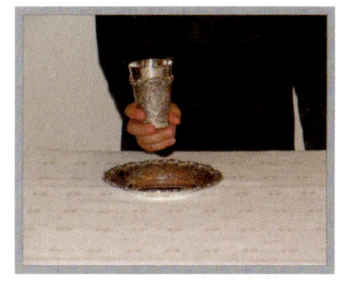

Surrounding the cup with one's fingers.

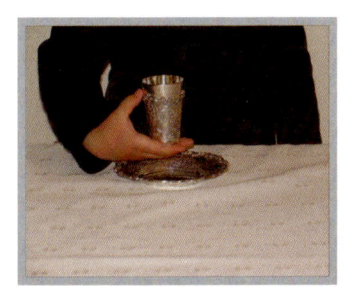

Holding the cup from the bottom and grasping it on top with one's thumb.

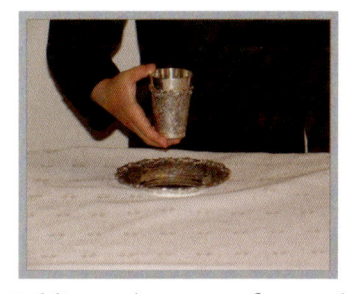

Holding the cup from the bottom and one's thumb is near the rim of the cup.

Kiddush Cup

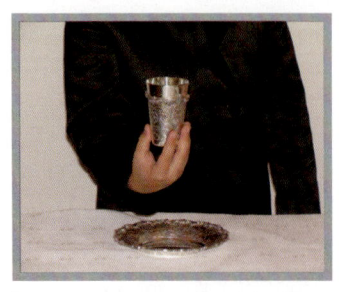

The upper part of one's fingers are bent and the cup is only slightly above one's palm.
(*Eifoh Shleimah*)

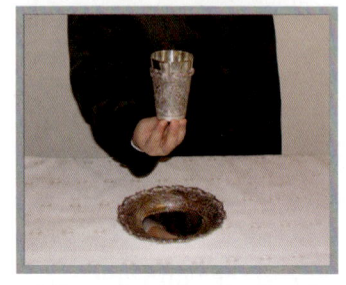

Holding the cup on the tip of the fingers of one's right hand.
(*Shaar Hamitzvos, Eikev*)

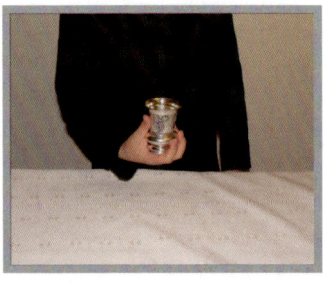

A Stemmed Kiddush Cup
The foot of the cup rests on the palm of one's hand and the five fingers surround the cup.
(*Tzvi Latzaddik*, Ziditchoiv)

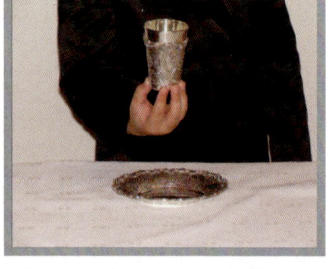

Holding the cup while one's fingers are straight and there is a larger space between the cup and one's palm.
(*Shemen Sason* on *Shaar Hamitzvos*)

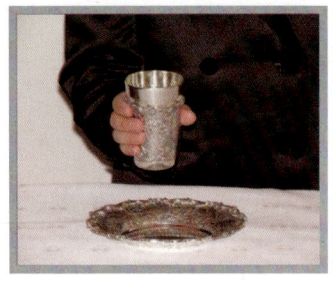

Holding the cup in the usual manner. (*Magen Avraham* 183:6)

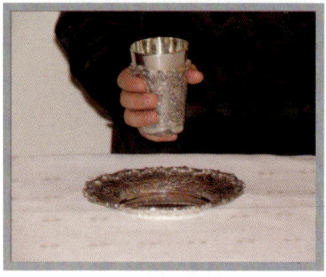

Holding the cup in the usual manner with one's little finger underneath the cup.
(*Magen Avraham* 183:6)

Kiddush Cup

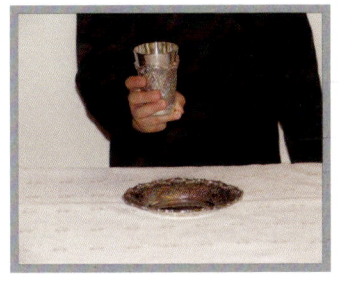

Holding the cup while forming Hashem's name of *Shakei*.

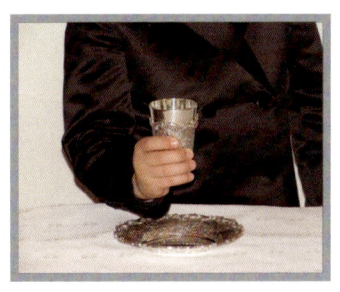

Grasping the surface of the cup. (*Magen Avraham* 183:6)

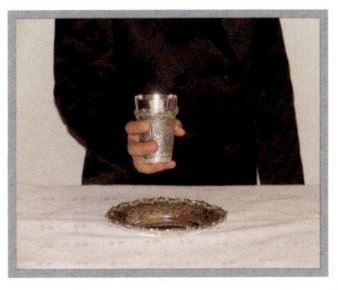

Two fingers surround the cup and two fingers are on the bottom of the cup.

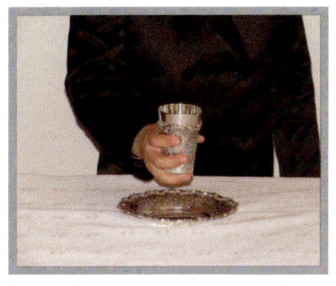

Three fingers surround the cup with one's little finger on the bottom.

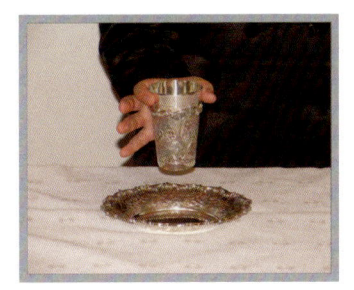

Holding the cup by placing two fingers around the rim of the cup.

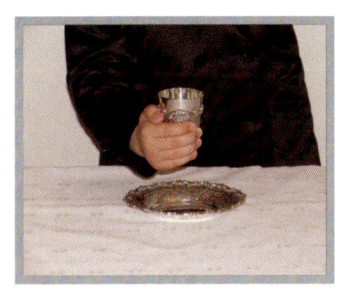

Grasping the surface of the cup with five fingers around it.

Kiddush Cup

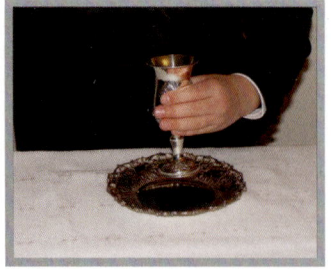

A Stemmed Kiddush Cup

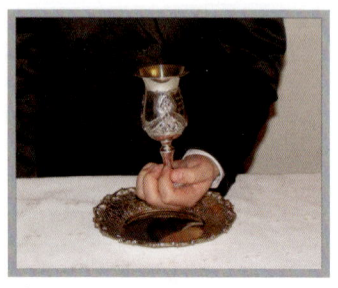

Holding the cup itself.

Holding the foot of the cup.

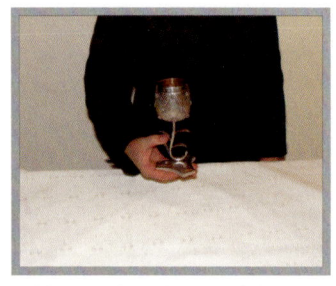

Holding the foot of the cup, partially on one's palm and partially on the four bent fingers. One's thumb is on the highest leaf that originates from the stem.

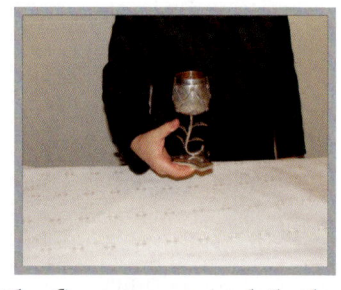

The fingers surround the base of the cup on the bottom and one's thumb is on the highest leaf so that one forms the letter *dalet* with his palm and the part that remains forms the letter *yud*.

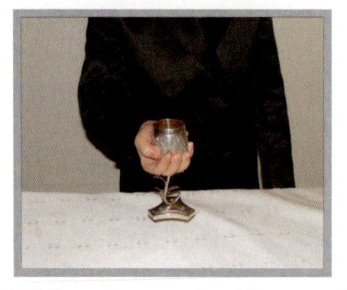

Holding the cup itself on one's fingers and palm.

(*Siddur Tefillah Yesharah* [Boston])

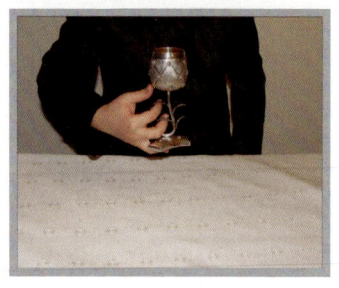

Holding the cup with five fingers on the leaves.

Kiddush Cup

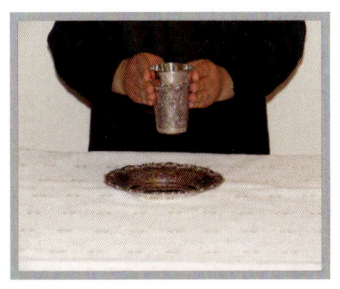

The Teimani custom is to grasp the cup from the top with both hands.

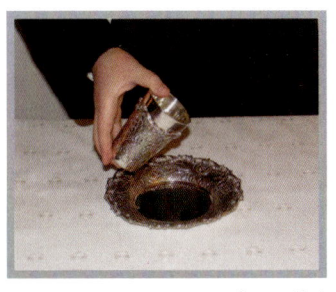

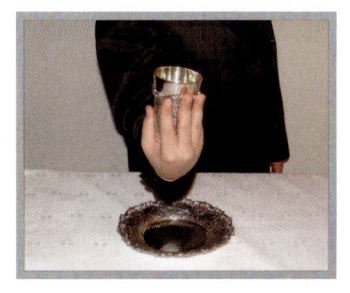

The cup rests on the right palm and the fingers are bent upwards.

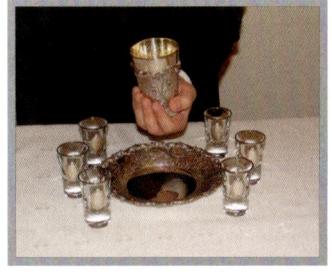

Some are accustomed to tilting the cup. In this way they fulfill both opinions of how full the cup should be since one side is full and one side is partially empty. *(Tur* 183:4)

Surrounding the Kiddush Cup

Rav Chisda would surround the Kiddush cup with small cups. *(Brachos* 51a)

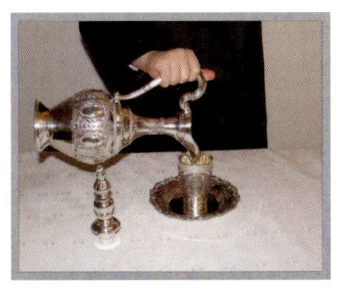

Pouring Wine into the Bottle

After Kiddush one should add some wine from the bottle to his cup so that the remaining wine in the cup should not be considered defective (*pagum*).

(Shulchan Aruch 182:5)

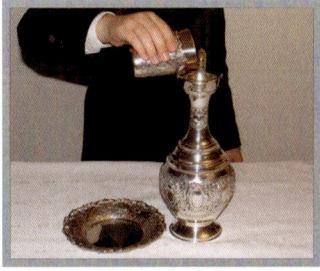

Pouring from the Cup into the Bottle

Some of the Kiddush wine is poured back into the bottle and is then used for Havdalah.

Shabbos Challos

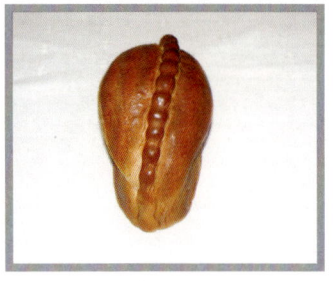

For the Friday night *suedah* many use a challah that is not braided, which is in the form of the letter *vav*. (*Likutei Maharin*)

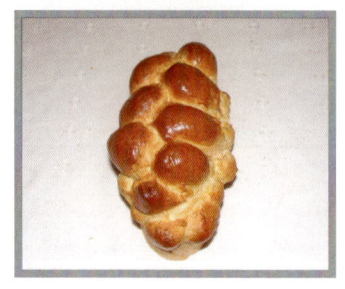

Braided challos are used for the Shabbos day *suedah*.

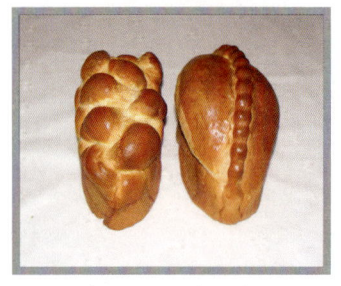

Lechen Mishneh on Friday Night

On Friday night, the challah that is not braided, which is placed on the right side, is cut open.

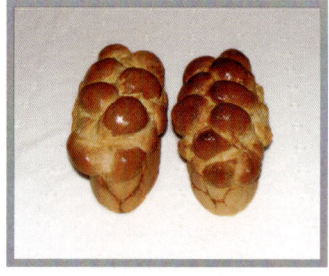

Lechem Mishneh on Shabbos Day

On Shabbos day, the braided challah that is on the right side is cut open.

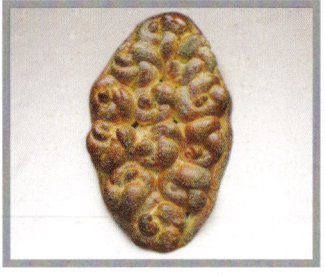

A Challah with Twelve Parts

The challah consists of six rows forming the shape of two triangles which appear like the shape of two *segels*, a Hebrew vowel. (Lelov)

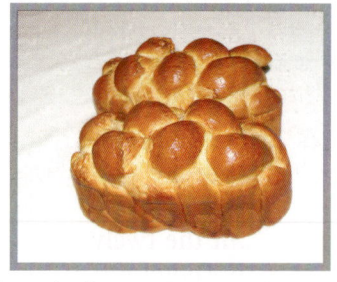

The challos are placed in the width. (*Taz*, 274)

Order of the Twelve Challos

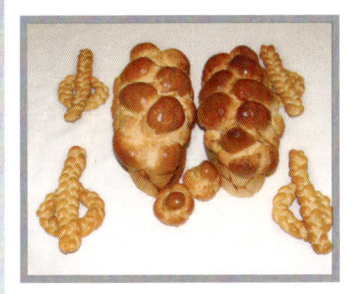

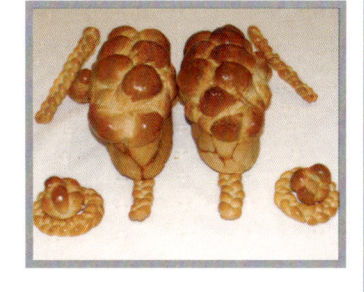

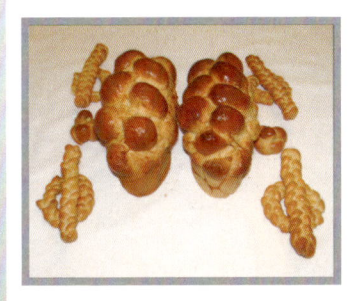

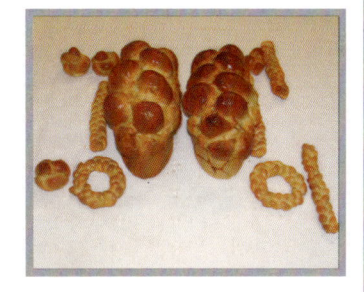

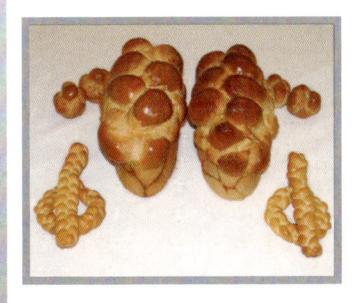

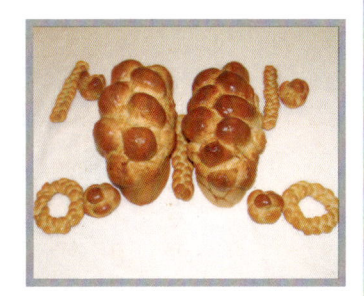

Twelve Challos

According to the Arizal, one should place twelve challos—corresponding to the twelve *Lechem Hapanim* in the Beis Hamikdash—on the table at all three *seudos*. (*Shaar Hakavanos, Inyan Hashulchan*, p. 84)

It is told in the name of the Baal Shem Tov that the twelve challos correspond to the *Trei Asar* of the *sefer* of Tanach. Other *nevi'im* have their name immortalized by the name of their *sefer* (e.g. Yechezkel, Yirmiyah) but the twelve *nevi'im* of *Trei Asar* have no complete *sefer* in their name. Therefore, to ensure that their names should be mentioned, we take twelve challos, corresponding to their twelve names. Indeed, the Arizal would call the twelve challos by the names of the *nevi'im* of Trei Asar. (*Peninim V'avnei Chefetz, Beshalach*)

Cutting the Challah

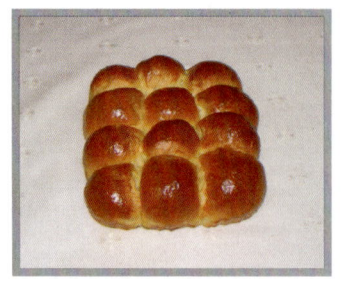

Twelve challos in the form of the *choshen*.

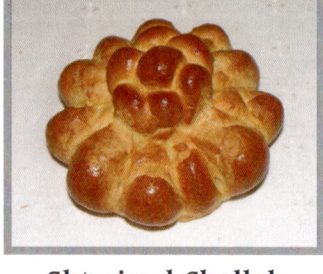

Shtreimel Challah
Some make a round challah with twelve small challos in it. This is called a "*shtreimel* challah." (*Sefer Kehillah*)

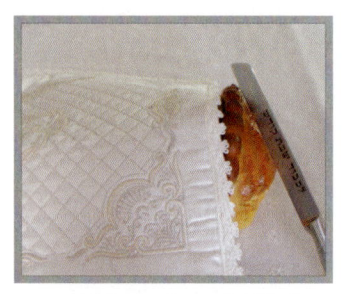

Marking the Challah
Before reciting *Hamotzi*, one should uncover the challah and mark the spot that he is planning to cut. (*Magen Avraham*)

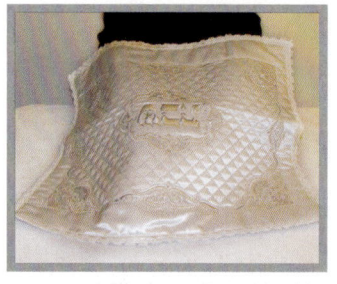

Two Hands on the Challos
During the recitation of *Hamotzi* one should place two hands on the two challos.
(*Levush, Orach Chaim* 167:4)

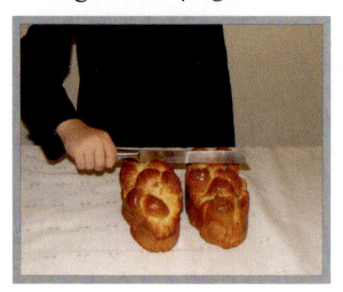

The mark should be made on the side where the challah is the most well baked so that one is reciting the *brachah* on the choicest part of the challah.
(*Shulchan Aruch* 167:1)

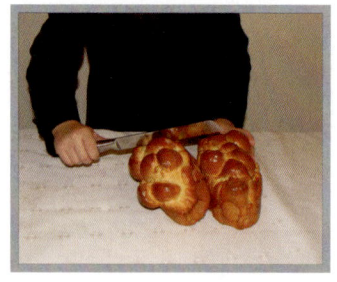

Some are accustomed to uncovering the challos prior to reciting *Hamotzi* and marking both of them. (Lelov)

Cutting the Challah

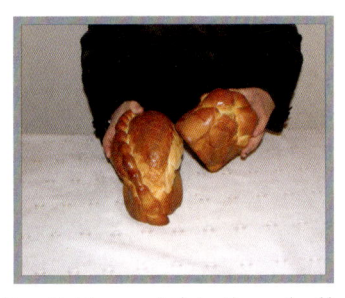

On Friday night the challah that is not braided is on the right side and beneath the braided challah, closer to the person.

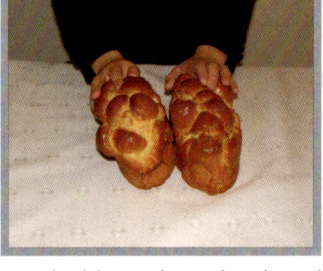

On Shabbas day the braided challah on the right side is on top on the left challah.

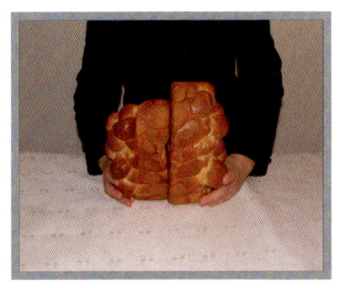

After reciting *Hamotzi*, some set the challos upright on the table so that they appear to have two "faces," one on either side, which alludes to the *Lechem Hapanim*.
(*Devar Tzvi Shabbos*)

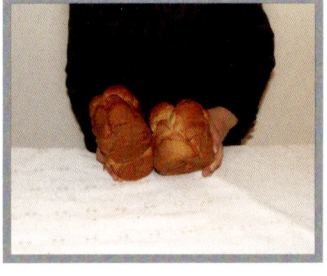

Lifting the Challos
While reciting the *brachah* one should lift the challos a bit so that the edge of the challah touches the table and the rest of the challah is in the air.
(*Zemiros Shirei Hamalchus*)

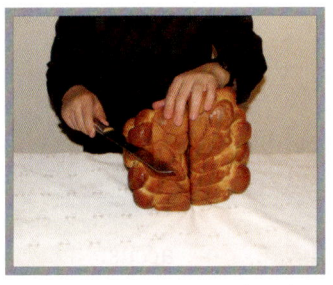

Many are accustomed to begin cutting the challah either in the middle of the challah or above that. (*Zemiros Shirei Hamalchus*)

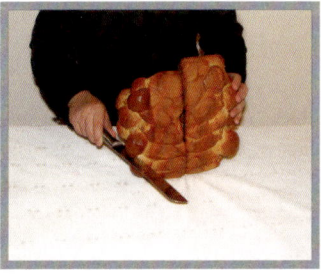

Some begin cutting the challah in the lower third of the challah, from the side that is closer to the person.

Cutting the Challah

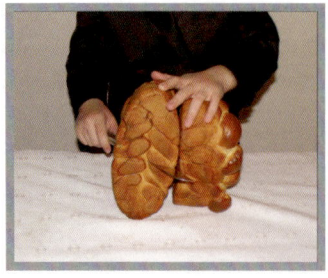

When cutting the challah, one should be careful not to cut it straight on the table but to circle the challah with one's knife. (*Zemiros Shirei Hamalchus*)

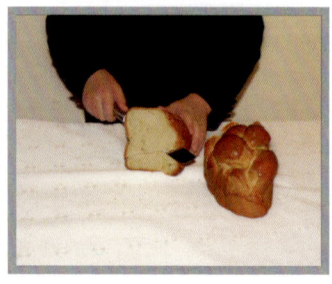

One should cut from the bottom towards the top, diagonally, in the form of a crown.

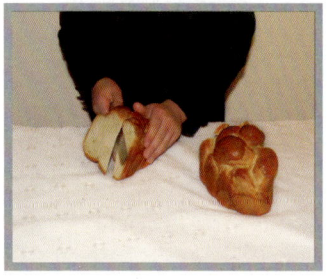

It is a mitzvah to cut a large slice of challah which is enough for the entire *seudah*. Doing so demonstrates that the mitzvah is beloved to us and therefore one wishes to eat a lot of it.
(*Shulchan Aruch, Orach Chaim* 274)

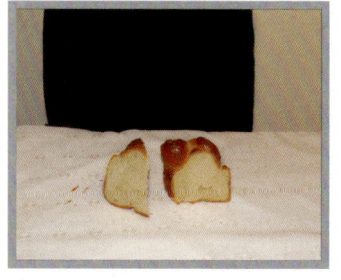

The slice that a person cuts for himself is only half of the width of the challah. However for a woman, one should cut a slice the entire width of the challah.
(*Zemiros Raza Deuvda*)

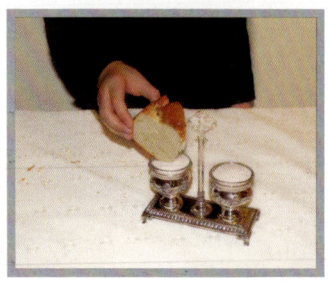

Dipping the middle of the slice of challah in salt three times.
(*Or Tzaddikim, Derech Seudah*)

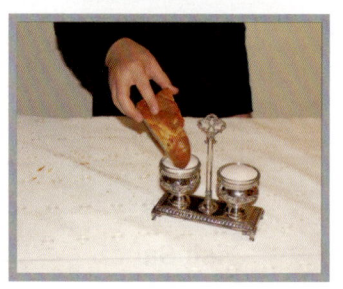

One should dip the challah into salt three times.
(*Be'er Heitav* 167:8)

Friday Night Seudah

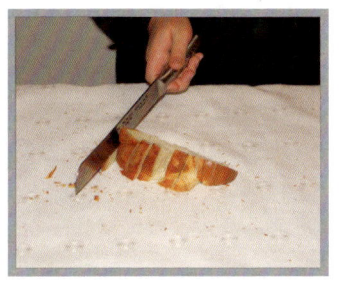

Seven Pieces of Challah

On Shabbos we cut seven pieces of challah corresponding to the seven Torah portions that are read.

(*Elyah Rabbah, Orach Chaim* 176:2)

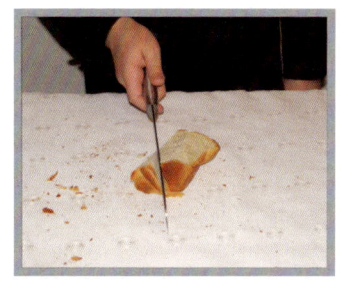

Three Pieces of Challah

At *seudah shlishis* the challah is cut into three pieces, corresponding the to the three Torah portions read at Minchah.

(*Elyah Rabbah, Orach Chaim* 176:2)

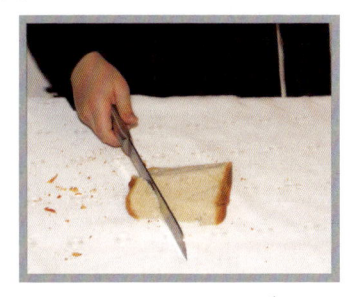

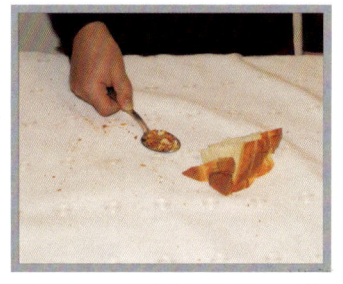

Some are accustomed to cut off the piece of challah that was dipped into the salt, and then eat it. (*Shulchan Aruch* 170:7)

It is a *segulah* for wealth to eat the crumbs of the slice of challah upon which *Hamotzi* was recited.

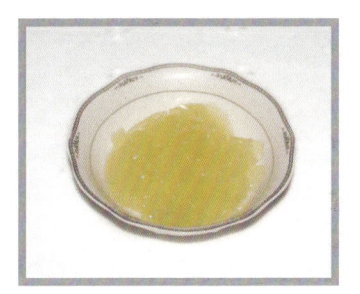

Fish Sauce

Some take seven pieces of challah upon which *Hamotzi* was recited and dip them into the fish sauce.

(*Piskei Teshuvos* 274:4)

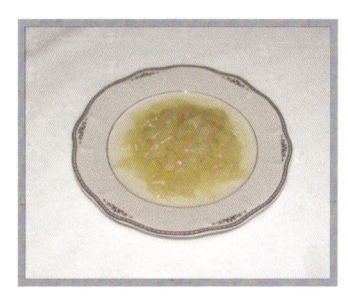

Onions That Were Cooked with the Fish

Some first eat the onions (*betzeil*) that were cooked with the fish prior to eating the fish.

Friday Night Seudah

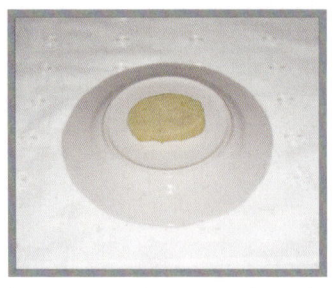

The custom in many locations is to eat the fish on the back of a plate. (*Darkei Hayashar V'hatov*)

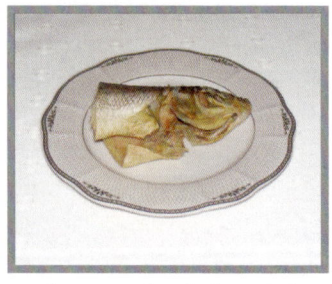

The Head of the Fish
Many *tzaddikim* begin eating the fish by eating the head and the eyes of the fish.
(*Taamei Haminhagim* sec. 306)

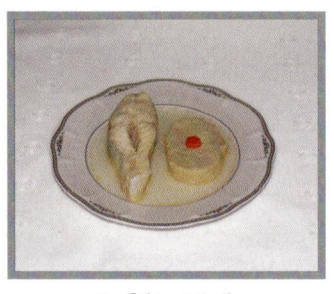

Gefilte Fish
Many are accustomed to first eating the gefilte fish and then other fish.
(*Zechor L'Avraham* p. 309)

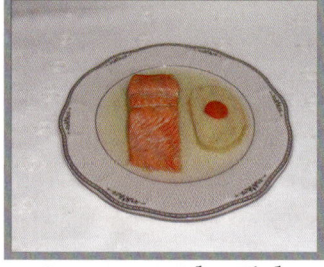

Carrots on the Fish
Many people put carrots on fish (called *mehren* in Yiddish, which means to increase), to allude to the fact that we should be numerous.

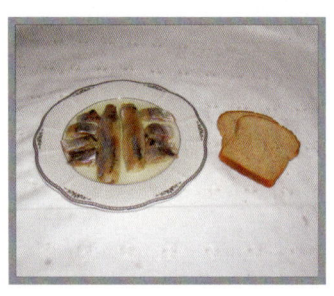

Some people are accustomed to eating herring at each *seudah*.
(*Seudasa D'Malka* p. 32)

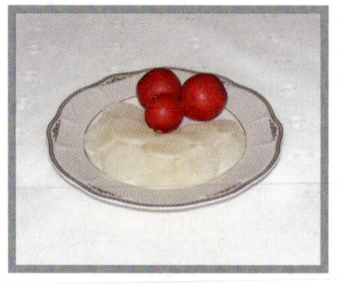

Radishes
Some people eat radishes with fish and some with the soup, since radish is a food eaten only on Shabbos. (*Maggid Meisharim*)

Friday Night Seudah

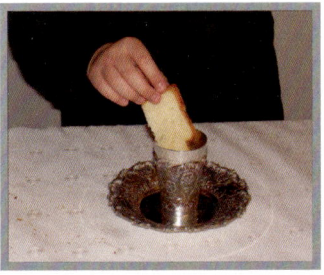

Dipping Challah into Wine
Dipping challah into the wine from Kiddush is a *segulah* against chest pains.

(*Hilchasa Rabasa L'Shabbata*)

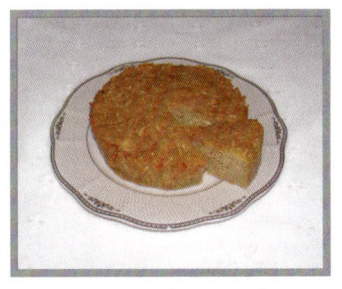

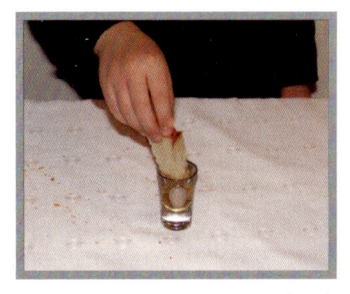

Dipping Challah into Whiskey
After eating the fish, challah is dipped into whiskey and eaten in order to rinse one's mouth between the fish and the meat.

(*Shulchan Aruch, Yoreh Deah* 116:3)

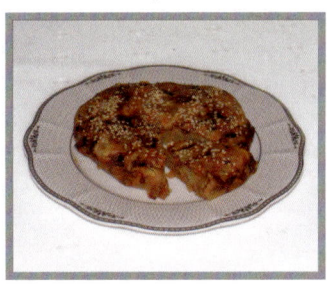

Challah Kugel
Some are accustomed to eating challah kugel before eating the soup. (*Minhag* Shedlitz)

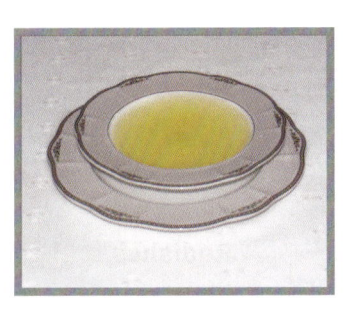

Onion Kugel
Some eat onion kugel with the soup to allude to Hashem's holy Name of Yabak which is an acronym for *yoch* (soup) and *batzeil kugel* (onion kugel).

(*Minhag* Chernobyl)

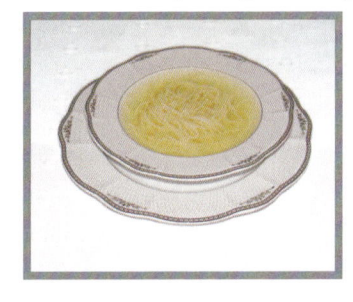

Soup
The soup is first placed in a bowl and then the noodles are added.

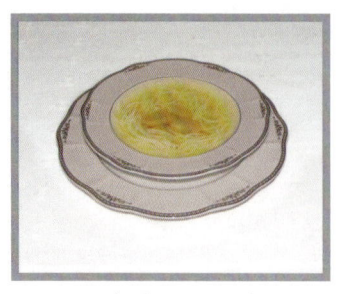

Friday Night Seudah

Soup, Lokshen, and Beans
Sanzer chassidim are accustomed to eating long noodles and beans in the soup.
(see p. 222)

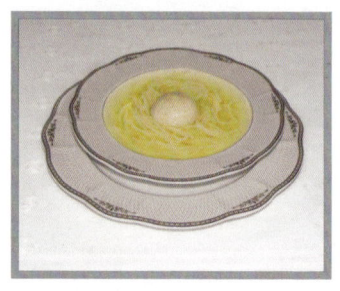

Kneidel in the Soup
Some people eat *kneidlach* in the soup to allude to the holy Name of Hashem, *Yabak*. *Yabak* is an acronym for *yoch* (soup), *bebelach* (beans), and *kneidlach*.

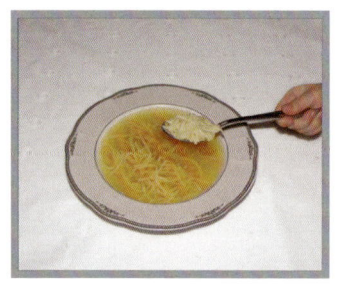

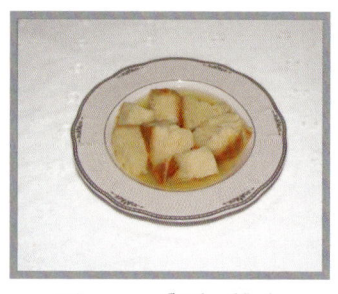

One should be careful to eat the noodles in a refined manner.

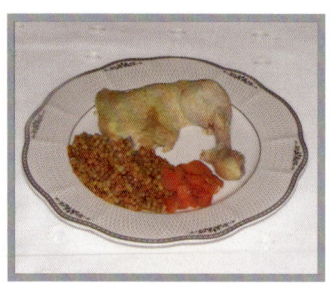

Pieces of Challah
Some put seven pieces of challah in the soup. (*Magen Avos*)

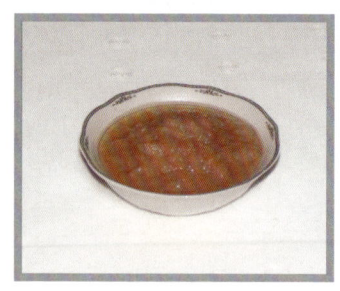

Chicken
Chicken with *tzimmes* (carrots and *farfel*) on one plate. Some make sure to put the carrots on the right side and the *farfel* on the left side. (*Magen Avos*)

Compote
After the *seudah*, compote is served as dessert for the sake of Torah, to enhance one's Torah study. (*Midrash Rabbah, Rus* 5:15)

Friday Night Seudah

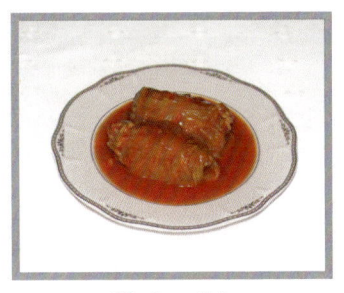

Stuffed Cabbage
Some eat cabbage filled with chicken to fulfill the words of the Rema (242:1) to eat a filled food on Shabbos.

(*Minhagei Kamarna* sec. 234)

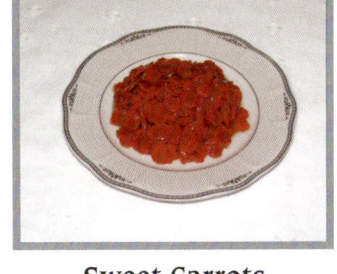

Sweet Carrots
Some eat carrots before the *farfel* and some eat the *farfel* first. This is because *farfel* alludes to *sur meira*, turning away from the bad, and carrots allude to *va'ase tov*, doing good.

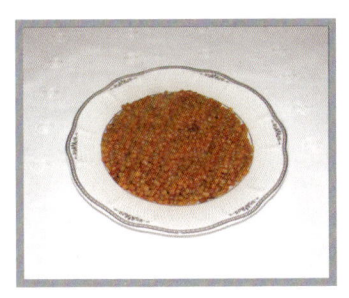

Farfel
The Baal Shem Tov instituted the custom that *farfel* should be eaten. (*Imrei Pinchas Shaar* 4)

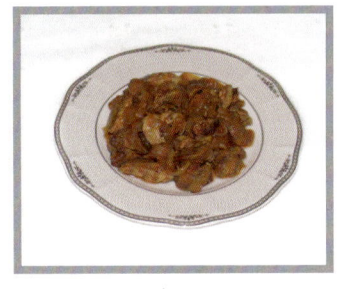

Liver
Some eat liver at the very end of the *seudah*. (*Chullin* 111)

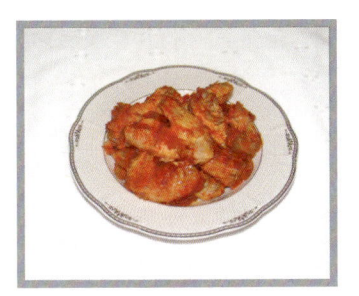

Gedishachts
A dish made of wings and necks of chicken. This is a Satmar *minhag*.

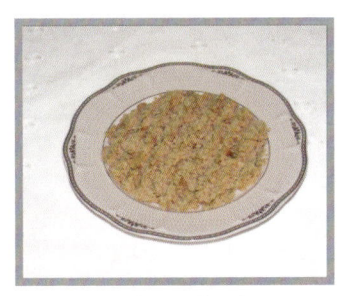

Gelingelach
A Satmar *minhag*.

Friday Night Seudah

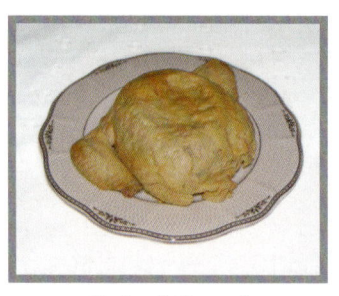

Helzel Kugel

Some eat *helzel kugel* on Friday night since that is the original kugel mentioned in the Rema (242:1). (*Shiras HaShabbos*)

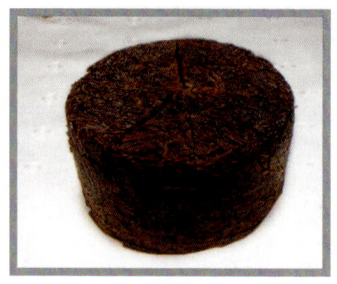

Yerushalmi Kugel

In some locations kugel is also eaten at night.

(Rema, *Orach Chaim*, 242:1)

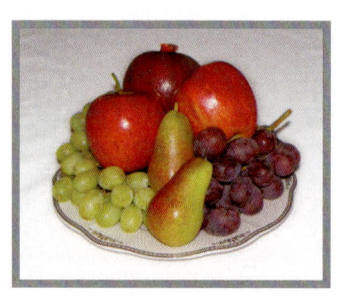

Fruits

Fruits are eaten after the *seudah* to complete 100 *brachos*. (*Shulchan Aruch* 290:1)

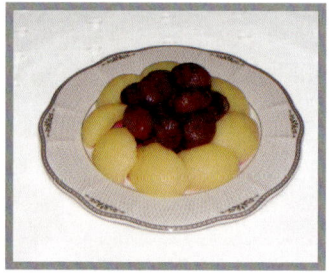

Compote

Whole cooked fruit upon which a *brachah* is recited in order to complete 100 *brachos*.

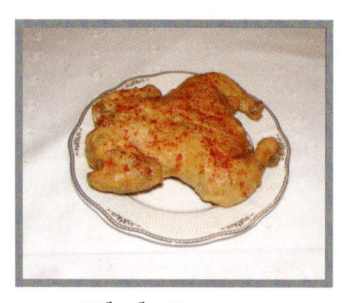

Whole Rooster

In Sanz, they brought a cold, whole, baked rooster to the Shabbos table prior to *Birkas Hamazon*. (*Darkei Chaim*, Sanz)

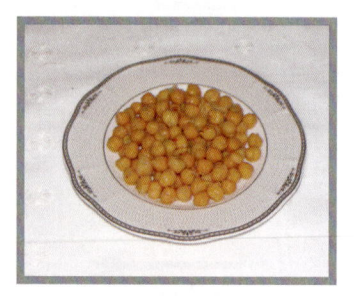

Zachor Beans

Chickpeas are traditionally eaten at a *shalom zachar*.

Shabbos Day Seudah

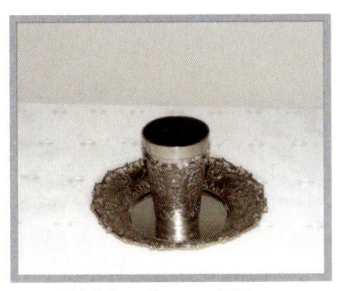

Kiddush on Wine

There are those who recite Kiddush on wine.

(*She'eilos Uteshuvos Chasam Sofer, Orach Chaim* 17)

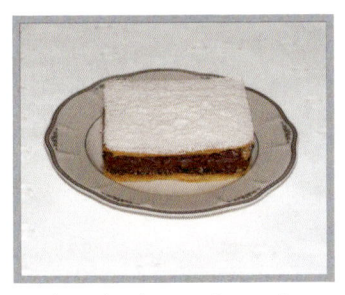

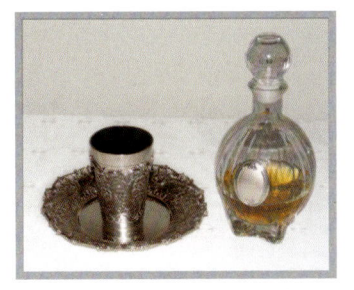

Kiddush over Whiskey

Many of the *gedolim* preferred to recite Kiddush on whiskey so that they can recite the *brachah* of *Shehakol*.

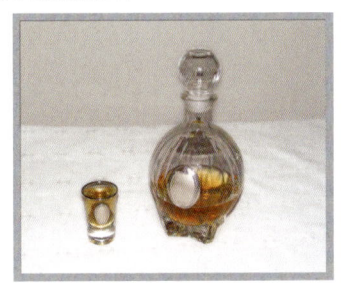

A cake which consists of pastry on top and on the bottom and a filling in the center. The white top alludes to the *mann* which is described in the *pasuk* as white.

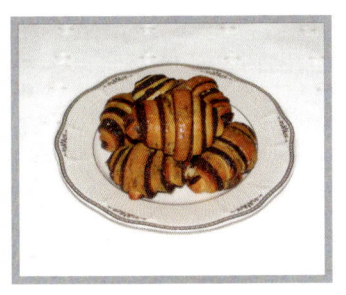

Kiddush in a Small Cup

Many people recite Kiddush on less than a *revi'is* of whiskey, based on the ruling of the Taz.

(*Taz* 210:1)

A Whole Cookie

Ideally, one should recite a *Mezonos* on a whole cookie, since it is preferable to recite Hashem's Name on something whole.

(*Levush* 167)

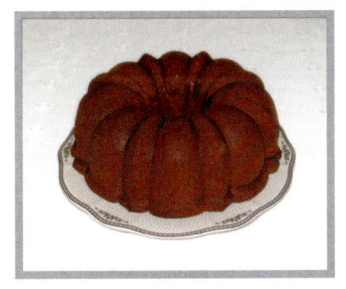

Lekach (Honey Cake)

Lekach alludes to the Torah since the *pasuk* states "*Ki lekach tov nasati lachem*," and honey is compared to the Torah as well.

21

Shabbos Day Seudah

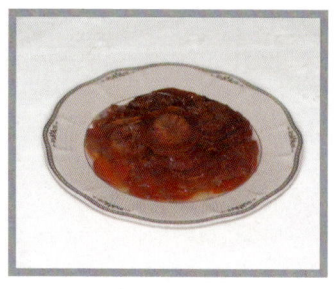

Fruit Preserves

Many people eat fruit preserves after the morning Kiddush.

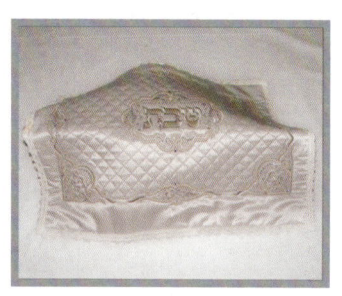

Shalom Bayis Kugel

Kugel is eaten after Kiddush and is referred to as "Shalom Bayis Kugel." (*Minhag* Kozhnitz)

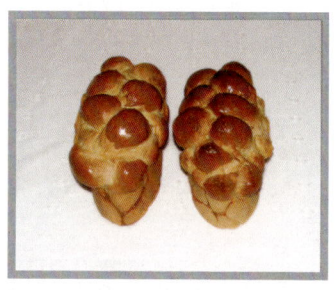

Covering the Challos

Some are accustomed to covering the challos during Kiddush that is recited by day.

(Chozeh of Lublin)

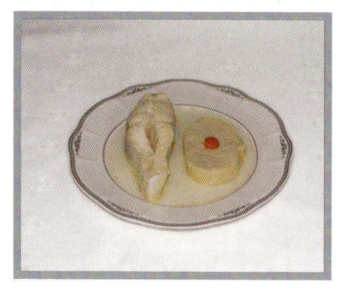

There are those who do not cover the challos during Kiddush that is recited by day.

(*Minhag* of Reb Mendel of Riminov and the Ropshitzer Rav)

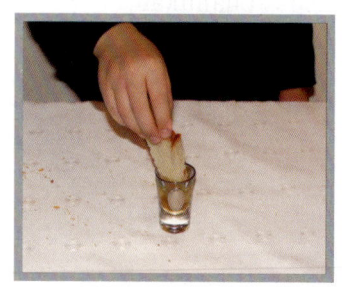

Fish

Some eat fish only after Kiddush. Some eat the fish at the beginning of the *seudah*, and some eat it at the end of the *seudah*.

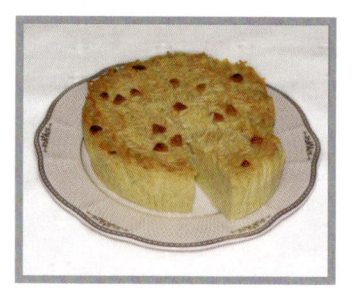

Drinking Whiskey

After eating fish many people drink whiskey and wish each other "*L'chaim*." (*Minhag* Kozhnitz)

Shabbos Day Seudah

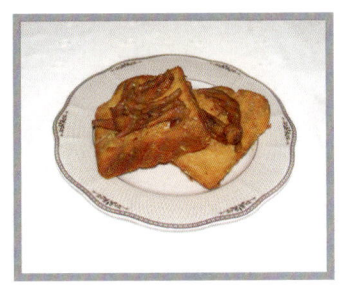

Petcha
A dish made of chicken feet and challah. (see p. 296)

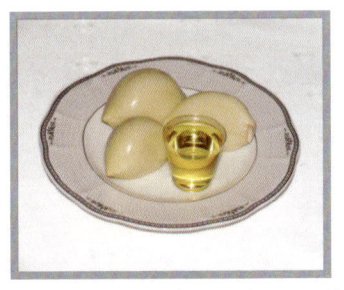

Galareta
A dish made from chicken or calf feet. (see p. 297; *Imrei Pinchas*)

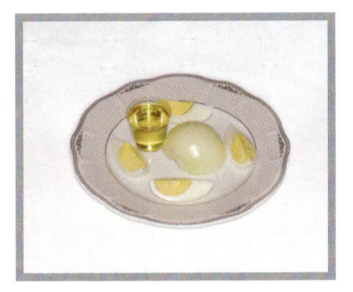

Garlic Dipped in Olive Oil
A dish made of garlic and the olive oil that is set aside for the Chanukah menorah is eaten after the eggs with onions on Shabbos Chanukah.

Cutting the Eggs
There are those who cut (*chatoch*) the egg into four parts to allude to *Chatoch*, the holy Name of Hashem that is associated with livelihood.

(*Even Yisrael* vol. 2)

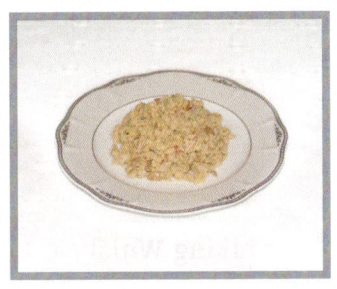

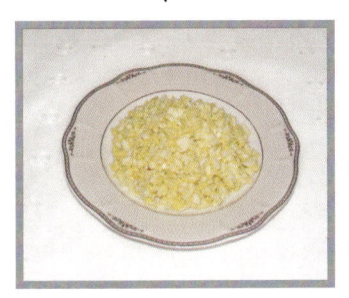

Eggs with Cholent
Many are accustomed to eating some of the eggs with the cholent. (*Divrei Tzaddikim* 2:4)

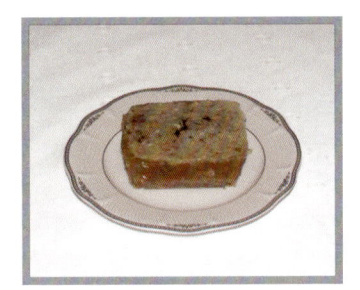

Eggs and Onions
The eggs and onions are cut into small pieces during the *seudah*, and eaten with a slice of challah.

Shabbos Day Seudah

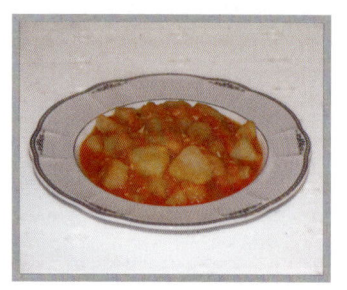

Potato Cholent

Eating cholent is a *segulah* for having complete *emunah* in Hashem and *emunah* in our *tzaddikim*.

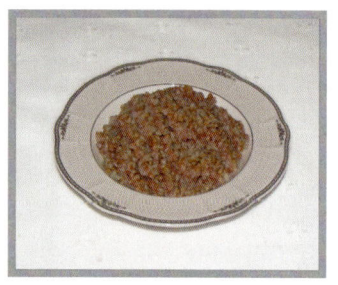

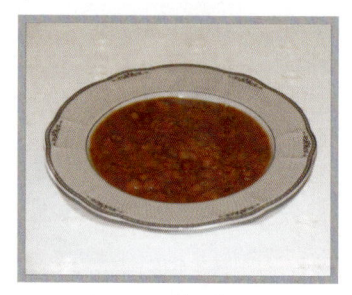

Bean Cholent

Tzaddikim have said that there is an angel appointed over every bean in the cholent.

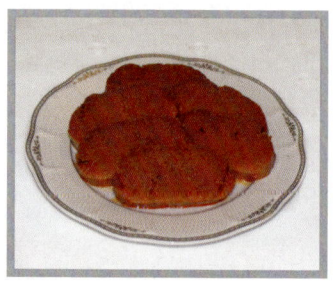

Kasha Cholent

Some eat kasha cholent as a *segulah* for finding their spouse and having livelihood since it says, "**Kasheh** *zivugo shel adam*" and "**Kasheh** *mezonosov shel adam*." We hope that by eating kasha cholent these difficulties will be eased.

Geknetene (Kneaded) Kugel

Some call it Ganav Kugel since it "steals" the fat from the cholent. It is said that this kugel drips fat like the tears of Leah, is pretty like Rochel, tastes good like Yaakov, and is red like Eisav.

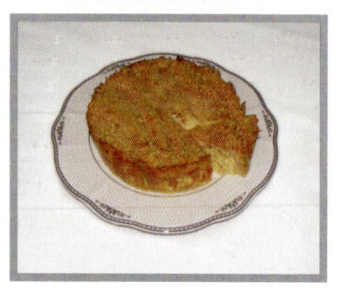

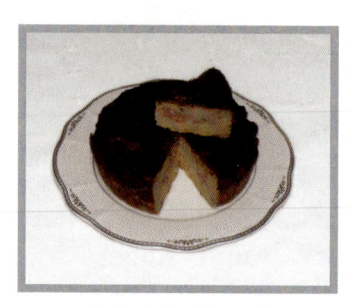

Cornflakes Kugel

A Kiviashed *minhag*.

Yabchik Kugel

A Polish/Gur *minhag*.

Shabbos Day Seudah

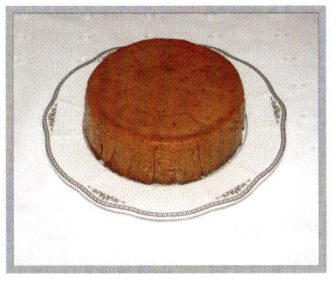

Flipping Over the Kugel

A whole kugel is served, turned over, to signify that we should succeed in turning over the *middas hadin* to *middas harachamim*. (Chozeh of Lublin)

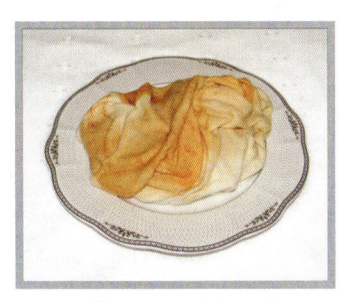

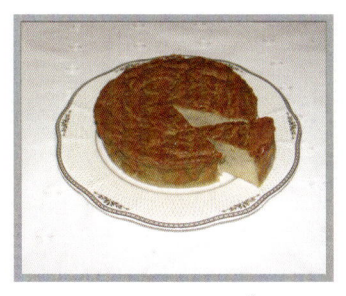

Potato Kugel

Potatoes in Yiddish can be called "*erd eppel*" (lit. apples of the earth). The sphere of Earth in Yiddish is called "*erd kuge*l" (lit. "earth kugel"). The word kugel is also related to the word *k'igul*, which also means Earth. So we eat potato kugel on Shabbos is to remind us of Hashem's creation of the world.

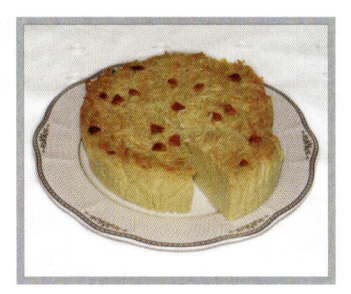

Shmatte Kugel

A Bluzhover *minhag*.

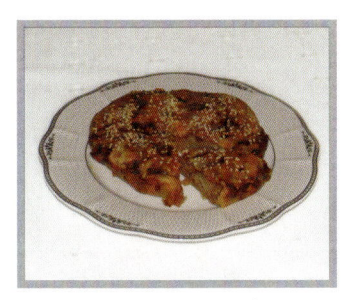

Sweet Lokshen Kugel

On Shabbos day a sweet kugel is eaten.

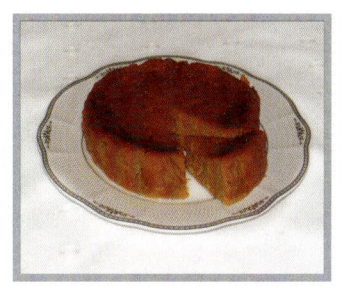

Onion Kugel

A Skver and Rachmastrivka *minhag*.

Carrot Kugel

In honor of Shabbos Shuvah.

Shabbos Day Seudah

Apple Kugel
Kugel made out of grated apples. Apples allude to our closeness to Hashem, as stated in *Shir Hashirim*.

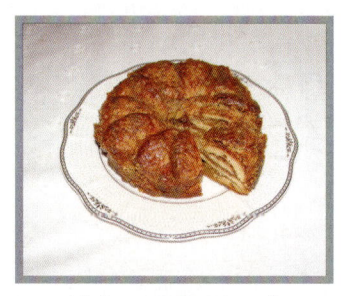

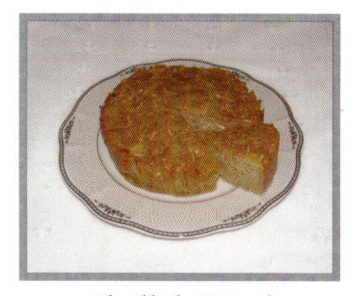

Challah Kugel
Some use the leftover challah to prepare a kugel for the coming Shabbos. This is comparable to the *Lechem Hapanim*. (see p. 320)

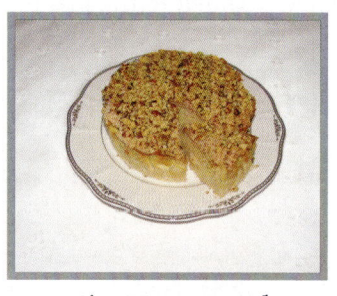

Tzip Mich Kugel
In honor of Shabbos Chanukah.

Nis (Nut) Kugel
Made in honor of Shabbos Chanukah to allude to *Al Hanissim*.

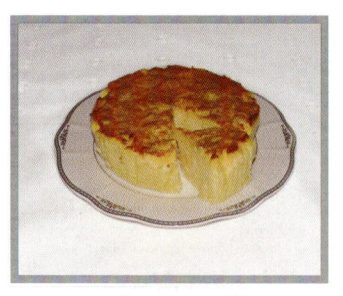

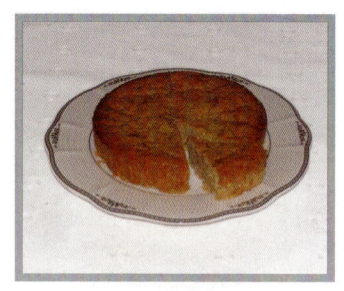

Rice Kugel
In honor of Shabbos Shirah.

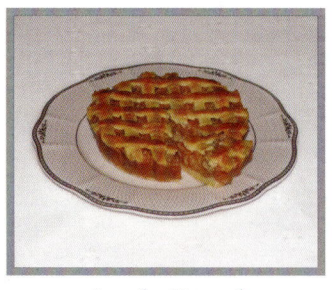

Kasha Kugel
Eaten in honor of Shabbos Shirah as a *segulah* for livelihood, as alluded to in the Chazal, "**Kasheh** *mezonosov shel adam…*"

Shabbos Day Seudah

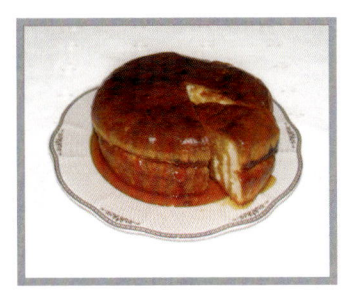

Honey Challah Kugel

In honor of Shabbos Mevorchim, challah kugel baked with a large amount of honey is added to the menu.

(*Minhag* Nadvorna)

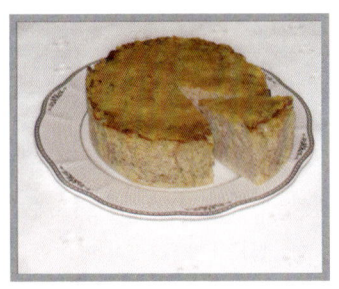

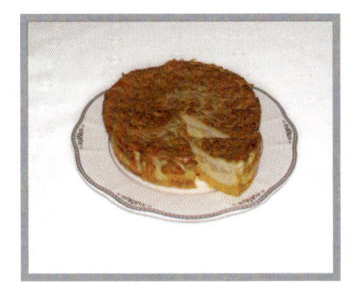

Amalek Kugel

It is eaten in honor of Shabbos Zachor. It contains *epel* (apples), *mehl* (flour), *lokshen* (noodles), and *kartafel* (potatoes), whose first letters spell *Amalek*.

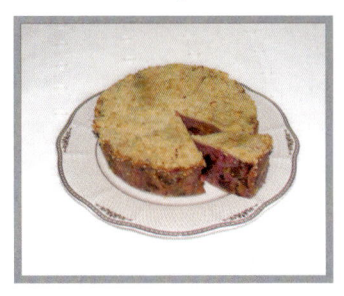

Rice Kugel

In honor of Shabbos Mevarchim.

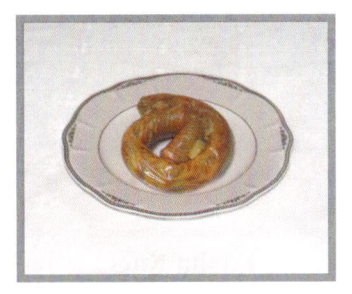

Shivas Haminim Kugel

In honor of Shabbos Tu B'Shevat.

Kishke

The intestines of the animal are cleaned and filled. This teaches us that a person's inside should match his outside.

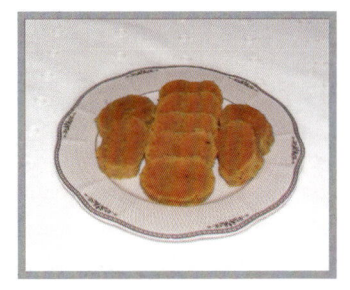

Maharshal's Mehl Kugel

A dish which is baked from the flour that was ground to be used for the Pesach matzos.

(*Mateh Moshe* 543)

Shabbos Day Seudah

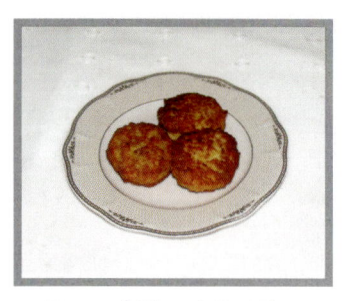

Round Meat Patties

This alludes to the words of Chazal that one who keeps the Shabbos is forgiven. (The word forgiven, *machul* can also mean *machol*—a dance in a circle.) (*Hadras Kodesh*, p. 22 sec. 100)

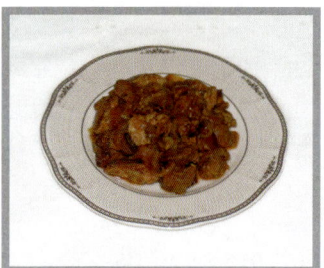

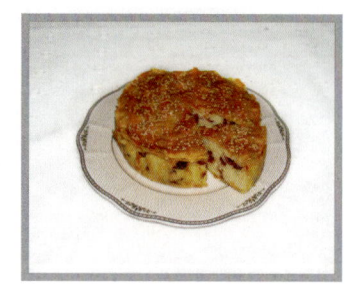

Mann Kugel

As a remembrance to the *mann* that was covered above and below it.

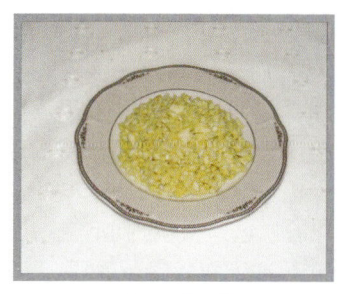

Leberlech—Liver

This alludes to the words "*leb ehrlich*"—live piously.

Bitterlach

A dish made of onions and oil that is eaten with the egg. This alludes to the words "*beht ehrlich*"—daven devoutly.

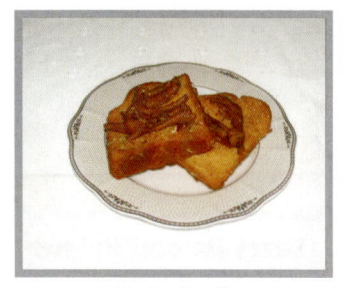

Zoierlach

A pickled ingredient that is put in to the *petcha* which alludes to "*zei ehrlich*"—be honest.

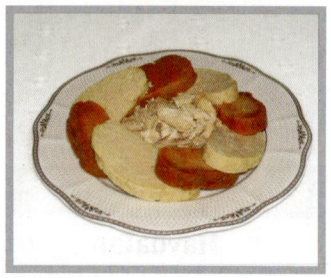

Kalte Oif (Cold Chicken)

If one honors the Shabbos properly, he receives *kol tuv*, everything good. (*Meir Hachaim*)

Shalosh Seudos

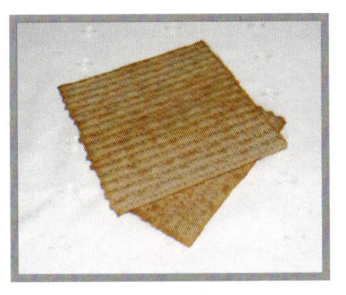

Matzah
There are those who eat matzah at *seudah shlishis*.

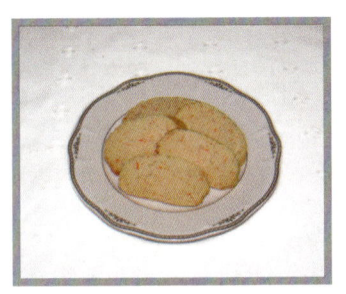

Lechem Mishneh
Lechem mishneh for *seudah shlishis*.

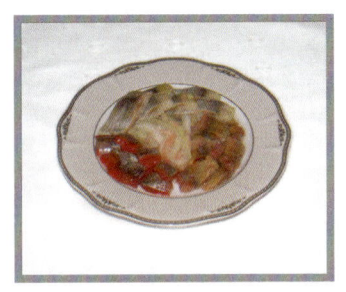

Gefilte Fish
There are those who eat only gefilte fish at *seudah shlishis*.

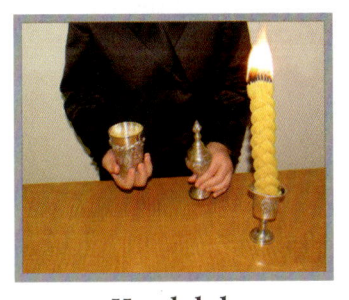

Herring
Many people eat herring, which are small fish, at *seudah shlishis*. This idea is mentioned in *Azameir B'shvuchin* with the words *nunin im rachashin*.

(see p. 344)

Havdalah
The person reciting Havdalah holds the wine in his right hand and the *besamim* in his left hand. (*Orach Chaim* 296:6)

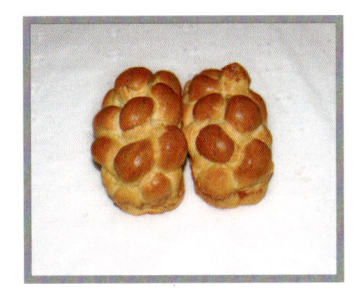

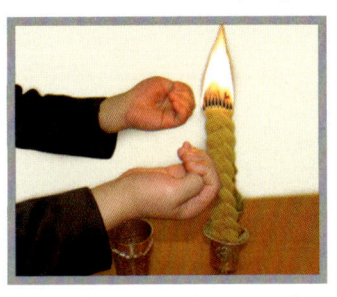

Borei Me'orei Ha'eish
Both palms are pointed upwards and one's fingers are bent over his thumbs. One should look at his palm and fingernails.

Havdalah

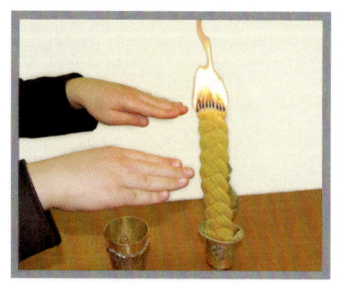

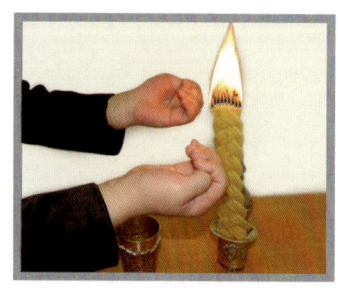

One should then turn over his hands and straighten them near the light. His thumbs should be under his palms. He should look at his fingernails. This should be done three times.

(*Magen Avraham* 298:5 and Ibid: *Machatzis Hashekel*)

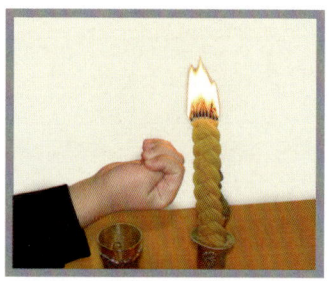

There are those who bend only the right hand. One's thumb should be under his palm.

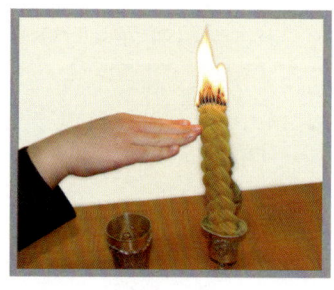

Then straighten the right hand against the light.

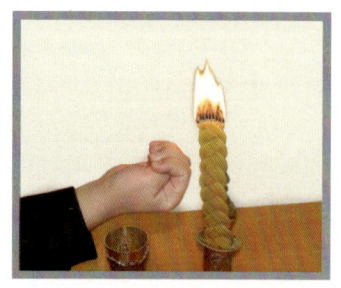

One performs the above three times.

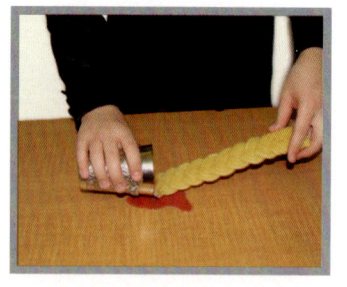

Extinguishing the Fire with Wine

One should extinguish the fire with wine that spilled during Havdalah together with the remaining wine from the cup.

Melaveh Malkah

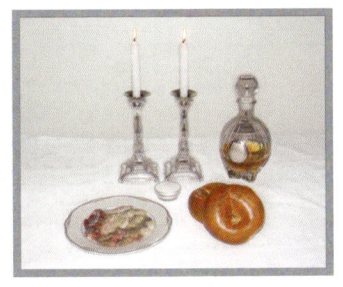

Bagel, Herring, and Whiskey

The Rebbe of Bichave would eat bagel, herring, and whiskey on Motza'ei Shabbos. He called it "*taanis bahab*" (an acronym for *broit*, herring, and *broinfen*).

(*Toras Hayehudi Hakadosh* p.44)

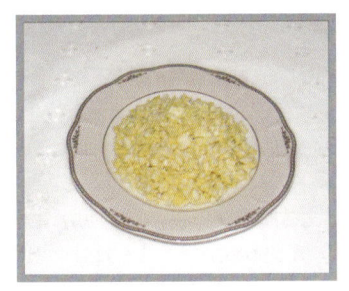

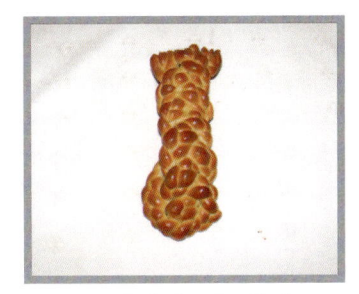

Havdalah Challah

A challah in the form of a Havdalah candle is used as a second challah for *lechem mishneh* for *shalosh seudos*. It is then eaten at *melaveh malkah*. (*Kitzur Halachos*, sec. 274)

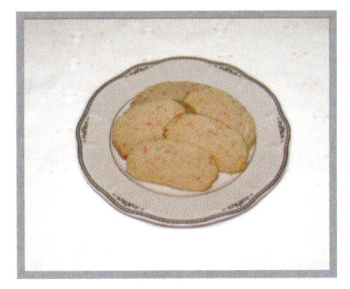

Eggs and Onion

Leftover eggs and onion dish.

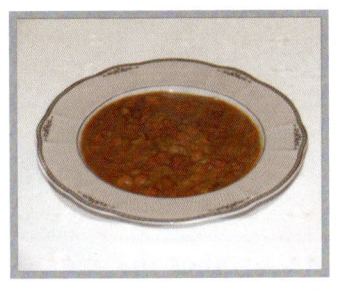

Gefilte Fish

There are those who eat gefilte fish to have a week full of goods.

Leftover Shabbos Food

There are those who eat leftover Shabbos food, since the holiness of Shabbos that is in it remains after Shabbos as well.

(*Vayedabeir Moshe*)

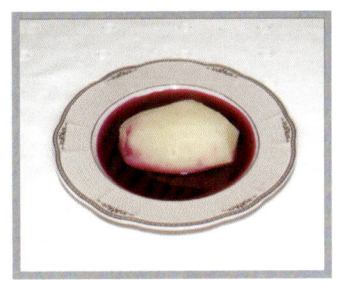

Borscht

Reb Yochonon of Stolin did not want someone who did not eat borscht at *melaveh malkah* to lead the davening on Sunday.

(*Pri Yesha Aharon* p. 105)

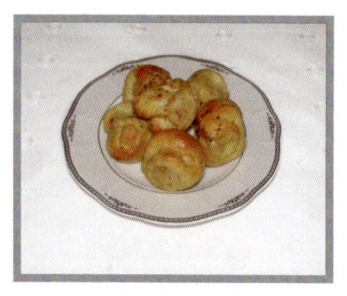

Melaveh Malkah

Hot Bread
Some eat hot bread that was baked on Motza'ei Shabbos.
(*Maharshu Shabbos* 119)

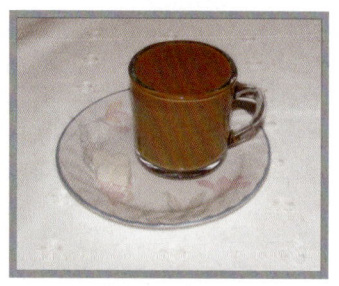

Garlic
Eating garlic on Motza'ei Shabbos is a *segulah* for livelihood. (Baal Shem Tov, *Yisro*)

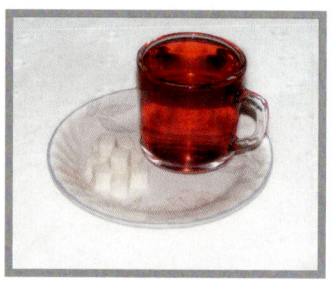

Hot Coffee
The Sanzer Rav said: "It's foolish to eat meat by *shalosh seudos* because one won't be able to drink coffee."
(*Zemiros Shabbos Shulem Imvoiruch*)

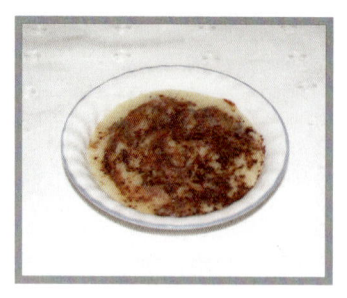

Drinking a Warm Drink on Motza'ei Shabbos
Drinking tea alludes to the *pasuk* "*Tehei hasha'ah hazos*." (Tea in Yiddish is *tei*.)
(*Tiferes Shebitiferes* p. 430)

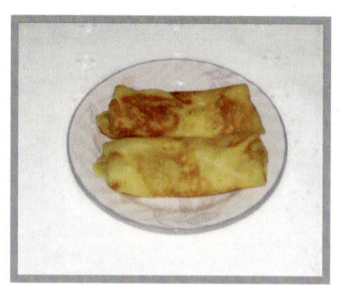

A New Dish
It is good to prepare a freshly cooked dish for *melaveh malkah*. (Maharsha, *Shabbos* 119)

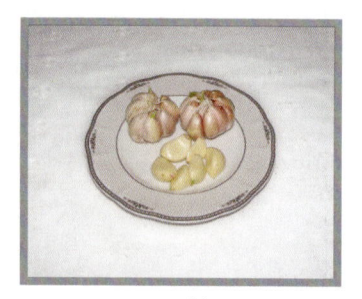

Dairy Food
Some eat dairy food at *melaveh malkah* so that the holiness of Shabbos should encompass dairy food as well. (*Magen Avos*)